Orthopedics for Medical Practitioners

Orthopedics for Medical Practitioners

Edited by Solomon Willis

hayle medical

New York

Hayle Medical,
750 Third Avenue, 9th Floor,
New York, NY 10017, USA

Visit us on the World Wide Web at:
www.haylemedical.com

ISBN: 978-1-63241-509-7

Cataloging-in-Publication Data

Orthopedics for medical practitioners / edited by Solomon Willis.
p. cm.
Includes bibliographical references and index.
ISBN 978-1-63241-509-7
1. Orthopedics. 2. Orthopedics--Practice. I. Willis, Solomon.
RD732 .O78 2018
617--dc23

Table of Contents

Preface

This book has been an outcome of determined endeavour from a group of educationists in the field. The primary objective was to involve a broad spectrum of professionals from diverse cultural background involved in the field for developing new researches. The book not only targets students but also scholars pursuing higher research for further enhancement of the theoretical and practical applications of the subject.

Orthopedics is the field of medical science that deals with diseases and disorders related to our musculoskeletal system. The doctors practicing this field apply surgical and non-surgical methods to treat diseases like congenital disorders, tumors, sports injuries, muscular dystrophy, soft tissue injuries, etc. This book unravels the recent studies in the field of orthopedics. It discusses in detail the methods and techniques used to diagnose and treat these diseases. The topics included in this book are of utmost significance and bound to provide incredible insights to readers. For all readers who are interested in orthopedics, the case studies included in this text will serve as an excellent guide to develop a comprehensive understanding.

It was an honour to edit such a profound book and also a challenging task to compile and examine all the relevant data for accuracy and originality. I wish to acknowledge the efforts of the contributors for submitting such brilliant and diverse chapters in the field and for endlessly working for the completion of the book. Last, but not the least; I thank my family for being a constant source of support in all my research endeavours.

Editor

1

Spontaneous Recurrent Hemarthrosis of the Knee: A Report of Two Cases with a Source of Bleeding Detected during Arthroscopic Surgery of the Knee Joint

Eisuke Nomura, Hisatada Hiraoka, and Hiroya Sakai

Department of Orthopaedic Surgery, Saitama Medical Center, Saitama Medical University, Kawagoe, Saitama, Japan

Correspondence should be addressed to Hiroya Sakai; hsakai@saitama-med.ac.jp

Academic Editor: John Nyland

We report two cases of the spontaneous recurrent hemarthrosis of the knee. In these cases lateral meniscus was severely torn and a small tubular soft tissue with pulsation was identified on the synovium in the posterolateral corner during arthroscopic surgery of the knee joint. Gentle grasping of this tissue by forceps led to pulsating bleeding, which stopped by electrocoagulation. This soft tissue was considered a source of bleeding, since no recurrence of hemarthrosis was observed for more than four years after surgery. It was highly probable that this soft tissue was the ruptured end of the lateral inferior genicular artery or its branch. This case report strongly supports the theory that the bleeding from the peripheral arteries of the posterior portion of the lateral meniscus is the cause of spontaneous recurrent hemarthrosis of the knee.

1. Introduction

Spontaneous recurrent hemarthrosis of the knee joint is relatively rare disorder mostly seen in the elderly with osteoarthritis. Since the first report of Wilson [1], synovium had been considered the origin of the bleeding [2, 3], and synovectomy was considered to be the most reasonable treatment. In 1994, however, Kawamura et al. [4] reported five cases of spontaneous recurrent hemarthrosis of the knee in which a degenerative flap tear of the posterior horn of lateral meniscus was revealed with arthroscopic examination. These patients did not experience the recurrent hemarthrosis after arthroscopic resection of the injured lateral meniscus, suggesting that the origin of the bleeding was the peripheral arteries of the posterior horn of the lateral meniscus [4]. Since this report, there have been some reports supporting this theory [5–8]. In some cases, bleeding from the posterior portion of the lateral meniscus was observed during arthroscopic examination [4, 6, 7]. Among these reports, Sasho et al. [7] detected throbbing bleeding indicating arterial bleeding in the process of debridement of lateral meniscus, which suggested direct bleeding from the lateral genicular artery. However, the arterial structure itself as a bleeding source was not detected in any case. We report two cases of the spontaneous recurrent hemarthrosis of the knee in which a pulsating soft tissue with a tubular structure as a source of bleeding was identified in the posterolateral corner during arthroscopic surgery of the knee joint.

2. Case Report

2.1. Case 1. A 64-year-old man presented with recurrent painful swelling of the left knee for one month without any traumatic episode. His medical history was unremarkable and only some anti-inflammatory drugs were taken sporadically for the knee pain after hemarthrosis occurred. He received knee joint puncture three times in one month and bloody fluid was aspirated each time. Radiographs of his left knee showed lateral-dominant osteoarthritis (Figure 1), and MRI showed that the posterior portion of the lateral meniscus was torn (Figure 2).

At four months after the onset of the symptom, surgery was performed without using tourniquet. Arthroscopic examination revealed that the lateral compartment had severe degenerative change and that almost no meniscal substance, including the meniscal rim, was observed in

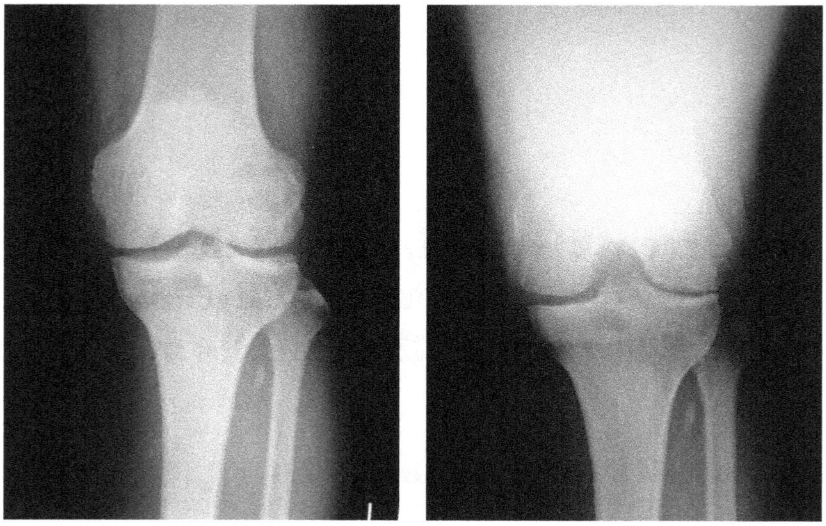

(a) (b)

Figure 1: Radiographs of Case 1. AP view (a) shows grade 3 osteoarthritis according to Kellgren and Lawrence scale and Rosenberg view (b) shows lateral-dominant osteoarthritis.

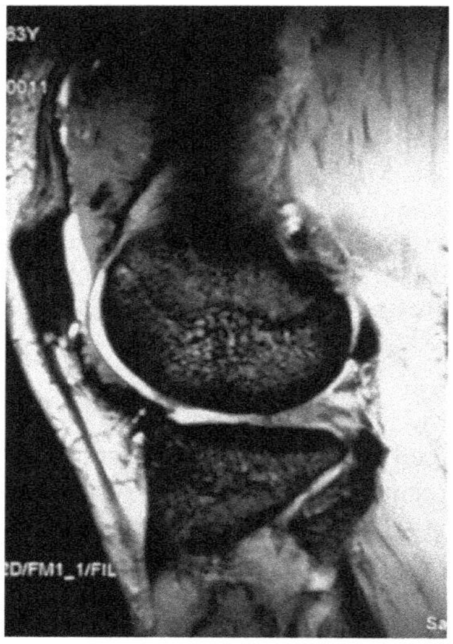

Figure 2: MRI of Case 1 (T2 weighted image). The posterior portion of the lateral meniscus is torn.

the middle and posterior portions of the lateral meniscus, although the posterior horn remained. On the exposed synovium behind this area, a 3-4 mm wide projecting tubular soft tissue was identified (Figure 3). It was pulsating, and when gently grasping this tissue with forceps, pulsating bleeding from the top of this soft tissue was shown, which stopped by electrocoagulation. No recurrence of hemarthrosis was observed at 54 months postoperatively.

2.2. Case 2. A 71-year-old woman presented with two-year history of recurrent swelling of the left knee. The swelling always occurred after sport activity, but she did not have clear history of trauma. She was hypertensive and took hypotensors, but her medical history was otherwise unremarkable. Within those two years, she had her left knee punctured four times with bloody fluid aspiration. Radiographs of her left knee showed lateral-dominant osteoarthritis (Figure 4), and MRI showed that the middle and posterior portions of the lateral meniscus were torn (Figure 5).

At 28 months after the onset of the symptom, surgery was performed without tourniquet. Arthroscopic examination demonstrated that the lateral compartment had remarkable degenerative change. And the middle and posterior portions of the lateral meniscus were degeneratively torn and almost no meniscal substance was left in these portions. On the exposed synovium behind this area, a 2-3 mm long projecting tubular soft tissue with a 3-4 mm diameter was identified (Figure 6). It was pulsating and on its top a red spot, suggesting coagulated blood clot, was observed. Gentle grasping with forceps led to pulsating bleeding from the top of this soft tissue, which ceased by electrocoagulation. There was no recurrence of hemarthrosis for 64 months after surgery.

3. Discussion

Regarding the etiology of the spontaneous recurrent hemarthrosis of the knee joint in elderly, synovium had been considered the origin of the bleeding until the report of Kawamura et al. [1–4]. Since the report of Kawamura et al. [4], the peripheral arteries of the posterior portion of the lateral meniscus have been recognized as the origin of the bleeding in most cases [5–8]. In some reports, the bleeding from the posterior portion of the lateral meniscus was observed during arthroscopic surgery [4, 6, 7]. This finding, together with the fact that the recurrence of the hemarthrosis did not occur after lateral meniscectomy alone [4–6, 8], or lateral meniscectomy followed by coagulation [7], was the

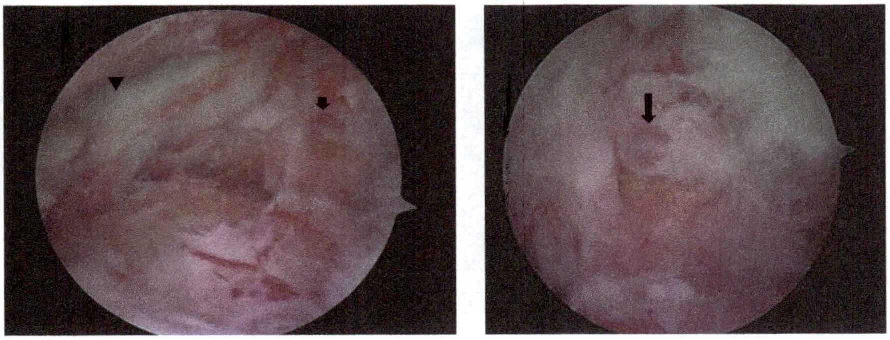

FIGURE 3: Arthroscopic findings of Case 1. The lateral compartment has severe degenerative change and almost no meniscal substance, including the meniscal rim, is observed in the middle and posterior portions of the lateral meniscus. Arrow head indicates the remaining posterior horn of the lateral meniscus (a). On the synovium behind this area, a small projecting tubular soft tissue with pulsation (arrows) is shown (a and b).

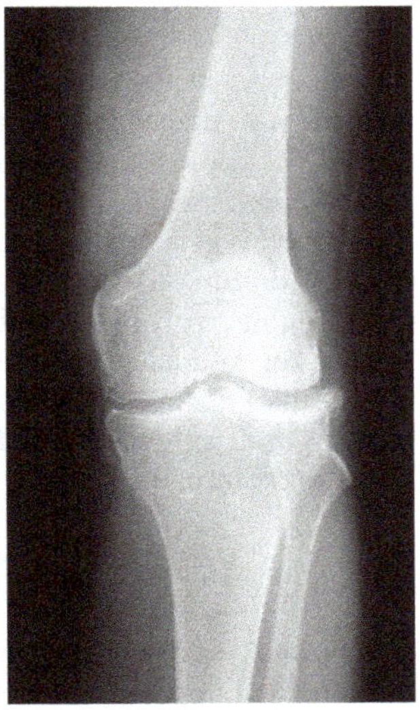

FIGURE 4: Radiograph of Case 2. AP view shows grade 3 lateral-dominant osteoarthritis according to Kellgren and Lawrence scale.

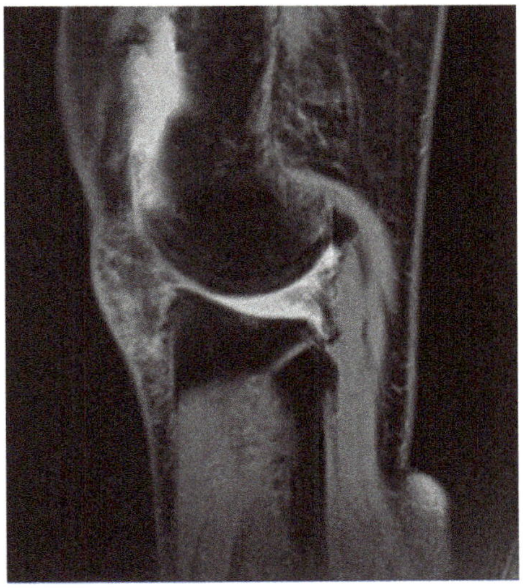

FIGURE 5: MRI of Case 2 (T2 weighted image). The middle and posterior portions of the lateral meniscus are torn.

ground of the theory that the origin of the bleeding was the peripheral arteries of the posterior portion of the lateral meniscus. In these reports, however, the arterial structure itself at the posterior portion of lateral meniscus, which would be the direct evidence of this theory, was not detected during surgery.

We reported two cases of the spontaneous recurrent hemarthrosis of the knee, in which a pulsating soft tissue with a tubular structure was identified on the exposed synovium in the posterolateral corner during arthroscopic surgery. Taking account of its shape, the existing of pulsation, and pulsating bleeding from the top by gentle grasping, it was highly probable that this soft tissue was a ruptured end of the artery. Electrocoagulation of this soft tissue led to no recurrence of hemarthrosis after surgery for more than four years, indicating that this was the source of bleeding in our cases. From the anatomical standpoint, it was the ruptured end of the lateral inferior genicular artery or its branch. Arnoczky and Warren [9] demonstrated that lateral inferior genicular artery was located very close to the peripheral border of the lateral meniscus. Sasho et al. [7] suggested that the throbbing bleeding during lateral meniscectomy was due to direct bleeding from lateral genicular artery.

The lateral inferior genicular artery and its branches supply the posterior portion of the lateral meniscus [9]. In our cases, the posterior portion of the lateral meniscus was severely torn and almost no meniscal substance, including the meniscal rim, was observed, suggesting that when the lateral meniscus was torn from its junction with the synovium, the artery was ruptured with its end left on the exposed synovium and was identified as a pulsating soft tissue during surgery. Therefore, our cases strongly support the theory that the bleeding from the peripheral arteries of the posterior portion of the lateral meniscus is the cause of spontaneous recurrent

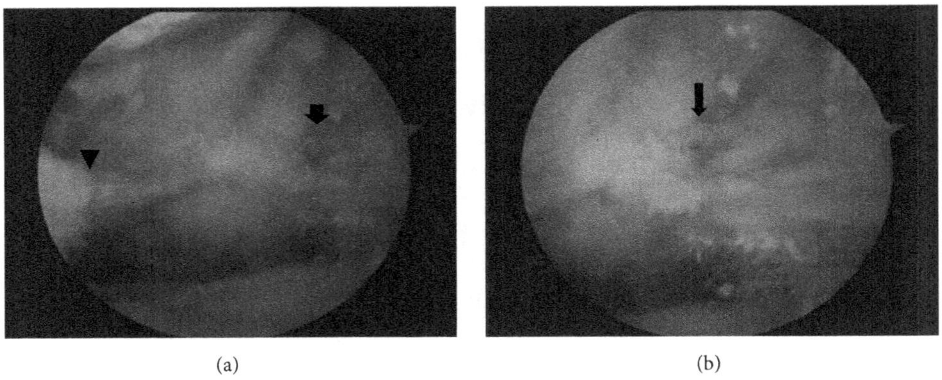

FIGURE 6: Arthroscopic findings of Case 2. Remarkable degenerative change is shown in the lateral compartment. The middle and posterior portions of the lateral meniscus are degeneratively torn (arrow head) and almost no meniscal substance was left in these portions (a). On the exposed synovium behind this area, a small projecting tubular soft tissue with pulsation (arrows) is shown (a and b).

hemarthrosis of the knee. Although Sasho et al. [7] observed throbbing bleeding indicating arterial bleeding during lateral meniscectomy, the arterial structure itself was not detected. As far as we know, there was only one case report showing the ruptured end of the pulsating vessel in the patient of the recurrent hemarthrosis of the knee [10]. In this report, the ruptured end of pulsating vessel behind the rim of lateral meniscus was observed during arthroscopic examination and the coagulation of the vessel led to no recurrence of the hemarthrosis [10]. The operative findings of this case were very similar to those of our cases.

Regarding the cause of the bleeding from the artery in spontaneous recurrent hemarthrosis, Kawamura et al. [4] suggested that the pulling and laceration into the branches of the genicular arteries supplying the peripheral rim of the lateral meniscus might be the direct cause of the hemorrhage into the joint. In our cases, however, the pulling of the artery was not likely to occur, because almost no meniscus substance was left, causing no continuity of the artery with the meniscus. In our cases, it was most likely that the thrombus created at the end of artery was detached due to mechanical irritation with knee motion, causing bleeding into the joint, that the increased intraarticular pressure caused by bleeding led to the stop of the bleeding with thrombus formation at the end of the artery, and that this thrombus was detached later, causing intraarticular bleeding again. This cycle was likely the cause of the recurrent hemarthrosis in our cases. In our two cases, it was likely that grasping the end of the artery during surgery caused the detachment of the thrombus, leading to the bleeding, and that the electrocoagulation was successful in permanent closing of the end of the artery.

Although medial-dominant osteoarthritis is more common than lateral-dominant osteoarthritis, most of the cases with spontaneous recurrent hemarthrosis of the knee are associated with lateral-dominant osteoarthritis and/or lateral meniscal injury [4–8]. This may be explained by the location and size of the genicular arteries. The lateral inferior genicular artery courses adjacent to the peripheral border of the lateral meniscus [9], whereas the medial genicular arteries do not course so close to the medial meniscus. Also the lateral inferior genicular artery is much larger than the medial genicular arteries [11, 12].

We did not use tourniquet from the beginning of the surgery, which enabled us to detect the pulsation of the soft tissue. If we had used the tourniquet, this might not have been detected in our cases. When a patient of recurrent hemarthrosis of the knee is encountered, especially when such a patient has lateral-dominant osteoarthritis and/or torn lateral meniscus, it is highly probable that the origin of the bleeding is the branch of lateral inferior genicular artery that penetrates and supplies the lateral meniscus. And in the beginning of the arthroscopic surgery for such a case, the use of the tourniquet is not recommended.

Consent

Written informed consent was provided by each patient regarding submission for publication.

Competing Interests

The authors declare that there is no conflict of interests regarding the publication of this paper.

References

[1] J. N. Wilson, "Spontaneous hemarthrosis in the osteoarthritis of the knee. A report of five cases," *British Medical Journal*, vol. 23, pp. 1327–1328, 1959.

[2] M. Burman, C. J. Sutro, and E. Guariglia, "Spontaneous hemorrhage of bursae and joints in the elderly," *Bulletin of the Hospital for Joint Diseases*, vol. 25, pp. 217–239, 1964.

[3] T. Morii, T. Koshino, K. Suzuki, A. Kobayashi, T. Kurosaka, and M. Shimaya, "Etiology and treatment of spontaneous hemarthrosis of knee in the elderly," *The Japanese Orthopaedic Association*, vol. 64, p. S195, 1990.

[4] H. Kawamura, K. Ogata, H. Miura, T. Arizono, and Y. Sugioka, "Spontaneous hemarthrosis of the knee in the elderly: etiology and treatment," *Arthroscopy*, vol. 10, no. 2, pp. 171–175, 1994.

[5] F. Pellacci and M. Lughi, "Spontaneous recurrent hemarthrosis of the knee with lesion of the lateral meniscus and arthrosis of the lateral compartment," *La Chirurgia Degli Organi di Movimento*, vol. 82, no. 1, pp. 69–72, 1997.

[6] H. Ogawa, M. Itokazu, Y. Ito, M. Fukuta, and K. Simizu, "An unusual meniscal ganglion cyst that triggered recurrent hemarthrosis of the knee," *Arthroscopy*, vol. 22, no. 4, pp. 455–e4, 2006.

[7] T. Sasho, S. Ogino, H. Tsuruoka et al., "Spontaneous recurrent hemarthrosis of the knee in the elderly: arthroscopic treatment and etiology," *Arthroscopy*, vol. 24, no. 9, pp. 1027–1033, 2008.

[8] K. Nagai, T. Matsumoto, T. Matsushita et al., "Spontaneous recurrent hemarthrosis of the knee joint in the elderly: a report of two cases," *Journal of Orthopaedic Science*, vol. 17, no. 5, pp. 649–653, 2012.

[9] S. P. Arnoczky and R. F. Warren, "Microvasculature of the human meniscus," *American Journal of Sports Medicine*, vol. 10, no. 2, pp. 90–95, 1982.

[10] M. Maruyama, M. Hariu, H. Satake, N. Hasuike, and Y. Urayama, "A case of idiopathic hemarthrosis of the knee caused by vessel injury with torn lateral meniscus," *Kansetsukyo*, vol. 34, pp. 36–41, 2009 (Japanese).

[11] S.-S. Shim and G. Leung, "Blood supply of the knee joint. A microangiographic study in children and adults," *Clinical Orthopaedics and Related Research*, vol. 208, pp. 119–125, 1986.

[12] M. Oshida and K. Shimada, "Anatomical study of the blood supply to the meniscus," *Seikeisaigaigeka*, vol. 44, pp. 725–731, 2001 (Japanese).

2

Delayed Reconstruction by Total Calcaneal Allograft following Calcanectomy: Is It an Option?

Benjamin Degeorge, Louis Dagneaux, David Forget, Florent Gaillard, and François Canovas

Department of Orthopedic Surgery, Division of Lower Limb Surgery, Lapeyronie University Hospital, 371 Avenue du Doyen Gaston Giraud, 34295 Montpellier Cedex 5, France

Correspondence should be addressed to Louis Dagneaux; louisdagneaux@gmail.com

Academic Editor: Kaan Erler

Many options are available in literature for the management of delayed reconstruction following calcanectomy. In cases of low-grade tumor lesions, conservative surgery can be considered. We describe a case of delayed reconstruction by calcaneal allograft after calcanectomy for low-grade chondrosarcoma. At 12-month follow-up, the patient had no pain; MSTS score and AOFAS score were satisfactory. Subtalar nonunion was observed with no secondary displacement or graft necrosis. The aim of conservative treatment for this patient was to restore normal gait with plantigrade locomotion and function of the Achilles tendon. Calcaneal reconstruction by total allograft is an alternative approach following calcanectomy for calcaneal tumors. We also discussed other options of calcaneal reconstruction.

1. Introduction

Delayed reconstruction is needed in rare cases, especially following calcanectomy. For example, conservative surgery can be considered in cases of low-grade tumors. The aim of this report was to make a functional assessment of delayed reconstruction of the calcaneus by total allograft and to discuss alternative treatments.

2. Clinical Case

A 58-year-old patient was referred to our University Hospital in June 2014 for a chronic wound of the left heel. Review of the patient's clinical history revealed total calcanectomy in 2007 with a cement spacer fixed by pins after bone cancer. Pathological examination showed a well-differentiated cartilaginous tumor with bone resorption and hyaline tumor matrix without myxoid reshuffle. Investigations were compatible with a low grade of calcaneal chondrosarcoma with involvement of the Achilles tendon (Figure 1).

In January 2015, delayed allograft bone reconstruction was performed using total calcaneus with the distal extremity of the Achilles tendon (Figure 2) retrieved during multiorgan removal and processed in the standard manner. Surgeon performed lateral approach of the calcaneus, avoiding the sural nerve and fibular tendons. After the spacer was extracted by fragmentation, bone scissors were used for joint cartilage removal. The calcaneus allograft was then calibrated with an oscillating saw to obtain a size appropriate for the morphology of the hindfoot. The graft was temporarily fixed by pins under scopic guidance. Double arthrodesis was then performed after spongy bone grafting from the iliac bone: subtalar arthrodesis with two screws of 6.5 mm diameter and calcaneocuboid arthrodesis with a Blount's staple (Figure 3). The plantar fascia and the extremities of the Achilles tendon were sutured at their respective insertion sites on the allograft with a Krackow-type suture using nonabsorbable suture PremiCron® USP 5 after removal. The Achilles peritendon was then sutured to itself to promote its vascularization. Postoperative recommendations were total rest for 3 months followed by gradual resumption of foot contact with the ground in a shoe with heel support. The patient started to walk on the full sole of the foot as from the 4th month, with the aid of two crutches.

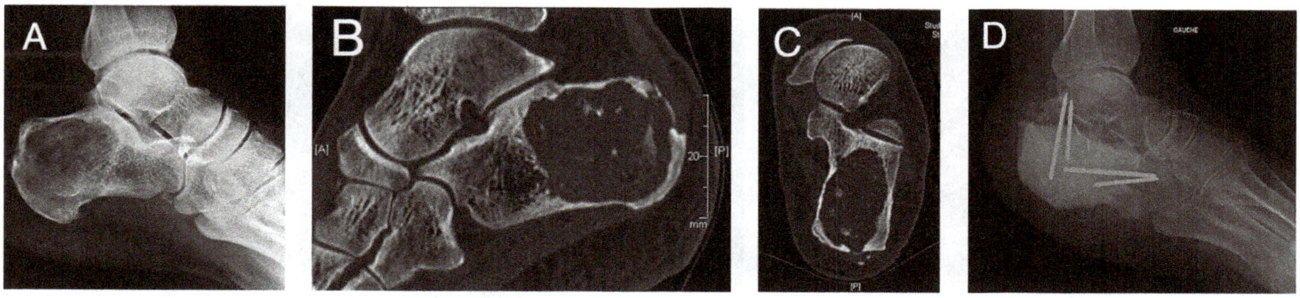

(a) (b) (c) (d)

FIGURE 1: Clinical history: X-ray (a) and CT-scan (b and c) images of calcaneal chondrosarcoma showing a heterogeneous, lytic picture with intracystic calcifications. Visualization of a cortical rupture of the greater tuberosity with involvement of the Achilles tendon. Lateral X-ray (d) showing the spacer following calcanectomy with talocalcaneal and calcaneocuboid fixation.

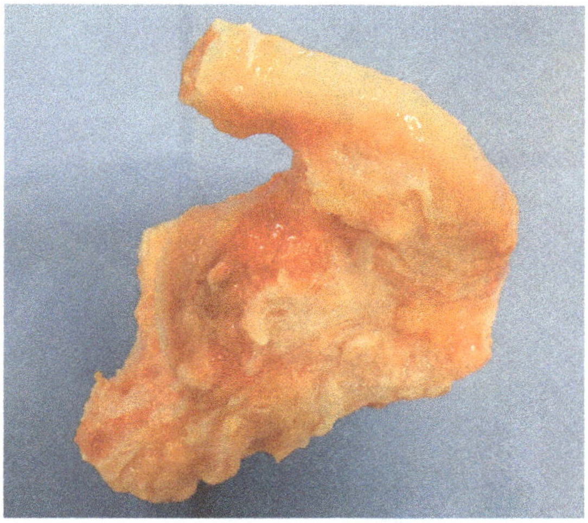

FIGURE 2: Photograph of the total calcaneal allograft with the distal extremity of the Achilles tendon.

At 12-month follow-up there were no signs of tumor relapse. The patient was pain-free and had returned to work (Figure 4), with an MSTS 93 score of 67% and an AOFAS score of 72 points. Dorsiflexion and plantar flexion were 15 and 30 degrees, respectively. Achilles tendon action was normal with muscle strength of 5/5, corresponding to similar contraction of the active plantar flexion compared to the contralateral side and a rise heel position allowed in single leg stance. Testing of subtalar and Chopart joints was painless. Podoscopic examination showed a hindfoot varus and defective medial support. The patient was able to walk barefoot without pain. He was prescribed pronation insoles for daily use over a walking distance of 500 m. X-rays showed a calcaneal varus of few degrees from Meary's method in weight-bearing and CT-scan highlighted a subtalar nonunion (Figure 4). The calcaneocuboid arthrodesis was healed. There was no evidence of secondary displacement, fracture, or graft necrosis.

3. Discussion

Chondrosarcomas develop very slowly in the young adult with no overt symptoms. A study by the Mayo Clinic reported a survival rate of 89% at 10-year follow-up [1] despite metastatic evolution in a quarter of the cases. The reference treatment is a surgical resection with satisfactory results. However, treatment by conservative surgery is not restricted to removal of the tumor in free margins [2], and the final aim is to restore normal gait. This involves several factors including bearing of weight without deformation of the hindfoot and normal movement of the Achilles tendon and plantar fascia to allow plantigrade locomotion. Our patient underwent delayed reconstruction 6 years after calcanectomy. There are few documented reports of the surgical procedure and approaches differ between authors (Table 1).

(i) Ottolenghi and Petracchi [3] and Muscolo et al. [4] were the first to study the possibility of a total calcaneal allograft. In both reports, osteointegration was successful with satisfactory functional results. However, the authors reported secondary osteonecrosis of the hindfoot at 4-year follow-up in both studies.

(ii) Li et al. [2, 5, 6] recommended the use of composite fibular flaps with or without allograft and achieved satisfactory functional and oncologic results. No information was given on postoperative foot statics.

(iii) Scoccianti et al. [7] and Kurvin et al. [8] used vascularized iliac crest bone graft. Owing to its greater volume and according to the size of the resection, the iliac bone graft allowed full weight-bearing and good-quality tissue for arthrodesis. However, the use of free flaps required microsurgical anastomosis including its complications. One case of bone graft fracture was observed in follow-up but without long-term functional consequences.

(iv) Imanishi and Choong [9] and Chou and Malawer [10] used a titan prosthesis after scan planning. Postoperative progress was similar to that following allograft, with successful functional recovery.

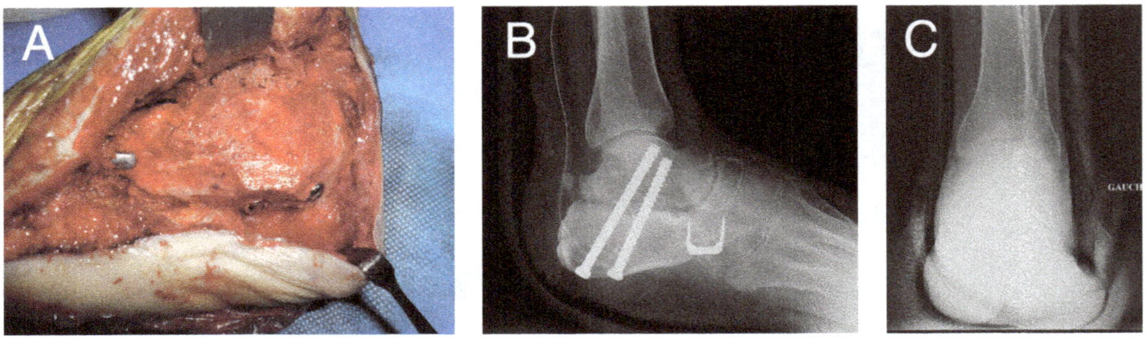

(a) (b) (c)

Figure 3: Intraoperative lateral view of the calcaneal allograft arthrodesis (a) and postoperative X-ray examination (b and c) of the calcaneal allograft and double arthrodesis.

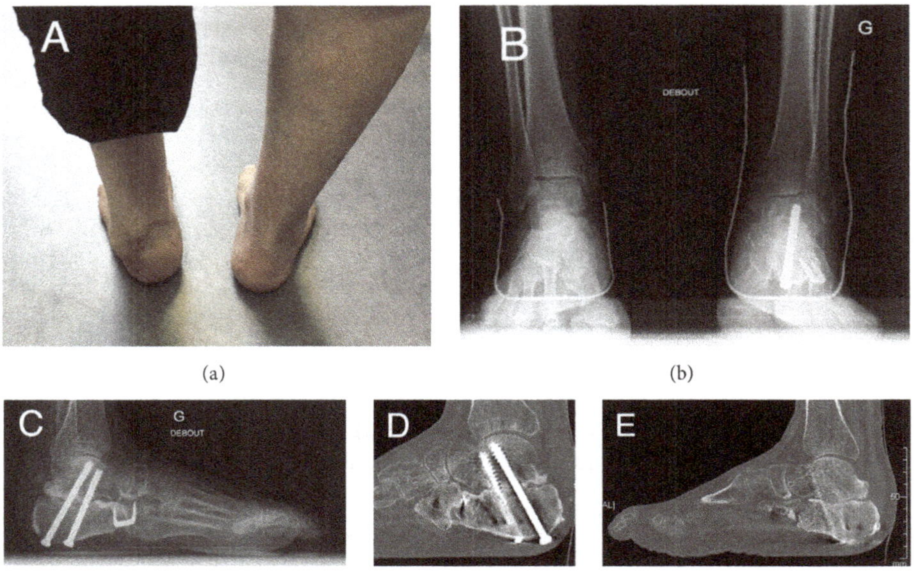

(a) (b)

(c) (d) (e)

Figure 4: Latest follow-up assessment: Photograph shows a slight varus of the hindfoot (a). X-ray (b) and scan (c) assessment at 12-month follow-up with Meary incidence showing the residual varus of the hindfoot.

Each technique had its specific problems with regard to fixation, soft tissue coverage, donor site morbidity, and functional recovery (Table 2). The use of Chopart's fixation was debatable. To our knowledge, there have been no biomechanical studies of the mode of fixation in calcaneal allografts. We attached the calcaneal allograft by double arthrodesis avoiding the talonavicular joint and using spongy autograft from the iliac bone [11]. The authors dealt with different fixation regarding the type of reconstruction: subtalar fixation [2, 5, 6] or double arthrodesis [4, 8]. Calcaneal prostheses [9, 10] were stable after ligament fixation and without bone fixation.

Soft tissue coverage is not always necessary and the decision to use flaps depends on tumor invasion. Several authors recommend the use of mixed flaps (pediculated fibular [2, 5, 6] or free iliac [7, 8]) for coverage. However, in more than a third of cases repeat surgery was required for local complications. Despite a reported success rate of 96%, microvascular anastomoses of the free flaps lead to further complications [12]. The use of flaps may be restricted by problems of tissue autonomization following calcaneal prosthesis. In calcaneal allografts, it is possible to include a sural pediculated flap and maintain epicritic plantar sensitivity.

Total calcaneal allograft is an alternative treatment of low-grade calcaneal tumors. We describe its use in delayed construction by allograft following calcanectomy. At 12-month follow-up, our patient had satisfactory clinical and functional scores. However, long-term monitoring is required to assess allograft survival in this indication.

TABLE 1: Review of the literature of the different options of reconstruction following calcanectomy.

Authors	Date	NC	Surgery	Characteristics	MSTS (%)	AOFAS	FU (y)
Imanishi and Choong [9]	2015	1	Calcaneal prosthesis	No tumor recurrence	/	82	0.4
Li and Wang [5]	2014	5-4	Allograft + pediculated composite fibular flap versus amputation	No local tumor recurrence	74–83	/	3.5
Li et al. [2]	2012	4	Allograft + pediculated composite fibular flap	2 local repeated surgeries No tumor recurrence	93	80–95	2
Li et al. [6]	2010	5	Pediculated composite fibular flap	2 local repeated surgeries No tumor recurrence	93	80–95	4.2
Scoccianti et al. [7]	2009	2	Free composite iliac flap	1 fracture No tumor recurrence	/	/	7.1
Kurvin et al. [8]	2008	1	Free composite iliac flap	/	/	/	2.6
Chou and Malawer [10]	2007	1	Calcaneal prosthesis	No tumor recurrence	/	67	12
Muscolo et al. [4] Ottolenghi and Petracchi [3]	2000	2	Calcaneal autograft + iliac autograft	1 osteonecrosis	/	/	9–32

NC: number of cases; MSTS: Musculoskeletal Tumor Society; AOFAS: American Orthopedic Foot and Ankle Society; FU: follow-up; y: years.

TABLE 2: Comparison of different reconstruction techniques following calcanectomy.

	Fixation	AT suture	Donor site morbidity	Foot statics	Complication at last follow-up (years)	Possibility of soft tissue coverage
Calcaneal allograft [3, 4]	Double arthrodesis	Yes	/	Restored	Osteonecrosis of the graft (32 and 9)	Yes*
Composite fibular flap [6]	Arthrodesis ST	No	None in the study Risk of lesions common PN, pain	Restored but strait calcaneal support	3 repeat flaps (4,2)	Yes
Allograft + pediculated composite fibular flap [2, 5]	Arthrodesis AT suture	Yes	None in the study Risk of lesions common PN, pain	Restored	2 repeat flaps (2 and 3,5)	Yes
Free composite iliac flap [7, 8]	Double arthrodesis (ST, CC, and TN)	Yes	Pain Scar	Restored Heel numbness	Graft fracture (7,1 and 2,6)	Yes
Calcaneal prosthesis [9, 10]	ST and CC avivement	Yes + plantar fascia and spring ligament	/	Restored	None (0,4 and 12)	To be assessed

ST: subtalar; CC: calcaneocuboid; AT: Achilles tendon; TN: talonavicular; PN: peroneal nerve; *associated or secondary sural flap.

Consent

The patient's consent was obtained before publication.

Disclosure

Level of evidence is level IV.

Competing Interests

The authors declare no conflict of interests.

References

[1] A. Itälä, T. Leerapun, C. Inwards, M. Collins, and S. P. Scully, "An institutional review of clear cell chondrosarcoma," *Clinical Orthopaedics and Related Research*, vol. 440, pp. 209–212, 2005.

[2] J. Li, G. Pei, Z. Wang, Z. Guo, M. Yang, and G. Chen, "Composite biological reconstruction following total calcanectomy of primary calcaneal tumors," *Journal of Surgical Oncology*, vol. 105, no. 7, pp. 673–678, 2012.

[3] C. E. Ottolenghi and L. J. Petracchi, "Chondromyxosarcoma of the calcaneus; report of a case of total replacement of involved

bone with a homogenous refrigerated calcaneus," *The Journal of Bone and Joint Surgery*, vol. 35-A, no. 1, pp. 211–214, 1953.

[4] D. L. Muscolo, M. A. Ayerza, and L. A. Aponte-Tinao, "Long-term results of allograft replacement after total calcanectomy. A report of two cases," *The Journal of Bone & Joint Surgery—American Volume*, vol. 82, no. 1, pp. 109–112, 2000.

[5] J. Li and Z. Wang, "Surgical treatment of malignant tumors of the calcaneus," *Journal of the American Podiatric Medical Association*, vol. 104, no. 1, pp. 71–76, 2014.

[6] J. Li, Z. Guo, G.-X. Pei, Z. Wang, G.-J. Chen, and Z.-G. Wu, "Limb salvage surgery for calcaneal malignancy," *Journal of Surgical Oncology*, vol. 102, no. 1, pp. 48–53, 2010.

[7] G. Scoccianti, D. A. Campanacci, M. Innocenti, G. Beltrami, and R. Capanna, "Total calcanectomy and reconstruction with vascularized iliac bone graft for osteoblastoma: a report of two cases," *Foot and Ankle International*, vol. 30, no. 7, pp. 716–720, 2009.

[8] L. A. Kurvin, C. Volkering, and S. B. Keßler, "Calcaneus replacement after total calcanectomy via vascularized pelvis bone," *Foot and Ankle Surgery*, vol. 14, no. 4, pp. 221–224, 2008.

[9] J. Imanishi and P. F. M. Choong, "Three-dimensional printed calcaneal prosthesis following total calcanectomy," *International Journal of Surgery Case Reports*, vol. 10, pp. 83–87, 2015.

[10] L. B. Chou and M. M. Malawer, "Osteosarcoma of the calcaneus treated with prosthetic replacement with twelve years of followup: a case report," *Foot and Ankle International*, vol. 28, no. 7, pp. 841–844, 2007.

[11] C. R. Lareau, M. E. Deren, A. Fantry, R. M. J. Donahue, and C. W. DiGiovanni, "Does autogenous bone graft work? A logistic regression analysis of data from 159 papers in the foot and ankle literature," *Foot and Ankle Surgery*, vol. 21, no. 3, pp. 150–159, 2015.

[12] R. Gao and S. Loo, "Review of 100 consecutive microvascular free flaps," *New Zealand Medical Journal*, vol. 124, no. 1345, pp. 49–56, 2011.

3

An Interesting Case of Intramuscular Myxoma with Scapular Bone Lysis

Jérôme Tirefort,[1] Frank C. Kolo,[2] and Alexandre Lädermann[1,3,4]

[1]*Division of Orthopaedics and Trauma Surgery, Department of Surgery, Geneva University Hospitals, Geneva, Switzerland*
[2]*Rive Droite Radiology Center, Geneva, Switzerland*
[3]*Faculty of Medicine, University of Geneva, Geneva, Switzerland*
[4]*Division of Orthopaedics and Trauma Surgery, La Tour Hospital, Geneva, Switzerland*

Correspondence should be addressed to Alexandre Lädermann; alexandre.laedermann@gmail.com

Academic Editor: Akio Sakamoto

Introduction. Intramuscular myxoma is a rare benign primitive tumor of the mesenchyme founded at the skeletal muscle level; it presents itself like an unpainful, slow-growing mass. Myxomas with bone lysis are even more rare; only 7 cases have been reported in the English literature, but never at the shoulder level. *Case Presentation.* We describe an 83-year-old patient with a growing mass in the deltoid muscle with unique scapular lysis, without any symptom. Magnetic resonance imaging (MRI) and a biopsy were performed and the diagnosis of intramuscular myxoma has been retained. In front of this diagnosis of nonmalignant lesion, the decision of a simple follow-up was taken. One year after this decision, the patient was still asymptomatic. *Conclusion.* In the presence of an intramuscular growing mass with associated bone lysis, intramuscular myxoma as well as malignant tumor should be evoked. MRI has to be part of the initial radiologic appraisal but biopsy is essential to confirm the diagnosis. By consensus, the standard treatment is surgical excision but conservative treatment with simple follow-up can be an option.

1. Introduction

Myxoma is a rare benign primitive tumor of the mesenchyme [1]; it presents itself like an unpainful, slow-growing mass. It is even more rare at the skeletal muscle level [2] and is named in this case "intramuscular myxoma." We describe here an exceptional case of intramuscular myxoma in the deltoid, which has the particularity to lyse the surrounding scapular bone. This bone lysis is almost unique; indeed, only 7 cases have been reported since the fifties, but never at the shoulder level.

2. Case Presentation

An 83-year-old woman presented with a slow-growing, palpable, painless mass in her left shoulder. She was known for auricular fibrillation, a type of hypothyroidism. The patient had no symptom; she just noticed the apparition of this mass two years earlier. At examination, no limitation in shoulder range motion was found and a mass of about 6 cm diameter was palpable.

Conventional X-rays were normal. CT scan and magnetic resonance imaging (MRI) were performed and showed an important prescapular necrotic cystic-like mass measuring 9.5 × 6.0 cm (Figures 1–3) with scapular encroachment (bony erosion) (Figure 4). Finally, a guided biopsy under ultrasonographic control was performed. Four samples were taken in the periphery of the lesion. They showed a cystic lesion with necrotic debris in its center. At histological examination, a myxoid aspect with few cells was noticed. Some fusiform cells of little size, regular, elongated aspect nuclei were found, without hyperchromasia or mitotic activity. The myxoid matrix was abundant and loose. The lesion was not vascularized (Figures 5–7). The diagnosis of a benign tumor of myxoma type was retained. Simple follow-up was decided due to the lack of symptoms and the age of the patient. One year later, she was still asymptomatic.

3. Discussion

Intramuscular myxomas are localized in skeletal muscles; they represent a distinct subtype of myxomas and have been described for the first time in 1965 by Enzinger [1], constituting only 17% of all soft tissue myxoma cases in his study. They occur more frequently in females and usually affect patients between 40 and 70 years of age [2].

In terms of localization, extracardiac myxomas are rare, and they occur most commonly in the head and skin tissue [3]. Regarding intramuscular myxomas, they have been exceptionally reported in shoulder muscles, thighs, buttocks, or upper extremities [4]. In the present case, the intramuscular myxoma was in the deltoid muscle. Such localization has only been published three times [5–7], but never in conjunction with bone lysis. This bone lysis is in fact very rare, and some odontogenic myxomas with gnathic bone lysis have been described [8] but they presented more aggressive proliferation with cortical lysis and the worst prognostics. To the best of our knowledge, there are only seven cases of extragnathic myxomas associated with bone lysis described in the English literature [9–13].

Histologically, myxoma is a primitive tumor of the mesenchyme composed of undifferentiated stellate cells in a loose mucoid stroma with reticulin fibers; vascularization is poor but focal hypervascularity may be seen and an abundant myxoid matrix is present [14]. The tumor is characterized by the absence of a true capsule but only possessed an incomplete pseudocapsule [8]. These criteria were met in our case (Figures 5–7). The etiology of myxomas remains elusive. Some authors suggested a traumatic origin [2]. It is also possible that growth of polysaccharide-producing cells is implicated in the neoplastic process [1, 15].

Under MRI examination, the myxoma presented a cystic-like aspect partly solid with thick rim enhancement (Figures 1–3) [16]. Usually, intramuscular myxomas appear hypointense on T1-weighted sequences with a characteristic perilesional fat rind and an increased signal in the adjacent muscle on T2-weighted and fluid-sensitive MR sequences can be found [17]. Unfortunately, in our case, these criteria were not all present. But the final diagnosis is always retained on a biopsy, especially to differentiate a simple intramuscular myxoma from a malignant tumor.

The differential diagnosis of intramuscular myxomas includes also aggressive angiomyxoma, myxoid neurofibroma, myxoid liposarcoma, cellular or juxta-articular myxoma, and nodular fasciitis [18, 19]. Because focal areas of hypervascularity and hypercellularity may be present, it is sometimes difficult to differentiate a simple intramuscular myxoma from a malignant tumor. Immunostain for S-100 protein and GNAS 1 mutations can distinguish myxoid liposarcoma and low-grade myxofibrosarcoma from intramuscular myxomas, respectively [20, 21]. In the present case, the diagnosis was clear and additional investigations were not necessary.

Clinically intramuscular myxomas usually present as a painless slow-growing mass; symptoms are due to the compression of surrounding structures [1]. In case of multiple intramuscular myxomas, the Mazabraud syndrome and the McCune-Albright syndrome should be considered, but the first is associated with fibrous dysplasia and the second with polyostotic bone dysplasia, café-au-lait spots, and precocious puberty [22, 23], conditions not present in our patient.

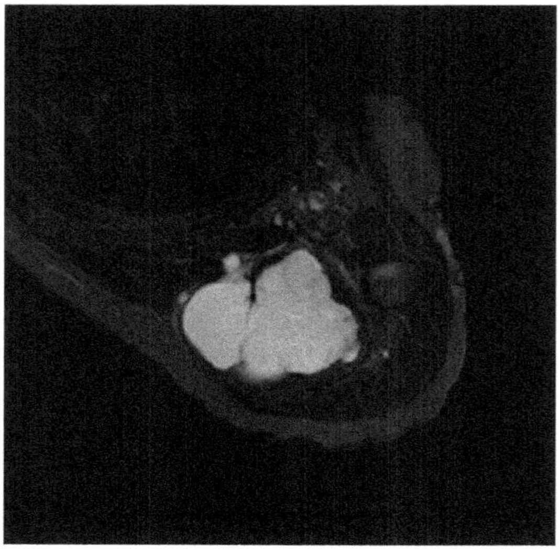

Figure 1: STIR and T2-weighted transverse MRI. Observe the huge cystic-like hyperintense mass growing inside the deltoid muscle and invading the scapula. The mass contains some septations but there is no apparent solid component.

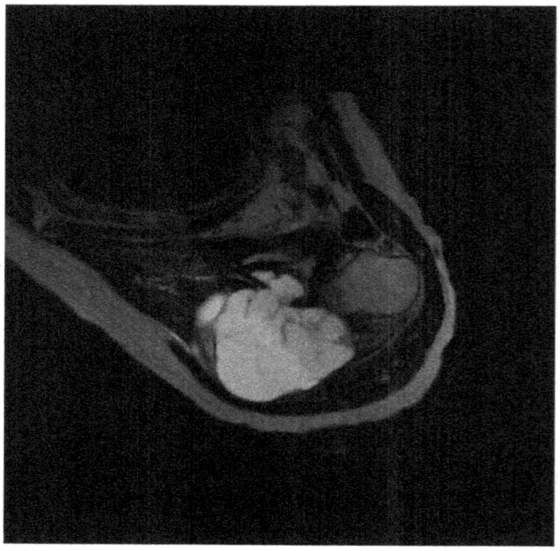

Figure 2: STIR and T2-weighted transverse MRI. Observe the huge cystic-like hyperintense mass growing inside the deltoid muscle and invading the scapula. The mass contains some septations but there is no apparent solid component.

By consensus, the recommended treatment of intramuscular myxomas is surgical excision. However, the recurrence of intramuscular myxomas is rare, restricted to isolated cases, and more commonly associated with syndromes [24–26]. In our case, the decision of a conservative treatment was taken

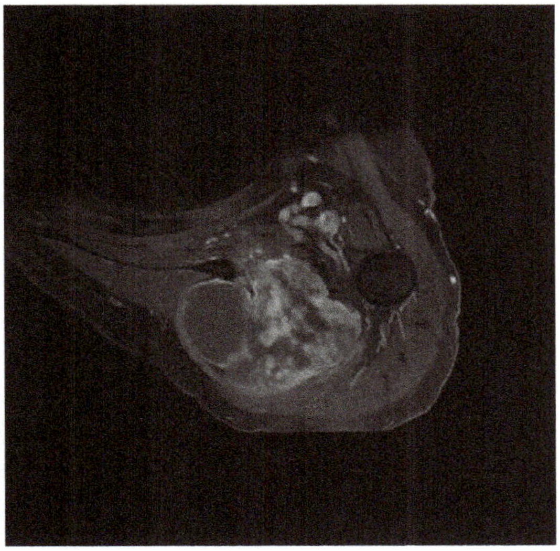

FIGURE 3: T1 transverse image with fat saturation after intravenous gadolinium injection. Note the enhancement indicating the presence of a solid component inside the mass which in consequence is a pseudocystic mass.

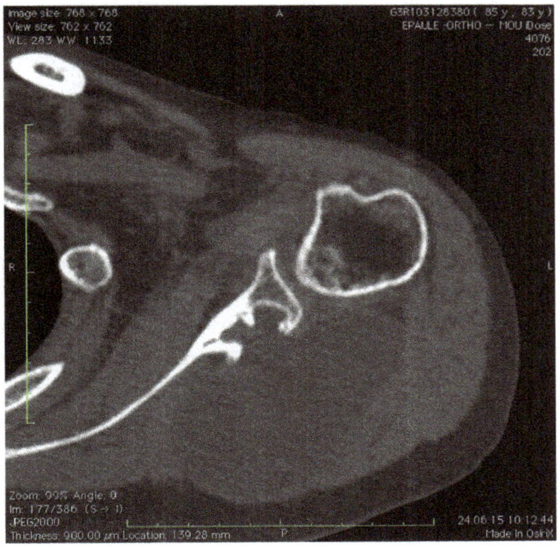

FIGURE 4: CT scan confirming the invasion of the scapula by the mass.

regarding age and lack of symptoms in our patient. One year after the biopsy, the patient was still asymptomatic.

4. Conclusion

In the presence of an intramuscular growing mass with associated bone lysis, myxoma as well as malignant neoplasm must be evoked. MRI with gadolinium injection and biopsy should be part of the initial appraisal to obtain a clear diagnosis. Surgical excision is the recommended treatment but every case should be discussed, and conservative treatment with simple follow-up can be an option for this benign tumor.

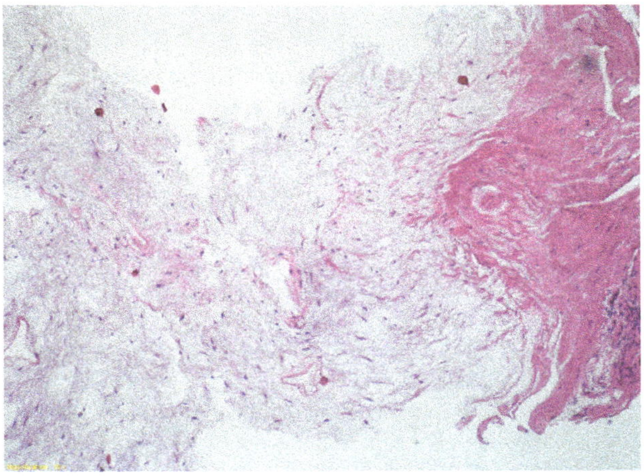

FIGURE 5: On histological examination, abundant myxoid matrix with few cells is observed. Notice the poor vascularization. Normal adjacent skeletal muscle is present on the left side of Figure 4.

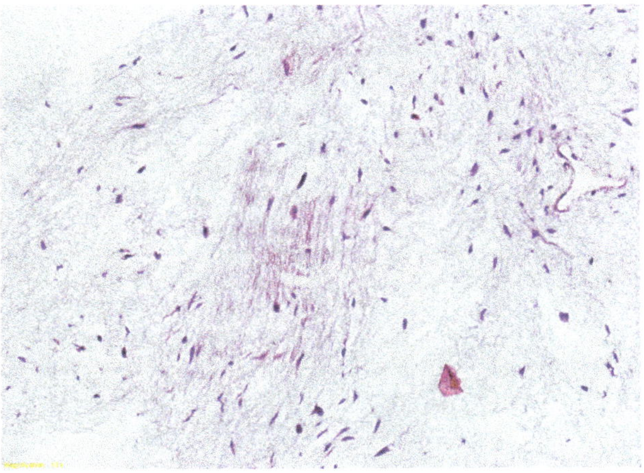

FIGURE 6: On histological examination, abundant myxoid matrix with few cells is observed. Notice the poor vascularization. Normal adjacent skeletal muscle is present on the left side of Figure 4.

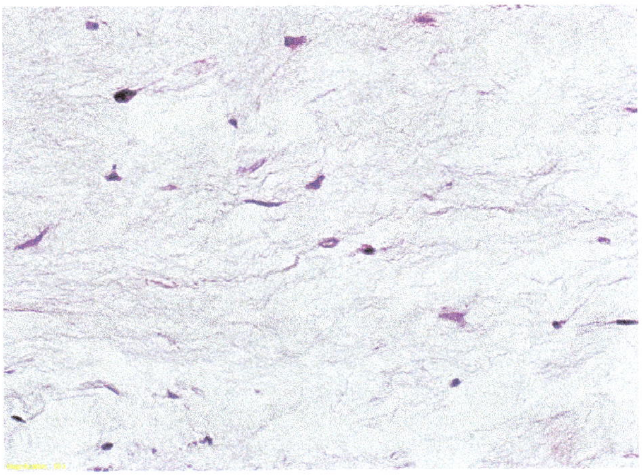

FIGURE 7: At higher magnification, fusiform cells of little size and regular shape are seen. Elongated aspect nuclei are present, without mitotic activity.

Competing Interests

The authors certify that they or any members of their immediate families have no funding or commercial associations (consultancies, stock ownership, equity interest, patent/licensing arrangements, etc.) that might pose a conflict of interests in connection with the submitted article.

References

[1] F. M. Enzinger, "Intramuscular myxoma; a review and follow-up study of 34 cases," *American Journal of Clinical Pathology*, vol. 43, pp. 104–113, 1965.

[2] S. Rachidi, A. J. Sood, T. Rumboldt, and T. A. Day, "Intramuscular myxoma of the paraspinal muscles: a case report and systematic review of the literature," *Oncology Letters*, vol. 11, no. 1, pp. 466–470, 2016.

[3] A. P. Stout, "Myxoma, the tumor of primitive mesenchyme," *Annals of surgery*, vol. 127, no. 4, pp. 706–719, 1948.

[4] P. W. Allen, "Myxoma is not a single entity: a review of the concept of myxoma," *Annals of Diagnostic Pathology*, vol. 4, no. 2, pp. 99–123, 2000.

[5] B. Kemah, M. S. Soylemez, B. Ceyran, S. Şenol, S. Mutlu, and K. Özkan, "A case of intramuscular myxoma presenting as a swollen shoulder: a case report," *Journal of Medical Case Reports*, vol. 8, no. 1, article no. 441, 2014.

[6] D. Costamagna, S. Erra, and R. Durando, "Intramuscular myxoma of the deltoid muscle: report of a case," *BMJ Case Reports*, vol. 2009, 2009.

[7] S. Monga, S. K. Shukla, S. Bhargava, and L. S. Bhatnagar, "Intramuscular myxoma of deltoid—a case report," *Indian Journal of Pathology and Microbiology*, vol. 20, no. 3, pp. 189–190, 1977.

[8] Z. Chaudhary, P. Sharma, S. Gupta, S. Mohanty, M. Naithani, and A. Jain, "Odontogenic myxoma: report of three cases and retrospective review of literature in Indian population," *Contemporary Clinical Dentistry*, vol. 6, no. 4, pp. 522–528, 2015.

[9] W. H. Bauer and A. Harell, "Myxoma of bone," *The Journal of Bone and Joint Surgery. American Volume*, vol. 36, no. 2, pp. 263–266, 1954.

[10] S. S. Santhanam, V. Goni, B. Saibaba, and A. Das, "Myxoma of the femur: an unusual site of origin," *BMJ Case Reports*, vol. 2015, 2015.

[11] D. K. McClure and D. C. Dahlin, "Myxoma of bone; report of three cases," *Mayo Clinic Proceedings*, vol. 52, no. 4, pp. 249–253, 1977.

[12] P. B. Chacha and K. K. Tan, "Periosteal myxoma of the femur. A case report," *Journal of Bone and Joint Surgery A*, vol. 54, no. 5, pp. 1091–1094, 1972.

[13] J. A. Hill, T. A. Victor, W. J. Dawson, and J. W. Milgram, "Myxoma of the toe: a case report," *Journal of Bone and Joint Surgery A*, vol. 60, no. 1, pp. 128–130, 1978.

[14] A. Luna, S. Martinez, and E. Bossen, "Magnetic resonance imaging of intramuscular myxoma with histological comparison and a review of the literature," *Skeletal Radiology*, vol. 34, no. 1, pp. 19–28, 2005.

[15] D. C. R. Ireland, E. H. Soule, and J. C. Ivins, "Myxoma of somatic soft tissues: a report of 58 patients, 3 with multiple tumors and fibrous dysplasia of bone," *Mayo Clinic Proceedings*, vol. 48, no. 6, pp. 401–410, 1973.

[16] M. D. Murphey, G. A. McRae, J. C. Fanburg-Smith, H. T. Temple, A. M. Levine, and A. J. Aboulafia, "Imaging of soft-tissue myxoma with emphasis on CT and MR and comparison of radiologic and pathologic findings," *Radiology*, vol. 225, no. 1, pp. 215–224, 2002.

[17] L. W. Bancroft, M. J. Kransdorf, D. M. Menke, M. I. O'Connor, and W. C. Foster, "Intramuscular myxoma: characteristic MR imaging features," *American Journal of Roentgenology*, vol. 178, no. 5, pp. 1255–1259, 2002.

[18] P. Gavriilidis, G. Balis, A. Giannouli, and A. Nikolaidou, "Intramuscular myxoma of the soleus muscle: a rare tumor in an unusual location," *American Journal of Case Reports*, vol. 15, pp. 49–51, 2014.

[19] A. Lädermann, P. Kindynis, S. Taylor et al., "Articular nodular fasciitis in the glenohumeral joint," *Skeletal Radiology*, vol. 37, no. 7, pp. 663–666, 2008.

[20] S. Okamoto, M. Hisaoka, M. Ushijima, S. Nakahara, S. Toyoshima, and H. Hashimoto, "Activating Gsα mutation in intramuscular myxomas with and without fibrous dysplasia of bone," *Virchows Archiv*, vol. 437, no. 2, pp. 133–137, 2000.

[21] D. Delaney, T. C. Diss, N. Presneau et al., "GNAS1 mutations occur more commonly than previously thought in intramuscular myxoma," *Modern Pathology*, vol. 22, no. 5, pp. 718–724, 2009.

[22] L. Faivre, A. Nivelon-Chevallier, M. L. Kottler et al., "Mazabraud syndrome in two patients: clinical overlap with McCune-Albright syndrome," *American Journal of Medical Genetics*, vol. 99, no. 2, pp. 132–136, 2001.

[23] A. Diaz, M. Danon, and J. Crawford, "McCune-Albright syndrome and disorders due to activating mutations of GNAS1," *Journal of Pediatric Endocrinology and Metabolism*, vol. 20, no. 8, pp. 853–880, 2007.

[24] M. Szendrói, P. Rahóty, I. Antal, and J. Kiss, "Fibrous dysplasia associated with intramuscular myxoma (Mazabraud's syndrome): a long-term follow-up of three cases," *Journal of Cancer Research and Clinical Oncology*, vol. 124, no. 7, pp. 401–406, 1998.

[25] R. L. Caballes, "Fibromyxoma of bone," *Radiology*, vol. 130, no. 1, pp. 97–99, 1979.

[26] M. Kamiyoshihara, T. Hirai, O. Kawashima, S. Ishikawa, and Y. Morishita, "Fibromyxoma of the rib: report of a case," *Surgery Today*, vol. 29, no. 5, pp. 475–477, 1999.

4

Nontraumatic Myositis Ossificans of Hip: A Case Presentation

Yunus Oc,[1] Muhammed Sefa Ozcan,[1] Hasan Basri Sezer,[1] Bekir Eray Kilinc,[2] and Osman Tugrul Eren[1]

[1] *Sisli Hamidiye Etfal Training and Research Hospital, 19 Mayıs Mahallesi, Sisli, 34360 Istanbul, Turkey*
[2] *Igdir State Hospital Orthopaedics and Traumatology Department, Igdir, Turkey*

Correspondence should be addressed to Bekir Eray Kilinc; dreraykilinc@gmail.com

Academic Editor: Koichi Sairyo

In most of the cases trauma is the leading etiology and the nontraumatic myositis ossificans (MO) is a very rare condition. We present an MO case without any trauma occurring. A 36-year-old female patient with a history of pain and restriction of range of motion of the left hip was admitted. Hip motions were restricted with 10–60° of flexion, 10° of internal rotation, 20° of external rotation, 10° of abduction, and 10° of adduction. There was no history of trauma and familial involvement. The biopsy of the lesion revealed mature bone tissue confirming our diagnosis of MO. The mass was removed surgically and postoperatively the patient was treated with a single dose radiotherapy with 800 gyc. MO is a benign and well differentiated bone formation or in other words heterotopic ossification of the muscle tissue. It has a prevalence of less than 1/1 million. Trauma is the most frequent etiological factor seen in almost 60–75% of the cases. Nontraumatic MO is very rare in the literature. Our patient had no history of trauma or familial involvement. Combination of the surgical excision with radiotherapy in the treatment of the MO of the hip may give satisfactory results.

1. Introduction

Myositis ossificans (MO) is a nonneoplastic and benign condition in which there is an increased activity of periarticular tissues resulting in intramuscular bone formation [1]. In most of the cases trauma is the leading etiology and the nontraumatic MO is a very rare condition. It may affect any localization in the human body but selectively the areas which are susceptible to the trauma are involved such as hip, elbow, and wrist [2]. Biopsy may be required in some cases for differential diagnosis. This paper presents a very rare case of nontraumatic heterotopic ossification of hip.

2. Presentation of Case

A 36-year-old female patient with a history of the pain and the restriction of range of motion of the left hip admitted to our outpatient clinic. She complained of a mass in the left hip diagnosed by an orthopaedic surgeon 2 years ago and she was followed up with only clinical observation. Hip motions were restricted with a 10°–60° of flexion, 10° of internal rotation, 20° of external rotation, 10° of abduction, and 10° of adduction. There was no history of trauma or familial involvement.

Radiographic evaluation of the patient with X-ray revealed a 13 × 6 cm radiopaque mass extending from the anterior border of acetabulum to the trochanter minor medially and the trochanter major laterally (Figure 1).

The CT revealed a mass which was bridging from anterior aspect of coxofemoral joint to the trochanter minor with a large attachment (Figure 2). CT was applied at 2-year follow-up to show the removal of the mass (Figure 3).

The MRI revealed a mass which was broader in the intertrochanteric line where it was in a close relation to the bone. It was 11 cm long and 3 cm wide at the broadest part (Figure 4). The mass was osseous in character which was located along the lateral border of the iliopsoas muscle in its craniocaudal extension. Intraoperatively, the mass was seen starting from the superoanterior edge of the acetabulum with a small portion in the rectus femoris muscle and ending with a large attachment part to the anterior aspect of femur on the trochanter minor level. Furthermore, it was building an osseous bridge from anterior aspect of coxofemoral joint that

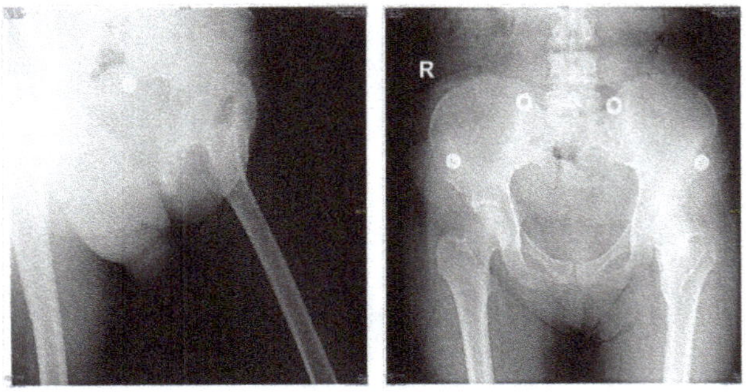

FIGURE 1: Preoperative radiographic evaluation with X-ray.

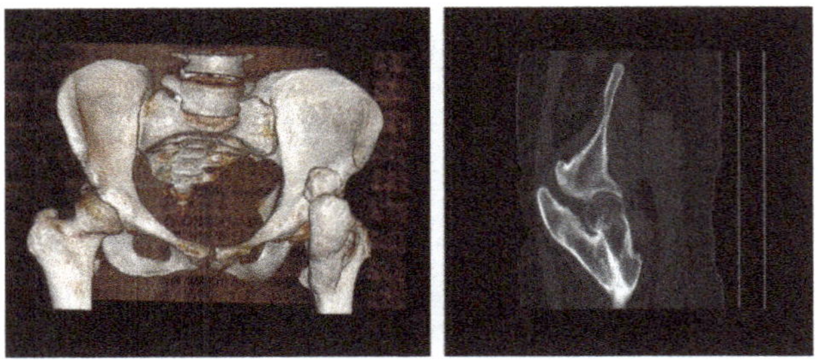

FIGURE 2: Preoperative radiographic evaluation with 3D and sagittal view of CT.

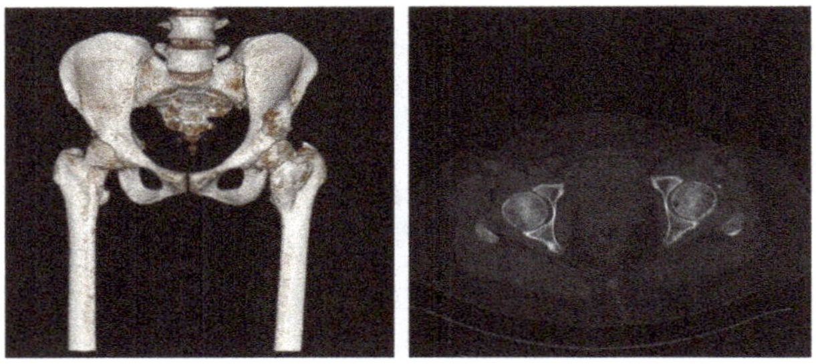

FIGURE 3: Post-op 2nd-year radiographic evaluation with 3D and axial view of CT.

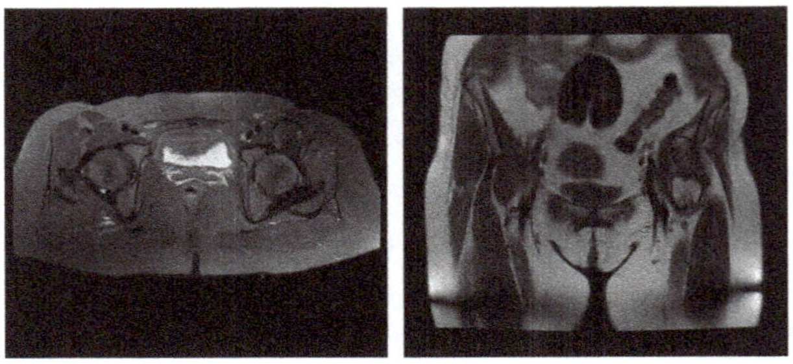

FIGURE 4: Preoperative radiographic evaluation MRI.

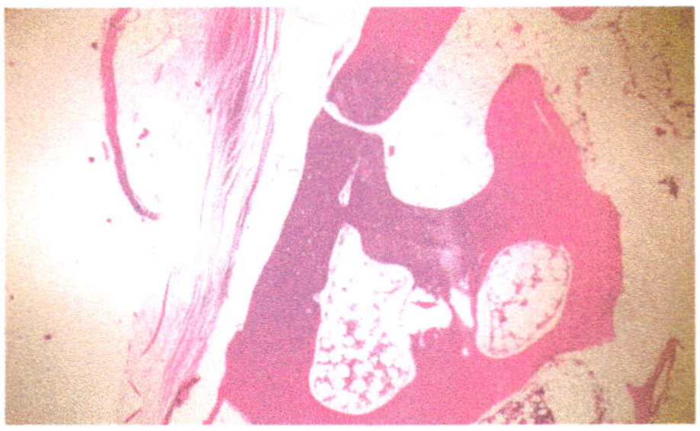

FIGURE 5: Histological examination of the specimen showing mature osteoid under 40x magnification.

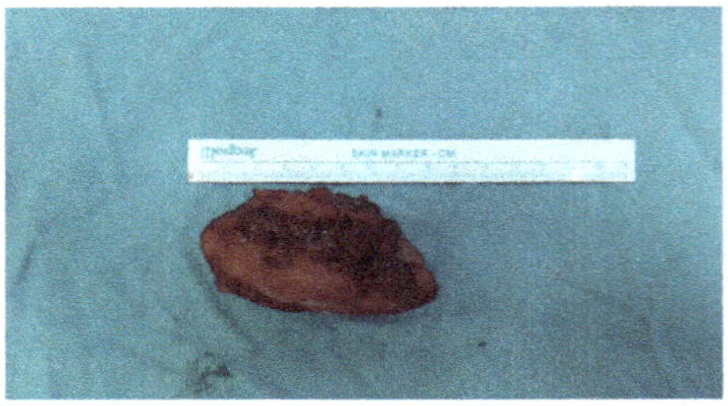

FIGURE 6: Surgically excised mass.

was limiting the range of motion of the hip. We realized that after removal of the mass the range of motion of the hip was totally released.

There was another mass sized 35 × 19 mm located superiorly close to the iliac bone anterior to the acetabulum. The soft tissue between 2 masses was edematous and inflammatory in character resembling the MO.

The biopsy of the lesion revealed mature bone tissue confirming our diagnosis of MO (Figure 5). The mass was removed surgically (Figure 6) and postoperatively the patient was treated with a single dose radiotherapy with 800 gyc.

There was a dramatic decrease in the pain and increase in the range of motion postoperatively. In the last follow-up examination the hip was able to reach 120° of flexion, 10° of extension, 30° of internal rotation, 40° of external rotation, 40° of abduction, and 30° of adduction.

3. Discussion

Myositis ossificans is a benign and well differentiated bone formation or in other words heterotopic ossification of the muscle tissue [1]. It has a prevalence of less than 1/1 million. There is no sexual predominance [3]. Trauma is the most frequent etiological factor seen in almost 60–75% of the cases [4–8]. It is believed that after a distinguishable trauma there occurs a tissue necrosis or bleeding initiating an uncontrolled vascular and fibroblastic activity resulting with bone formation [7]. Although unproven, some other etiological mechanisms were also hypothesized. One of the theories claims osteoblasts that are freed from periost and trapped in the soft tissues as the provocateur of the MO [6]. The other mechanism is the "ectopic calcification islands" theory which accuses periosteal tissue itself to be displaced into the soft tissues because of the impact of the trauma causing MO [9]. Tabes dorsalis, syringomyelia, poliomyelitis, paraplegia, tetanus, and hemophilia may play a role as the underlying pathology [9–11]. In the presence of such conditions MO may occur even; passive range of motion exercises is carried out. Burns, infections, and drug abuse are other rare conditions which may cause MO [9, 10].

Nontraumatic MO is very rare in the literature [7, 8, 12, 13]. Repetitive microtrauma, tissue ischemia, and inflammation were addressed as the causal mechanisms of the nontraumatic MO [7, 12]. MO of the hip occurs more frequently in patients experiencing palsy, subdural or epidural bleeding, and hip operation. Our case is free of all of those conditions. Fibrodysplasia ossificans progressive is another disease which presents with nontraumatic MO. It is a rare disease of 5- to 25-year-old population expressing autosomal dominant inheritance [9]. Clinically it is a progressive disease and may present with thumb and toe anomalies [3, 9]. In our case there was no family history or concomitant hand or toe anomalies.

To our knowledge our case is unique of being nontraumatic and having no simultaneous predisposing factors.

The pattern of progression in MO is pathognomonic by expressing a peripheral to central manner [3, 7, 10, 13]. Histologically collagen producing cells are located in the center and increased osteoblastic activity and immature bone lies in the intermediate zone and lamellar bone in the peripherally [13].

Clinically there is a formation of a painful mass at the region of trauma within 7–10 days [4]. Between 10 days and 6 weeks there appear to be irregular osseous fragments in this mass [4, 6, 8]. Cortical bone production takes place between 6 and 8 weeks [10]. From 10 weeks to 6 months the typical egg shell appearance of central zone is visible [4, 10]. Maturation of the mass takes place between 6 and 8 months and the mass may shrink to some degree [4, 6, 8]. Some lesions decrease in volume and some disappear within 1-2 years [4, 6].

MRI findings demonstrate heterogeneity due to the histological structure of the MO lesions [8, 10]. In the early period of the disease in T2 MRI section there is a dark and nonhomogenous intensity distribution in the central zone [8, 10]. The emergence of a hyperintensive ring around a hypointensive core is the sign of maturation of the mass [8, 10, 11]. There is no specific radiological finding of the nontraumatic MO.

MO is generally self-limited pathology [10]. There is a possibility of the spontaneous regression; thus surgical excision is not the primary choice of treatment by most of the surgeons [3]. Typical lesions may be followed with clinical and radiological observation [10]. Surgical indications include pain, increasing diameter of the mass, deteriorating local tendon or muscle function, and decreasing functional ability of the patient [10, 13, 14]. Such lesions may be excised after maturation.

Radiotherapy (RT) may decrease the diameter of the mass and may increase the maturation of the mass [14]. In the treatment of MO, one low dose RT was performed in many cases and it was seen very effective. Gokkus et al. reported that 24 hours after operation one low dose RT was effective in their case [15]. In another case report, Pakos et al. showed that RT treatment with combined indomethacin protocol was an effective treatment in MO [16]. Our case had a 3-year history with no regression and progressive deterioration of the left hip function. Our diagnosis was confirmed with the biopsy of the lesion. After excision of the mass one dose of radiotherapy (800 gyc) was administered. Postoperatively, there was a dramatic decrease in the pain and the patient had closely normal hip range of motion. There was no recurrence at 2-year follow-up proved by CT scan.

4. Conclusion

Nontraumatic MO is very rare and our case is the first case in the literature with no trauma or predisposing factors. Biopsy may be required to verify diagnosis. Combination of the surgical excision with radiotherapy in the treatment of the MO of the hip may give satisfactory results.

Competing Interests

The authors declare that there are no competing interests regarding the publication of this paper.

References

[1] A. L. Folpe and C. Y. Inwards, "Osteocartilaginous tumors," in *Bone and Soft Tissue Pathology*, J. X. O'Connell, Ed., A Volume in the Foundations in Diagnostic Pathology Series, pp. 239–254, Saunders-Elsevier, Philadelphia, Pa, USA, 2010.

[2] M. Yazici, B. Etensel, M. H. Gürsoy, A. Aydoğdu, and M. Erkuş, "Nontraumatic myositis ossificans with an unusual location: case report," *Journal of Pediatric Surgery*, vol. 37, no. 11, pp. 1621–1622, 2002.

[3] J. Aneiros-Fernandez, M. Caba-Molina, S. Arias-Santiago, F. O'Valle, P. Hernandez-Cortes, and J. Aneiros-Cachaza, "Myositis ossificans circumscripta without history of trauma," *Clinical Medicine & Research*, vol. 2, no. 3, pp. 142–144, 2010.

[4] T. Baysal, O. Baysal, K. Sarac, N. Elmali, R. Kutlu, and Y. Ersoy, "Cervical myositis ossificans traumatica: a rare location," *European Radiology*, vol. 9, no. 4, pp. 662–664, 1999.

[5] H. Hatano, T. Morita, H. Kobayashi, T. Ito, and H. Segawa, "MR imaging findings of an unusual case of myositis ossificans presenting as a progressive mass with features of fluid-fluid level," *Journal of Orthopaedic Science*, vol. 9, no. 4, pp. 399–403, 2004.

[6] S. W. Kim and J. H. Choi, "Myositis ossificans in psoas muscle after lumbar spine fracture," *Spine*, vol. 34, no. 10, pp. E367–E370, 2009.

[7] J. Nishio, K. Nabeshima, H. Iwasaki, and M. Naito, "Nontraumatic myositis ossificans mimicking a malignant neoplasm in an 83-year-old woman: a case report," *Journal of Medical Case Reports*, vol. 4, article 270, 2010.

[8] S. Saussez, C. Blaivie, M. Lemort, and G. Chantrain, "Nontraumatic myositis ossificans in the paraspinal muscles," *European Archives of Oto-Rhino-Laryngology*, vol. 263, no. 4, pp. 331–335, 2006.

[9] R. Merchant, N. I. Sainani, M. A. Lawande, S. A. Pungavkar, D. P. Patkar, and A. Walawalkar, "Pre- and post-therapy MR imaging in fibrodysplasia ossificans progressiva," *Pediatric Radiology*, vol. 36, no. 10, pp. 1108–1111, 2006.

[10] J. Parikh, H. Hyare, and A. Saifuddin, "The imaging features of post-traumatic myositis ossificans, with emphasis on MRI," *Clinical Radiology*, vol. 57, no. 12, pp. 1058–1066, 2002.

[11] M. J. Kransdorf, J. M. Meis, and J. S. Jelinek, "Myositis ossificans: MR appearance with radiologic-pathologic correlation," *American Journal of Roentgenology*, vol. 157, no. 6, pp. 1243–1248, 1991.

[12] S. S. Mann, P. M. Som, and J. P. Gumprecht, "The difficulties of diagnosing myositis ossificans circumscripta in the paraspinal muscles of a human immunodeficiency virus-positive man: magnetic resonance imaging and temporal computed tomographic findings," *Archives of Otolaryngology—Head and Neck Surgery*, vol. 126, no. 6, pp. 785–789, 2000.

[13] C. Zoccali, G. Chichierchia, and R. Covello, "An unusual case of lumbar paravertebral miositis ossificans mimicking muscular skeletal tumor," *Musculoskeletal Surgery*, vol. 97, no. 3, pp. 251–253, 2013.

[14] I. Findlay, P. R. Lakkireddi, R. Gangone, and G. Marsh, "A case of myositis ossificans in the upper cervical spine of a young child," *Spine*, vol. 35, no. 25, pp. E1525–E1528, 2010.

[15] K. Gokkus, E. Sagtas, F. E. Suslu, and A. T. Aydin, "Myositis ossificans circumscripta, secondary to high-velocity gunshot and fragment wound that causes sciatica," *BMJ Case Reports*, vol. 2013, 2013.

[16] E. E. Pakos, E. J. Pitouli, P. G. Tsekeris, V. Papathanasopoulou, K. Stafilas, and T. H. Xenakis, "Prevention of heterotopic ossification in high-risk patients with total hip arthroplasty: the experience of a combined therapeutic protocol," *International Orthopaedics*, vol. 30, no. 2, pp. 79–83, 2006.

5

Pectoralis Major Tear with Retracted Tendon: How to Fill the Gap? Reconstruction with Hamstring Autograft and Fixation with an Interference Screw

L. Baverel,[1] K. Messedi,[1] G. Piétu,[1] V. Crenn,[1] and F. Gouin[1,2]

[1]*CHU de Nantes, Clinique Chirurgicale Orthopédique et Traumatologique, Hôtel-Dieu, Place A. Ricordeau, 44093 Nantes Cedex, France*
[2]*LPRO, Inserm UI957, Laboratoire de la Résorption Osseuse et des Tumeurs Osseuses Primitives, Faculté de Médecine, Université de Nantes, 44000 Nantes, France*

Correspondence should be addressed to L. Baverel; l.baverel@gmail.com

Academic Editor: Kaan Erler

Rupture of the pectoralis major tendon is considered an uncommon injury and a significant number of ruptures are missed or diagnosed late, leading to a chronic tear. We report an open reconstruction technique and its outcomes in a case of chronic and retracted PM tear. At the last follow-up (12 months), the patient was pain-free, with a visual analogic scale at 0 all the time. He was very satisfied concerning the cosmetic and clinical results. The constant score was 93%, the SST value 95%, and the Quick DASH score 4.5. MRI performed one year postoperatively confirmed the continuity between PM tendon and graft, even if the aspect of the distal tendon seemed to be thinner than normal PM tendon. The excellent clinical outcomes at one-year follow-up suggest that PM tear with major tendon retraction can be reliably reconstructed with hamstring autograft, using a bioabsorbable screw to optimize the fixation device. This technique has proven its simplicity and efficiency to fill the gap.

1. Introduction

Rupture of the pectoralis major (PM) tendon is considered an uncommon injury occurring in male patients between 20 and 40, most being of military population and athletes [1, 2]. The incidence seems to increase with both weight lifting practice and use of anabolic steroids [3]. Nonspecific clinical signs are ecchymosis and pain, but more specific is a loss or thinning of the anterior axillary fold [4]. Magnetic resonance imaging (MRI) is the gold standard to confirm diagnosis, localize and grade the tear, and measure the stump retraction and the muscle fatty degeneration [5]. Surgical repair during the acute phase is recommended, regarding excellent outcomes and low number of operative complications [6–12].

Pectoralis Major is well described as a two-head muscle, according to its clavicular and sternocostal heads [13]. Its humeral tendon insertion is just lateral to the bicipital groove and measures approximately 5 centimeters in length and 3 to 4 millimeters in width, with U-shape (anterior and posterior layers inferiorly continuous) [14]. According to Bak, complete tears are more common than partial tears, with, respectively, reported rates of 91% and 9%. However, significant number of PM injuries are missed or diagnosed late, leading to a chronic tear [4, 15, 16]. Some authors reported good clinical outcomes after direct sutures of chronic PM tears, once tendon was released and mobilized [12].

Otherwise, tendon graft is necessary in presence of chronic tear with significant tendon retraction and altered tissue quality [17]. Various graft techniques have been described: hamstrings autograft [16], bone-patellar bone-tendon autograft [18], fascia lata allograft [19], Achilles tendon allograft [4], and dermal allograft [15]. In the literature, numerous fixation devices have been reported and compared, as suture anchor [4], unicortical button [20, 21], bone trough [12], or transosseous suture [6]. Authors found no significant biomechanical difference between these fixation devices [22–24]. However, interference screw seems to be equal or superior to theses other modes of fixation for subpectoral tenodesis of the long head of the biceps [25–29].

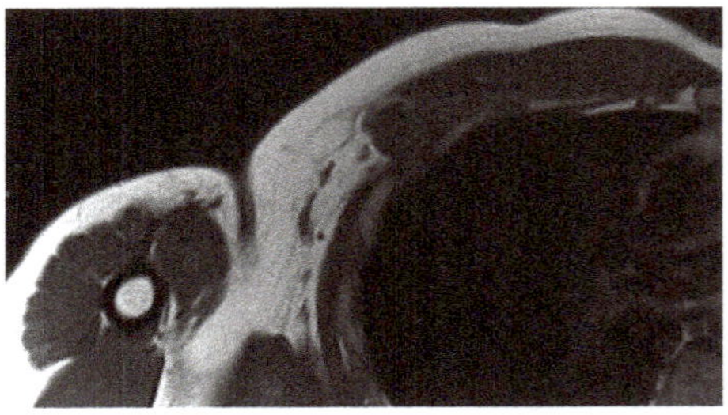

FIGURE 1: MRI axial T1 showing full-thickness PM tear at the humeral tendon-bone junction.

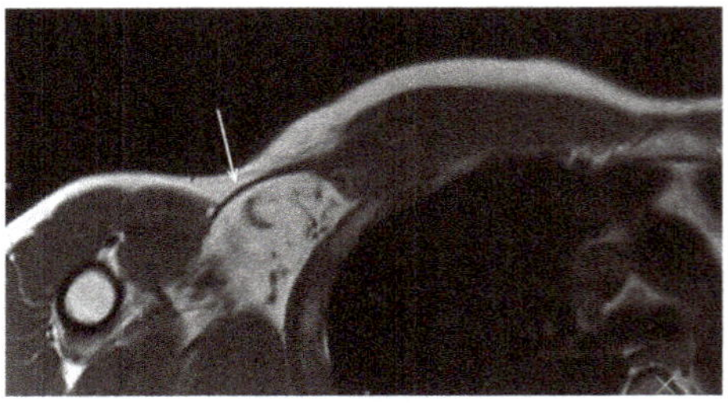

FIGURE 2: MRI axial T1 showing tendon retracted medial to the anterior chest wall and absence of any muscle fatty infiltration.

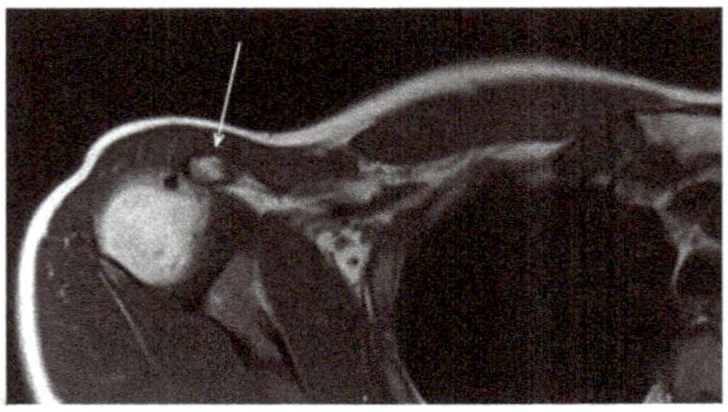

FIGURE 3: MRI axial T1 showing calcification inside the conjoint tendon immediately under its coracoid insertion.

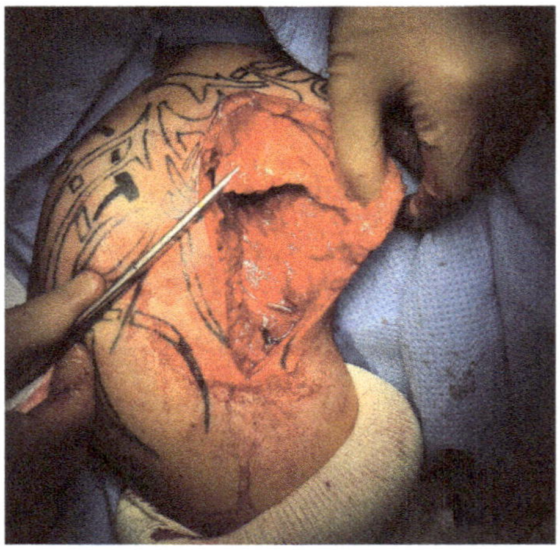

FIGURE 4: Intraoperative photograph demonstrating the gap between the footprint and the stump.

We report an open reconstruction technique and its outcomes in a case of chronic and retracted PM tendon tear. The tendon reconstruction was performed with hamstrings autograft fixed with a humeral interference screw. To the best of our knowledge, this technique has not been reported in the literature.

2. Case Report

A 30-year-old male, street-cleaner-worker, sustained a right (dominant) shoulder injury in a motorcycle accident. He was heavy manual worker and did not practice any sport. In the emergency department, an acromioclavicular joint dislocation was initially diagnosed, and the patient was treated in a conservative manner. One year later he presented to the senior author (LB) with complaints of pectoral pain and cramps and deformity of the chest. He had significant functional limitations; mainly return to work was impossible. Physical exam revealed an abnormal anterior axillary contour and reduced adduction and internal rotation strength. The shoulder range of motion was however complete. The constant shoulder score was 51 [30], the simple shoulder test 30% [31], and the quick DASH score 52.3 [32].

Standard shoulder X-ray did not reveal any abnormality. MRI identified (1) full-thickness PM tear at the humeral tendon-bone junction including both pectoral heads (Figure 1), (2) tendon retracted medial to the anterior chest wall (Figure 2), (3) absence of any muscle fatty infiltration, and (4) a calcification inside the conjoint tendon immediately under its coracoid insertion (Figure 3). The lesion corresponded to C2/F/C after ElMaraghy and Devereaux [33]. Surgical management was considered regarding major daily activity impairment. The patient consented to surgical procedure once detailed explications were given about PM repair with autograft hamstring tendon to fill the gap.

3. Operative Technique

An interscalene block was performed before surgery, and the patient was operated under general anaesthesia in the beach-chair position. Ipsilateral knee was positioned in 90° flexion with an air tourniquet applied to the limb and draped free. A deltopectoral approach was first performed. The proximal part of the incision was more medial than the standard approach to ease pectoral muscle release. The distal part of the incision was enlarged to the PM footprint. The operative findings confirmed both the full-thickness PM tendon tear and the retraction of the tendon that was positioned more medial than the anterior chest wall. Despite extensive muscle release, the tendon could not be approximated to its anatomic insertion. The gap between the footprint and the stump was more than 5 cm (Figure 4).

Tendon reconstruction with hamstrings was confirmed. Semitendinous and Gracilis tendon were harvested through an oblique anteromedial approach, [34] using a tendon stripper (Smith & Nephew). The tendons were cleaned of soft tissue and folded to form 7 cm length 6 strands. It was stitched along its distal part to obtain a fan-shape tendon. The diameter at the distal part of the graft was calibrated

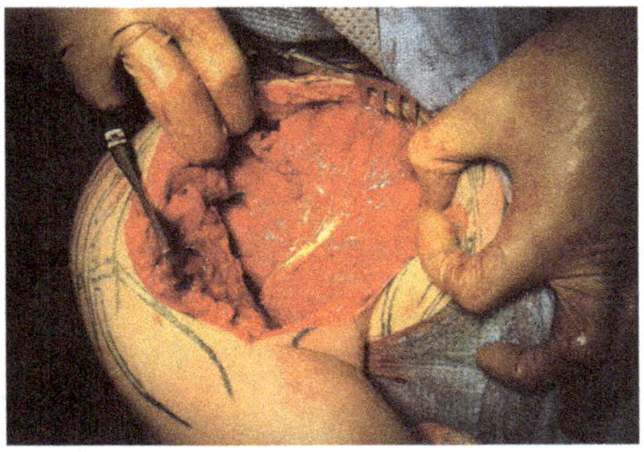

FIGURE 5: Intraoperative photograph, with the free border of the graft sutured at the PM.

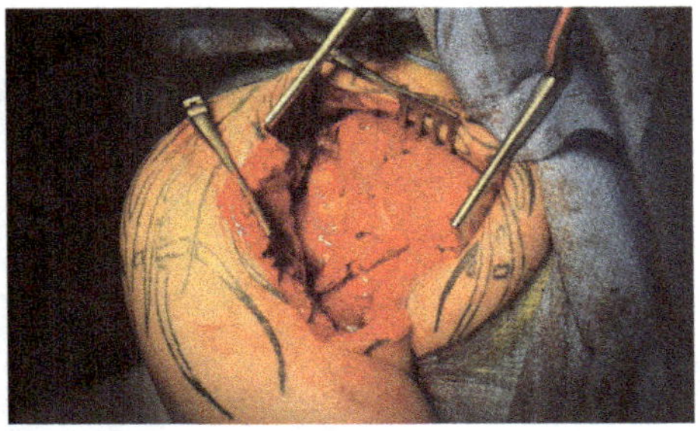

FIGURE 6: Intraoperative photograph with Vicryl plate wrapped around the graft.

at 9 mm. The lateral aspect of the bicipital groove was exposed, while the biceps tendon was carefully protected. The humeral tunnel was performed at the PM center footprint. The humeral tunnel was matched size for size with the graft diameter and had a depth of 25 mm to be bicortical. Two centimeters of hamstring graft was fixed within the bone tunnel with a 9 mm * 25 mm bioabsorbable screw (Biosure, Smith & Nephew). The fan-shaped free border of the graft was sutured into the muscle belly with Mason-Allen and Krachow stitches using nonabsorbable suture (Ultrabraid, Smith & Nephew) arm in neutral rotation (Figure 5). A Vicryl plate (Ethicon) was wrapped around the graft, in order to secure the sutures (Figure 6). The calcification in the conjoint tendon was removed.

4. Postoperative Care and Rehabilitation

The arm was immobilized postoperatively in a sling for 6 weeks. Passive closed chain pendulum exercises were initiated immediately after the surgical procedure, until 45° of abduction during 21 days and 90° for the three weeks later. No external rotation was allowed for six weeks. Active range of motion, stretching exercises, and external rotation were then initiated. Dynamic strengthening was delayed past three months, once complete range of motion was obtained. Return to heavily activities at work was allowed after 6 months.

5. Results

The drain was removed 2 days after surgery and then the patient was discharged. There was no early complication regarding the PM reconstruction and no morbidity at the donor site. At two months postoperatively, the anterior axillary contour was restored (Figure 7(a)), and the shoulder range of motion was 130° in anterior elevation, 110° in lateral elevation, 10° in external rotation, and 5° in internal rotation at 90° of abduction (Figure 7(b)). X-ray confirmed the correct position of the screw and the absence of osteolysis around it. Six months after surgical reconstruction, the patient was pain-free. The axillary anatomy was restituted and shoulder range of motion was complete. Therefore, return to work was authorized.

At the last follow-up (12 months), the patient was pain-free, with a visual analogic scale at 0 all the time. He was very satisfied concerning the cosmetic and clinical results (Figures 8(a)–8(c)). The constant score was 93%, the SST value 95%, and the Quick DASH score 4.5. After Bak's criteria [7], the patient was classified as excellent: no symptoms, normal range of motion, no cosmetic modifications, no adduction weakness, and work without restriction. MRI performed one year postoperatively confirmed the continuity between PM tendon and graft, even if the aspect of the distal tendon seemed to be thinner than normal PM tendon.

6. Discussion

To our knowledge, this is the first description of a full-thickness PM tendon tear with gap, successfully filled with hamstring autograft fixed with interference screw. PM tears are uncommon and can be easily missed during initial presentation, leading to delayed diagnosis and treatment [4, 15, 16]. In a meta-analysis of 112 cases, Bak et al. reported that acute tears were consensually repaired, and the earlier the surgery was performed, the better the clinical outcomes were observed [7]. In contrast, chronic tears are more difficult to manage, regarding alteration of tissue quality and tendon retraction [17]. However, surgical repair seems to be the preferred option as excellent or good outcomes occur in more than 90% of operated patients, versus 17% of conservatively treated patients (best choice for elderly/sedentary patients or in muscle belly tears) [9, 11, 35].

Previous studies reported that patients with chronic PM tears managed with direct repair obtain similar clinical outcomes than acute repairs [6, 9, 12]. However, a graft is required when extensive surgical release of the PM belly muscle does not allow direct repair [15]. Fascia lata or Achilles tendon allografts are widely used for reconstruction of PM tendon [10, 19, 35, 36]. Allografts avoid donor-site morbidity and can be easily tailored to fill the gap. Drawbacks are disease transmission, delayed graft incorporation, and increased risk of retear [37]. Previous studies reported that sterilization with gamma irradiation could result in impaired biomechanical properties [38]. Thus, recent publications do not advocate irradiated tendon allograft for anterior cruciate ligament reconstruction [39, 40]. Sherman et al. demonstrated the high load to which PM tendon is exposed [23]. As for

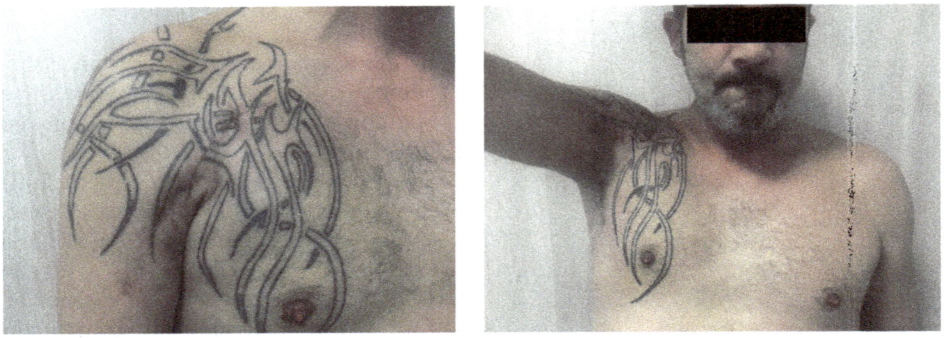

(a) (b)

FIGURE 7: At two months postoperatively, the anterior axillary contour was restored (a), and the range of motion was 110° in lateral elevation (b).

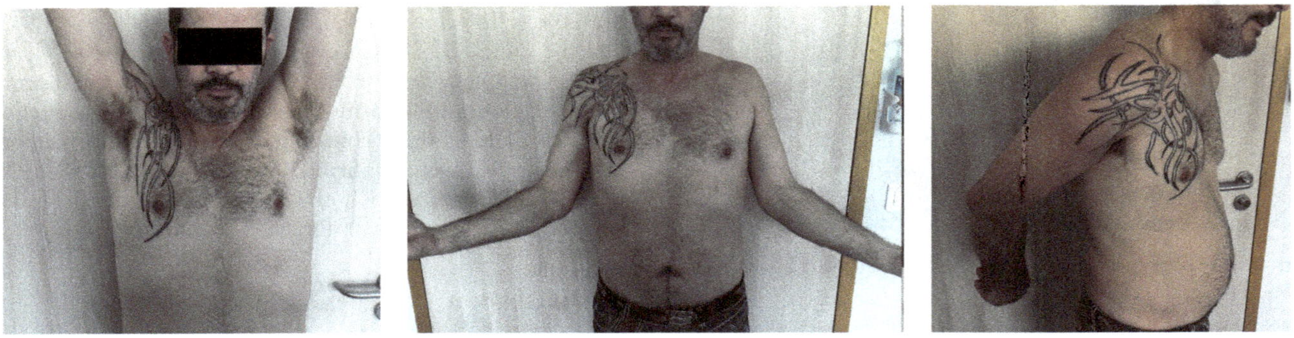

(a) (b) (c)

FIGURE 8: Complete range of motion in elevation (a) and in external rotation (b) and negative lift-off test (c).

biomechanical properties, autograft seems therefore to be more adapted for PM reconstruction.

Dehler et al. reported a reconstruction technique with Human extracellular matrix scaffold device [15]. The use of dermal allograft has been successfully reported in rotator cuff augmentation [41], arthroscopic superior capsule reconstruction [42], and open revision repair [43] in patients with irreparable rotator cuff tears. This graft eliminates donor-site morbidity and the time to prepare the autograft and could have a better biologic incorporation than tendon allograft. However, studies reporting this technique have short clinical follow-up and indication being limited to rotator cuff repair. A graft thickness of 1 mm could be insufficient for PM tendon reconstruction.

For the tendon reconstruction and to fill the gap, ipsilateral hamstrings autograft was our graft choice. The advantages of this technique are (1) using autograft leads to both complete biocompatibility and safety regarding diseases transmission, (2) hamstring graft allows filling a significant gap, and (3) it is tailored to restore the anatomy of the PM tendon (fan-shape). The drawbacks are donor-site morbidity including injuries of the saphenous nerve [44]. A recent systematic review seems to suggest lower rate of neurological impairment adopting an oblique incision [45], which corresponded to our harvesting method.

The success of PM tendon reconstruction requires solid incorporation of the tendon graft within the bone tunnel to enable its histological remodeling. Numerous graft fixation devices are reported in the literature. To optimize graft incorporation, interference screw was our choice, with 2 cm autograft driven in the bone tunnel. This fixation technique was easy to perform, resulting in a solid fixation of the graft in tubular bone of the humerus, as described in subpectoral tenodesis of the long head of the biceps. Drawbacks using an interference screw could be the risk of humeral fracture [46, 47], screw migration, and cyst formation [48] as described with anterior cruciate ligament reconstruction. Furthermore, this tendon reconstruction was not anatomical, the native humeral insertion of the PM measuring near 5 cm. In our case, regarding the gap, there was no possibility of using a superior second screw to perform a more anatomical double bundle tendon reconstruction with hamstring autograft.

Pectoral Major tears are mainly described in young male weight lifters and in high-performance athletes. We recognize that this profile did not correspond entirely to our case, who did not practice sport. However, this young patient had to be considered as a heavy manual worker who had a high demand corresponding to his return to work. The excellent clinical outcomes at one-year follow-up suggest that PM tear with major tendon retraction can be reliably managed with hamstring autograft reconstruction, using an interference screw for fixation device. This technique has proven its simplicity and efficiency to fill the gap. Biomechanical studies, although already validated for subpectoral tenodesis, could be considered for this technique.

Consent

The authors declare that they obtained the patient's written consent for the inclusion of his photo in the manuscript.

Competing Interests

The authors declare that there is no conflict of interests regarding the publication of this paper.

References

[1] G. C. Balazs, A. M. Brelin, M. A. Donohue et al., "Incidence rate and results of the surgical treatment of pectoralis major tendon ruptures in active-duty military personnel," *American Journal of Sports Medicine*, vol. 44, no. 7, pp. 1837–1843, 2016.

[2] A. De Castro Pochini, B. Ejnisman, C. V. Andreoli et al., "Pectoralis major muscle rupture in athletes: A Prospective Study," *American Journal of Sports Medicine*, vol. 38, no. 1, pp. 92–98, 2010.

[3] P. D. Inhofe, W. A. Grana, D. Egle, K.-W. Min, and J. Tomasek, "The effects of anabolic steroids on rat tendon: an ultrastructural, biomechanical, and biochemical analysis," *The American Journal of Sports Medicine*, vol. 23, no. 2, pp. 227–232, 1995.

[4] T. A. Joseph, M. J. DeFranco, and G. G. Weiker, "Delayed repair of a pectoralis major tendon rupture with allograft: a case report," *Journal of Shoulder and Elbow Surgery*, vol. 12, no. 1, pp. 101–104, 2003.

[5] J. A. Carrino, V. P. Chandnanni, D. B. Mitchell, K. Choi-Chinn, T. M. DeBerardino, and M. D. Miller, "Pectoralis major muscle and tendon tears: diagnosis and grading using magnetic resonance imaging," *Skeletal Radiology*, vol. 29, no. 6, pp. 305–313, 2000.

[6] V. Äärimaa, J. Rantanen, J. Heikkilä, I. Helttula, and S. Orava, "Rupture of the pectoralis major muscle," *The American Journal of Sports Medicine*, vol. 32, no. 5, pp. 1256–1262, 2004.

[7] K. Bak, E. A. Cameron, and I. J. P. Henderson, "Rupture of the pectoralis major: a meta-analysis of 112 cases," *Knee Surgery, Sports Traumatology, Arthroscopy*, vol. 8, no. 2, pp. 113–119, 2000.

[8] A. De Castro Pochini, C. V. Andreoli, P. S. Belangero et al., "Clinical considerations for the surgical treatment of pectoralis major muscle ruptures based on 60 cases: a prospective study and literature review," *American Journal of Sports Medicine*, vol. 42, no. 1, pp. 95–102, 2014.

[9] C. M. Hanna, A. B. Glenny, S. N. Stanley, and M. A. Caughey, "Pectoralis major tears: comparison of surgical and conservative treatment," *British Journal of Sports Medicine*, vol. 35, no. 3, pp. 202–206, 2001.

[10] G. Merolla, P. Paladini, S. Artiaco, P. Tos, N. Lollino, and G. Porcellini, "Surgical repair of acute and chronic pectoralis major tendon rupture: clinical and ultrasound outcomes at a mean follow-up of 5 years," *European Journal of Orthopaedic Surgery and Traumatology*, vol. 25, no. 1, pp. 91–98, 2014.

[11] J. Petilon, D. R. Carr, J. K. Sekiya, and D. V. Unger, "Pectoralis major muscle injuries: evaluation and management," *Journal of the American Academy of Orthopaedic Surgeons*, vol. 13, no. 1, pp. 59–68, 2005.

[12] A. A. Schepsis, M. W. Grafe, H. P. Jones, and M. J. Lemos, "Rupture of the pectoralis major muscle. Outcome after repair of acute and chronic injuries," *The American Journal of Sports Medicine*, vol. 28, no. 1, pp. 9–15, 2000.

[13] M. T. Provencher, K. Handfield, N. T. Boniquit, S. N. Reiff, J. K. Sekiya, and A. A. Romeo, "Injuries to the pectoralis major muscle: diagnosis and management," *The American Journal of Sports Medicine*, vol. 38, no. 8, pp. 1693–1705, 2010.

[14] L. Fung, B. Wong, K. Ravichandiran, A. Agur, T. Rindlisbacher, and A. Elmaraghy, "Three-dimensional study of pectoralis major muscle and tendon architecture," *Clinical Anatomy*, vol. 22, no. 4, pp. 500–508, 2009.

[15] T. Dehler, A. L. Pennings, and A. W. ElMaraghy, "Dermal allograft reconstruction of a chronic pectoralis major tear," *Journal of Shoulder and Elbow Surgery*, vol. 22, no. 10, pp. e18–e22, 2013.

[16] A. K. Schachter, B. J. White, S. Namkoong, and O. Sherman, "Revision reconstruction of a pectoralis major tendon rupture using hamstring autograft: a case report," *American Journal of Sports Medicine*, vol. 34, no. 2, pp. 295–298, 2006.

[17] J. H. Flint, A. M. Wade, J. Giuliani, and J.-P. Rue, "Defining the terms acute and chronic in orthopaedic sports injuries: a systematic review," *American Journal of Sports Medicine*, vol. 42, no. 1, pp. 235–241, 2014.

[18] M. Zafra, F. Muñoz, and P. Carpintero, "Chronic rupture of the pectoralis major muscle: report of two cases," *Acta Orthopaedica Belgica*, vol. 71, no. 1, pp. 107–110, 2005.

[19] R. S. Sikka, M. Neault, and C. A. Guanche, "Reconstruction of the pectoralis major tendon with fascia lata allograft," *Orthopedics*, vol. 28, no. 10, pp. 1199–1201, 2005.

[20] Y. Uchiyama, S. Miyazaki, T. Tamaki et al., "Clinical results of a surgical technique using endobuttons for complete tendon tear of pectoralis major muscle: report of five cases," *Sports Medicine, Arthroscopy, Rehabilitation, Therapy & Technology*, vol. 3, article no. 20, 2011.

[21] M. J. Wheat Hozack, B. Bugg, K. Lemay, and J. Reed, "Tears of pectoralis major in steer wrestlers: a novel repair technique using the endobutton," *Clinical Journal of Sport Medicine*, vol. 23, no. 1, pp. 80–82, 2013.

[22] S. J. Rabuck, J. L. Lynch, X. Guo et al., "Biomechanical comparison of 3 methods to repair pectoralis major ruptures," *American Journal of Sports Medicine*, vol. 40, no. 7, pp. 1635–1640, 2012.

[23] S. L. Sherman, E. C. Lin, N. N. Verma et al., "Biomechanical analysis of the pectoralis major tendon and comparison of techniques for tendo-osseous repair," *The American Journal of Sports Medicine*, vol. 40, no. 8, pp. 1887–1894, 2012.

[24] W. Thomas, S. Gheduzzi, and I. Packham, "Pectoralis major tendon repair: a biomechanical study of suture button versus transosseous suture techniques," *Knee Surgery, Sports Traumatology, Arthroscopy*, vol. 23, no. 9, pp. 2617–2623, 2014.

[25] A. S. Arora, A. Singh, and R. C. Koonce, "Biomechanical evaluation of a unicortical button versus interference screw for subpectoral biceps tenodesis," *Arthroscopy*, vol. 29, no. 4, pp. 638–644, 2013.

[26] A. D. Mazzocca, J. Bicos, S. Santangelo, A. A. Romeo, and R. A. Arciero, "The biomechanical evaluation of four fixation techniques for proximal biceps tenodesis," *Arthroscopy*, vol. 21, no. 11, pp. 1296–1306, 2005.

[27] A. D. Mazzocca, M. P. Cote, C. L. Arciero, A. A. Romeo, and R. A. Arciero, "Clinical outcomes after subpectoral biceps tenodesis with an interference screw," *The American Journal of Sports Medicine*, vol. 36, no. 10, pp. 1922–1929, 2008.

[28] A. D. Mazzocca, C. G. Rios, A. A. Romeo, and R. A. Arciero, "Subpectoral biceps tenodesis with interference screw fixation," *Arthroscopy—Journal of Arthroscopic and Related Surgery*, vol. 21, no. 7, pp. 896.e1–896.e7, 2005.

[29] P. M. Sethi, A. Rajaram, K. Beitzel, T. R. Hackett, D. M. Chowaniec, and A. D. Mazzocca, "Biomechanical performance of subpectoral biceps tenodesis: a comparison of interference screw fixation, cortical button fixation, and interference screw diameter," *Journal of Shoulder and Elbow Surgery*, vol. 22, no. 4, pp. 451–457, 2013.

[30] C. R. Constant, C. Gerber, R. J. H. Emery, J. O. Søjbjerg, F. Gohlke, and P. Boileau, "A review of the Constant score: modifications and guidelines for its use," *Journal of Shoulder and Elbow Surgery*, vol. 17, no. 2, pp. 355–361, 2008.

[31] T. S. Roddey, S. L. Olson, K. F. Cook, G. M. Gartsman, and W. Hanten, "Comparison of the University of California—Los Angeles Shoulder Scale and the Simple Shoulder Test with the shoulder pain and disability index: single-administration reliability and validity," *Physical Therapy*, vol. 80, no. 8, pp. 759–768, 2000.

[32] D. E. Beaton, J. N. Katz, A. H. Fossel, J. G. Wright, V. Tarasuk, and C. Bombardier, "Measuring the whole or the parts? Validity, reliability, and responsiveness of the disabilities of the arm, shoulder and hand outcome measure in different regions of the upper extremity," *Journal of Hand Therapy*, vol. 14, no. 2, pp. 128–146, 2001.

[33] A. W. ElMaraghy and M. W. Devereaux, "A systematic review and comprehensive classification of pectoralis major tears," *Journal of Shoulder and Elbow Surgery*, vol. 21, no. 3, pp. 412–422, 2012.

[34] H. Lanternier, J. B. de Cussac, and T. Collet, "Short medial approach harvesting of hamstring tendons," *Orthopaedics and Traumatology: Surgery and Research*, vol. 102, no. 2, pp. 269–272, 2016.

[35] U. Butt, S. Mehta, L. Funk, and P. Monga, "Pectoralis major ruptures: a review of current management," *Journal of Shoulder and Elbow Surgery*, vol. 24, no. 4, pp. 655–662, 2015.

[36] M. A. Zacchilli, J. T. Fowler, and B. D. Owens, "Allograft reconstruction of chronic pectoralis major tendon ruptures," *Journal of Surgical Orthopaedic Advances*, vol. 22, no. 1, pp. 95–102, 2013.

[37] S. A. Barbour and W. King, "The safe and effective use of allograft tissue—an update," *American Journal of Sports Medicine*, vol. 31, no. 5, pp. 791–797, 2003.

[38] T. A. Grieb, R.-Y. Forng, S. Bogdansky et al., "High-dose gamma irradiation for soft tissue allografts: high margin of safety with biomechanical integrity," *Journal of Orthopaedic Research*, vol. 24, no. 5, pp. 1011–1018, 2006.

[39] K. Sun, J. Zhang, Y. Wang et al., "Arthroscopic anterior cruciate ligament reconstruction with at least 2.5 years' follow-up comparing hamstring tendon autograft and irradiated allograft," *Arthroscopy—Journal of Arthroscopic and Related Surgery*, vol. 27, no. 9, pp. 1195–1202, 2011.

[40] S. Tian, B. Wang, L. Liu et al., "Irradiated hamstring tendon allograft versus autograft for anatomic double-bundle anterior cruciate ligament reconstruction: midterm clinical outcomes," *The American Journal of Sports Medicine*, vol. 44, no. 10, pp. 2579–2588, 2016.

[41] S. J. Snyder, S. P. Arnoczky, J. L. Bond, and R. Dopirak, "Histologic evaluation of a biopsy specimen obtained 3 months after rotator cuff augmentation with GraftJacket Matrix," *Arthroscopy*, vol. 25, no. 3, pp. 329–333, 2009.

[42] J. M. Tokish and C. Beicker, "Superior capsule reconstruction technique using an acellular dermal allograft," *Arthroscopy Techniques*, vol. 4, no. 6, pp. e833–e839, 2015.

[43] M. Petri, R. J. Warth, M. P. Horan, J. A. Greenspoon, and P. J. Millett, "Outcomes after open revision repair of massive rotator cuff tears with biologic patch augmentation," *Arthroscopy—Journal of Arthroscopic and Related Surgery*, vol. 32, no. 9, pp. 1752–1760, 2016.

[44] S. G. Papastergiou, H. Voulgaropoulos, P. Mikalef, E. Ziogas, G. Pappis, and I. Giannakopoulos, "Injuries to the infrapatellar branch(es) of the saphenous nerve in anterior cruciate ligament reconstruction with four-strand hamstring tendon autograft: vertical versus horizontal incision for harvest," *Knee Surgery, Sports Traumatology, Arthroscopy*, vol. 14, no. 8, pp. 789–793, 2006.

[45] A. Ruffilli, M. de Fine, F. Traina, F. Pilla, D. Fenga, and C. Faldini, "Saphenous nerve injury during hamstring tendons harvest: does the incision matter? A systematic review," *Knee Surgery, Sports Traumatology, Arthroscopy*, pp. 1–6, 2016.

[46] E. J. Dein, G. Huri, J. C. Gordon, and E. G. McFarland, "A humerus fracture in a baseball pitcher after biceps tenodesis," *The American Journal of Sports Medicine*, vol. 42, no. 4, pp. 877–879, 2014.

[47] S. A. Euler, S. D. Smith, B. T. Williams, G. J. Dornan, P. J. Millett, and C. A. Wijdicks, "Biomechanical analysis of subpectoral biceps tenodesis: effect of screw malpositioning on proximal humeral strength," *The American Journal of Sports Medicine*, vol. 43, no. 1, pp. 69–74, 2015.

[48] J. N. Watson, P. McQueen, W. Kim, and M. R. Hutchinson, "Bioabsorbable interference screw failure in anterior cruciate ligament reconstruction: a case series and review of the literature," *Knee*, vol. 22, no. 3, pp. 256–261, 2015.

6

A Surgical Opinion in a 36-Week Pregnant with Tibia Fracture: Intramedullary Nailing

Celal Bozkurt and Baran Sarikaya

Department of Orthopaedics and Traumatology, Faculty of Medicine, Harran University, Sanliurfa, Turkey

Correspondence should be addressed to Celal Bozkurt; bozkurt.celal@gmail.com

Academic Editor: Christian W. Müller

The operative treatment of tibial fractures in late pregnancy is a controversial issue that is rarely discussed in the literature. Here we present a case of a tibial diaphyseal fracture in a woman that was 36 weeks pregnant, which was treated with intramedullary nails under noninvasive foetal monitoring with cardiotocography. The patient underwent a successful surgery, and no harm or adverse events to either the mother or the foetus were reported during or after the procedure. Following surgery, the mother had a comfortable pregnancy and a normal spontaneous vaginal delivery with a healthy newborn.

1. Introduction

A fracture of the tibial shaft is one of the most common long bone fractures in the body [1]. Tibial diaphyseal fractures can be treated either surgically or conservatively; however, surgical treatment establishes a better union and rapid resumption of full weight-bearing activities [2, 3]. Conservative treatment consists of a closed reduction and an above-the-knee cast for at least two months. The patients are mobilized with crutches and are not allowed to bear weight during this period of time. Among the surgical treatment options, the three most common methods for fixation are plating, intramedullary nailing, and external fixation. Of these options, the literature suggests that intramedullary nails are most commonly indicated for midshaft fractures, while external fixation is generally indicated for damage control with open fractures or compromised soft tissues [4].

During the postoperative plating period, the patients bear partial weight until a union is achieved. External fixator may impede the natural delivery process [4]. After tibial nailing, weight-bearing mobilization in the early postoperative period is possible. In addition to a better fracture union, it is more comfortable and has less of an effect on the delivery choice.

After conservative treatment and tibial plating for at least for two months, the patients are mobilized as non-weight-bearing (plaster) or partial weight-bearing (plating) through crutches. However, this period is uncomfortable for the mother both before and after the delivery while caring for a baby, and there is an increased risk for deep venous thrombosis (DVT) due to decreased mobilization. Moreover, pregnancy designates a hypercoagulable status, and unfractionated heparin and low molecular weight heparin (LMWH) can be used for prophylaxis [5]. Because of the cast, vaginal delivery is difficult for the mother, which can affect the method of delivery [6].

Orthopaedic emergencies should be treated as such, regardless of the pregnancy status of the patient [7]. Closed extremity fractures can be managed nonoperatively or be delayed until postpartum, when appropriate [8]. However, an accelerated fracture union during pregnancy [9] will complicate a postponed surgery. In pregnancy, there is an increase in the level of steroid hormones, initially with progesterone in the first trimester, followed by the oestrogens and prolactin in the second and third trimesters. Oestrogen has well-documented effects on bone formation and remodelling during fracture healing [10, 11]. Other controversial issues are the anaesthetic agents used [12], radiation exposure [13], and probable thromboembolic events due to immobilization. On the basis of these adverse events, surgical management is a difficult decision for both the surgeon and the mother. Unfortunately, there are limited reports on the management of long bone fractures in late pregnancy.

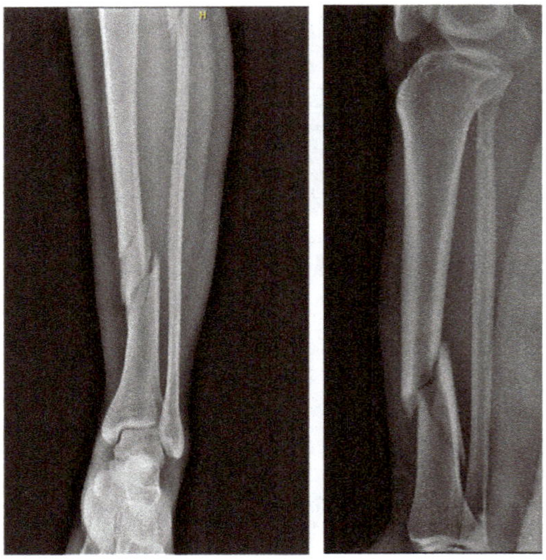

FIGURE 1: Radiographs showing the anteroposterior and lateral views of tibial shaft fracture.

Here we report the case of a patient with a tibial diaphyseal fracture at 36 weeks of gestation treated with tibial nailing.

2. Case Report

A 36-year-old pregnant woman presented to emergency department following an accidental fall down the stairs. She was evaluated by both an orthopaedic surgeon and an obstetrician. There was no history of any medical disorder, and she had had an uneventful pregnancy until this accident.

Upon examination, there was no evidence of a neurovascular deficit or compartment syndrome, and there were no open wounds. Radiographic imaging showed a left tibia and fibula diaphyseal fracture classified as 42-B1 according to the Arbeitsgemeinschaft für Osteosynthesefragen (AO) (Figure 1). The fracture was stabilized with an above-the-knee splint.

Following the orthopaedic examination, the obstetrician evaluated the foetus and the mother. According to the obstetric ultrasonography and cardiotocography (CTG), no pathologies were detected. There were no restraints for surgical treatment.

The patient was brought to the operating theatre after stabilization. Spinal anaesthesia was applied, and she was positioned supine on the operating table. She was tilted 15° by placing a wedge under her right buttock to reduce the inferior vena cava pressure [5]. A lead apron was placed over the patient's abdomen to minimise the radiation dose to the foetus. After spinal anaesthesia, the foetus was monitored with continuous CTG during the surgery. An obstetrician stood by in the theatre in case of an emergency caesarean section.

The tibial nail (manufactured by Tasarımmed®, Istanbul, Turkey) was inserted via a standard infrapatellar incision. During reamerization, the foetal wellbeing was monitored with CTG, which was reactive throughout the surgery, and no adverse reactions were observed. When encountering some resistance during the reamerization, we increased the reamer diameter size by one (1 mm increase) and then stopped reaming (we did not use additional fluoroscopy to decrease the radiation exposure) to decrease the operation time. We inserted a titanium tibial nail locked with four screws (Figure 1) and used the distal guide of the nail (Figure 2) to minimise the radiation dose.

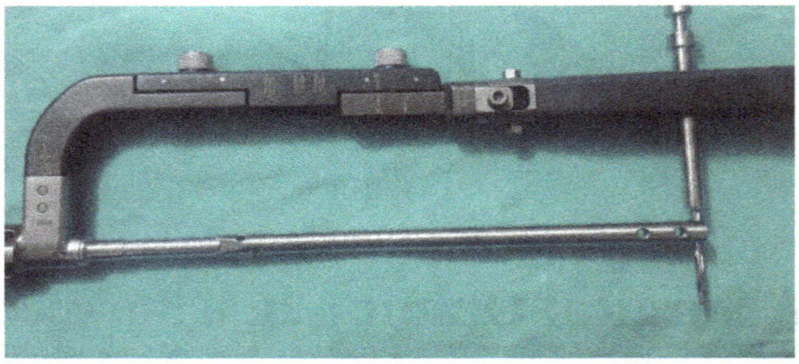

FIGURE 2: Distal guide.

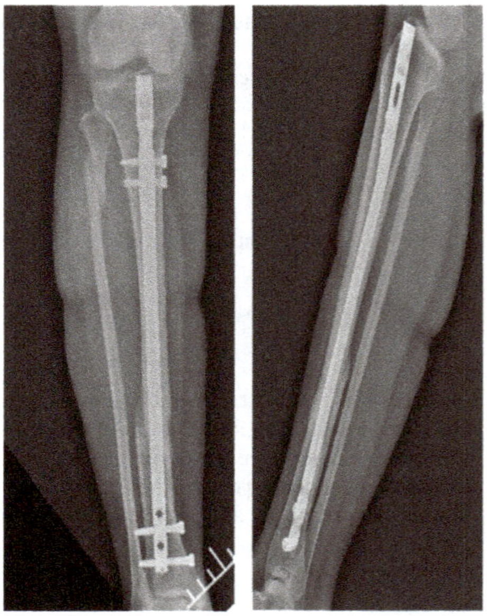

FIGURE 3: Radiographs showing united tibia at four months.

During the postoperative period, the mother and the foetus were evaluated serially by the obstetrician. The obstetric examination and CTG were normal throughout the postoperative period. This patient was administered analgesics, cold application, and 4000 IU/day subcutaneous enoxaparin for prophylaxis. On postoperative day one she was mobilized, permitting partial weight-bearing with crutches. She was discharged home on postoperative day three.

This mother had no problems during her final weeks of pregnancy. At the 40th week, she had a healthy newborn via vaginal delivery. Two days after delivery, the mother and newborn were discharged home. We saw fracture union in the fourth-month radiographs (Figure 3).

3. Discussion

The operative treatment of closed fractures in the third trimester of pregnancy remains controversial. The anaesthetic [12] and radiation exposure [13] to the foetus and probable embolic events [5] frighten both physicians and pregnant patients. We could find only a few cases in the literature regarding tibial fracture treatment in the third trimester of pregnancy [6, 8, 9, 14]. Since there are so few published case reports in the literature, there is no consensus on the appropriate management of maternal fractures during pregnancy.

Anaesthetics affect both the mother and the foetus; therefore, anaesthesia is more complex during pregnancy. Organogenesis occurs in the first trimester, and although there are no anaesthetic agents shown to be teratogenic, surgical treatments are usually delayed until the second trimester. From the second trimester until the end of pregnancy, the foetus will be less affected by anaesthesia [12].

Radiation exposure is another risk factor for the foetus. It affects the foetus more during the first trimester since the development of the central nervous system (CNS) is faster and more susceptible to radiation during this period. After 25 weeks of gestation, the CNS becomes more resistant to radiation; however, the cumulative radiation effects are still important. The foetus can absorb up to 100 mGy (milligray) of radiation safely, and, as long as this is not exceeded, X-rays can be used during surgery [13].

After conservative treatment for this type of fracture, the mother is non-weight-bearing, using crutches, so mobilization will be decreased. This period can be uncomfortable for the patient; an above-the-knee cast will affect the delivery, and a caesarean section should be planned [6]. After tibial nailing, there is no splint or cast, so the mother can choose vaginal delivery.

In the third trimester, a tibial fracture can be stabilized with an above-the-knee splint, and the surgery can be done following a caesarean section during the postpartum period [8]. In this situation, the mother's mobilization will be decreased, and she may not be able to choose a natural delivery [6]. In the literature, it has been reported that because of the changed hormonal status during pregnancy, the fracture union is accelerated [9]. In this case, a surgery planned later will be technically harder.

A gravid uterus can increase the pressure on the inferior vena cava, especially when the patient is in the supine position. The reduction in the preload caused by the compression of the inferior vena cava can lead to hemodynamic instability. If possible, the patient should be placed in the left lateral decubitus position. If there is any contraindication to lateral decubitus positioning, the patient should be tilted approximately 15° with a wedge under the right buttock, which displaces the uterus laterally. We chose the latter method for the surgery in this case, which was a more favourable position [5].

During tibial nailing, it has been shown that the distal locking process is responsible for at least 50% of the fluoroscopic exposure of the whole operative procedure [15, 16]. The average time for one distal locking screw is 17.9 minutes [17]. To decrease the operation time and radiation exposure, we used the distal locking system of the nail. Therefore, it took only five minutes to lock the nail distally, and we decreased the radiation exposure.

The stress on the foetus and mother may increase during surgery because of the anaesthetic exposure and surgical procedure, especially reamerization. Monitoring the foetus with CTG is important, and we did not detect any adverse activity during the surgical procedure while using CTG. Surgery and pregnancy increase the risk of DVT; however, heparin and LMWH are safe to use during pregnancy, so they can be used for prophylaxis [5, 18].

While reviewing the literature, we encountered only one case report on the surgical treatment of a tibial fracture during pregnancy [14]. The few other reports were on conservative management and the surgical treatment after a caesarean section [8]. For example, Ahmad et al. reported an accelerated tibial fracture union and no need for surgical treatment in the third trimester of pregnancy [9].

When deciding on the appropriate management for a fracture during pregnancy, the gestational age, type of the fracture, best way to obtain an acceptable fracture union, probable harm, risks to the mother and foetus, and the comfort of the mother and newborn should all be taken into consideration.

After obstetric ultrasonography, obstetric examination, and evaluation of the foetus, if the mother and foetus are stable, surgery can be planned. The surgical treatment chosen should not only be important for achieving appropriate bone alignment and union, but also for the comfort of the mother and newborn. Surgery after the delivery can negatively affect a mother's care of her baby, since she will be hospitalized and immobilized for at least few days. Moreover, a second surgery will add to the psychological stress of a mother who has already undergone a caesarean section. We believe that this approach may negatively affect mother-newborn bonding, decrease the care given by the mother to her baby, and adversely influence the emotional status of the mother.

Fracture management in a pregnant patient should be multidisciplinary, including orthopaedic surgeon, obstetrician, anaesthetist, and neonatologist. Before deciding on a treatment, one should consider not only the fracture, but also the comfort of the mother and foetus before and after delivery.

Competing Interests

The authors declare that they have no competing interests.

References

[1] M. Ferguson, C. Brand, A. Lowe et al., "Outcomes of isolated tibial shaft fractures treated at level 1 trauma centres," *Injury*, vol. 39, no. 2, pp. 187–195, 2008.

[2] B. Littenberg, L. P. Weinstwin, M. McCarren et al., "Closed fractures of the tibial shaft. A meta-analysis of three methods of treatment," *The Journal of Bone & Joint Surgery—American Volume*, vol. 80, no. 2, pp. 174–183, 1998.

[3] C. P. Coles and M. Gross, "Closed tibial shaft fractures: management and treatment complications. A review of the prospective

literature," *Canadian Journal of Surgery*, vol. 43, no. 4, pp. 256–262, 2000.

[4] W. Rudge, K. Newman, and A. Trompeter, "Fractures of the tibial shaft in adults," *Orthopaedics and Trauma*, vol. 28, no. 4, pp. 243–255, 2014.

[5] N. P. Mcgoldrick, C. Green, N. Burke, C. Quinlan, and D. Mccormack, "Pregnancy and the orthopaedic patient," *Orthopaedics and Trauma*, vol. 26, no. 3, pp. 212–219, 2012.

[6] R. Bharathan, J. Duckett, and S. Jain, "An unusual indication for caesarean section: lower limb fracture," *Journal of Obstetrics and Gynaecology*, vol. 28, no. 6, pp. 648–649, 2008.

[7] R. D. Barraco, W. C. Chiu, T. V. Clancy et al., "Practice management guidelines for the diagnosis and management of injury in the pregnant patient: the EAST Practice Management Guidelines Work Group," *The Journal of Trauma*, vol. 69, no. 1, pp. 211–214, 2010.

[8] F. Sorbi, G. Sisti, M. Di Tommaso, and M. Fambrini, "Traumatic tibia and fibula fracture in a 36 weeks' pregnant patient: a case report," *The Ochsner Journal*, vol. 13, no. 4, pp. 547–549, 2013.

[9] M. A. Ahmad, D. Kuhanendran, I. W. Kamande, and C. Charalambides, "Accelerated tibial fracture union in the third trimester of pregnancy: a case report," *Journal of Medical Case Reports*, vol. 2, article 44, 2008.

[10] M. H. Johnson and B. J. Everitt, *Essential Reproduction*, Blackwell Science, Hoboken, NJ, USA, 5th edition, 2000.

[11] C. C. Burnett and A. H. Reddi, "Influence of estrogen and progesterone on matrix-induced endochondral bone formation," *Calcified Tissue International*, vol. 35, no. 1, pp. 609–614, 1983.

[12] K. M. Kuckowski, "Nonobstetric surgery during pregnancy: what are the risks of anesthesia?" *Obstetrical & Gynecological Survey*, vol. 59, no. 1, pp. 52–56, 2004.

[13] J. K. Timins, "Radiation during pregnancy," *New Jersey Medicine*, vol. 98, no. 6, pp. 29–33, 2001.

[14] G. Walsh, G. Mustafa, S. C. Halder, and J. A. Chapman, "Tibial nailing during pregnancy: a safe option," *European Journal of Trauma and Emergency Surgery*, vol. 34, no. 1, pp. 80–82, 2008.

[15] P. E. Levin, R. W. Schoen Jr., and B. D. Browner, "Radiation exposure to the surgeon during closed interlocking intramedullary nailing," *The Journal of Bone & Joint Surgery—American Volume*, vol. 69, no. 5, pp. 761–766, 1987.

[16] I. D. Sugarman, I. Adam, and T. D. Bunker, "Radiation dosage during AO locking femoral nailing," *Injury*, vol. 19, no. 5, pp. 336–338, 1988.

[17] N. Suhma, P. Messmera, I. Zunab, A. Ludwig Jacob, and P. Regazzonia, "Average 17.9 min for 1 distal locking of intramedullary implants. A prospective, controlled clinical study," *Injury*, vol. 35, pp. 367–374, 2004.

[18] I. Pabinger and H. Grafenhofer, "Pregnancy-associated thrombosis," *Wiener Klinische Wochenschrift*, vol. 115, no. 13-14, pp. 482–484, 2003.

7

Neuromuscular Coordination Deficit Persists 12 Months after ACL Reconstruction But Can Be Modulated by 6 Weeks of Kettlebell Training: A Case Study in Women's Elite Soccer

Mette K. Zebis,[1,2] Christoffer H. Andersen,[1] Jesper Bencke,[2] Christina Ørntoft,[3] Connie Linnebjerg,[4] Per Hölmich,[5] Kristian Thorborg,[5] Per Aagaard,[6] and Lars L. Andersen[7,8]

[1]*Department of Physiotherapy and Occupational Therapy, Faculty of Health and Technology, Metropolitan University College, Copenhagen N, Denmark*
[2]*Human Movement Analysis Laboratory, Copenhagen University Hospital, Amager-Hvidovre, Copenhagen, Denmark*
[3]*Department of Sports Science and Clinical Biomechanics, SDU Sport and Health Sciences Cluster (SHSC), University of Southern Denmark, Odense M, Denmark*
[4]*Clinic of Sports Medicine, Danish Elite Sports Organization Team Denmark, Copenhagen, Denmark*
[5]*Sports Orthopedic Research Center-Copenhagen, Arthroscopic Center, Department of Orthopaedic Surgery, Copenhagen University Hospital, Amager-Hvidovre, Copenhagen, Denmark*
[6]*Institute of Sports Science and Clinical Biomechanics, University of Southern Denmark, Odense, Denmark*
[7]*National Research Centre for the Working Environment, Copenhagen, Denmark*
[8]*Physical Activity and Human Performance, Center for Sensory-Motor Interaction, Department of Health Science and Technology, Aalborg University, Aalborg, Denmark*

Correspondence should be addressed to Mette K. Zebis; mzeb@phmetropol.dk

Academic Editor: Zbigniew Gugala

The aim of the present single-case study was to investigate the effect of 6 weeks' kettlebell training on the neuromuscular risk profile for ACL injury in a high-risk athlete returning to sport after ACL reconstruction. A female elite soccer player (age 21 years) with no previous history of ACL injury went through neuromuscular screening as measured by EMG preactivity of vastus lateralis and semitendinosus during a standardized sidecutting maneuver. Subsequently, the player experienced a noncontact ACL injury. The player was screened again following postreconstruction rehabilitation, then underwent 6-week kettlebell training, and was subsequently screened again at 6-week follow-up. Prior to and after postreconstruction rehabilitation the player demonstrated a neuromuscular profile during sidecutting known to increase the risk for noncontact ACL injury, that is, reduced EMG preactivity for semitendinosus and elevated EMG preactivity for vastus lateralis. Subsequently, the 6-week kettlebell training increased semitendinosus muscle preactivity during sidecutting by 38 percentage points to a level equivalent to a neuromuscular low-risk profile. An ACL rehabilitated female athlete with a high-risk neuromuscular profile changed to low-risk in response to 6 weeks of kettlebell training. Thus, short-term kettlebell exercise with documented high levels of medial hamstring activation was found to transfer into high medial hamstring preactivation during a sidecutting maneuver.

1. Introduction

Anterior cruciate ligament (ACL) injuries in sports are of increasing concern for physicians and scientists worldwide [1]. In United States, between 100.000 and 300.000 ACL reconstructions are performed every year [2]. The enigmatic phenomenon "noncontact ACL injury" in sports has been objective for increasing preventative scientific research efforts in recent years. Across sports, noncontact ACL injuries account for about 60% of all ACL injuries registered [3]. A noncontact ACL injury is defined as an ACL injury sustained by the athlete without extrinsic contact to another player or object on the field [4]. Thus, the player performs a sports task, for example, a sidecutting maneuver, which has been executed numerous times before; only this time the ACL is ruptured. The mechanisms underlying this specific type of sports injury remain still in part a mystery, and identification of risk factors predisposing for noncontact ACL injury has high clinical relevance and priority in both injury prevention and rehabilitation therapy.

In the present case study, we report findings obtained in a 21-year-old female elite soccer player (Danish National Team), who sustained a noncontact ACL injury 3 years *after* being tested in our laboratory for neuromuscular performance during soccer relevant movements, including a sidecutting manoeuver. At the time of her ACL injury, we had identified a "high-risk" zone [5] for noncontact ACL injury based on a reduced EMG preactivity for m. semitendinosus (ST) and elevated EMG preactivity for m. vastus lateralis (VL), expressed as a large differential VL-ST EMG preactivity during standardized sidecutting maneuvers. The identification of a high-risk zone suggests that specific preventative efforts should be performed for players identified within this high-risk zone. Thus, we examined in retrospect the initial sidecutting test performed and found that the player displayed a neuromuscular high-risk profile for noncontact ACL injury as defined by Zebis et al. (2009) [5], that is, characterized by low semitendinosus (ST) EMG preactivity in combination with high vastus lateralis (VL) EMG preactivity. Thus, this case report represents an exclusive possibility of studying the plasticity of a motor program executed during a high-risk movement (sidecutting), from "prior to ACL injury" to "after ACL reconstruction and rehabilitation" and, finally, following specific neuromuscular training targeting the single most important ACL agonist, that is, the medial hamstring muscle (ST).

The aim of the present case study was to describe the effect of 6 weeks' kettlebell training on the neuromuscular profile for noncontact ACL injury during sidecutting in a high-risk elite athlete returning to sport after ACL reconstruction.

2. Case Presentation

August 2006. A 21-year-old female soccer player competing at elite level (Table 1) and with no previous history of knee injuries was engaged in a study examining functional performance during selected sports tasks. Among other tests, neuromuscular hamstring and quadriceps EMG preactivity was obtained during a standardized sidecutting maneuver. In 2009, a study identified a neuromuscular high-risk profile for noncontact ACL injury during sidecutting [5].

May 2009. The player sustains a documented (video recorded) noncontact ACL injury in the right knee during match play. Retrospectively examined, the initial test (2006) revealed that the female soccer player, in her uninjured state, displayed a high-risk profile during sidecutting consistent with the study reports by Zebis et al. (2009) [5].

Table 1: Physical activity scheme at time of testing.

Components	Test I: Before noncontact ACL injury	Test II: After surgery & rehabilitation	Test III: After kettlebell training
Soccer practice 90 min (/wk)	4-5	4-5	4-5
Match play 90 min (/wk)	1	1	1
Strength training (/wk)	2	2	2
Squat	3 × 8–10 RM	3 × 6 RM	3 × 6 RM
Leg press	3 × 4–6 RM	3 × 10 RM	3 × 10 RM
Lateral raise	—	3 × 10 RM	3 × 10 RM
Nordic hamstring	3 × 10 reps	—	—
Knee extension	3 × 8–10 RM	3 × 10 RM	3 × 10 RM
Leg curl	3 × 8–10 RM	3 × 10 RM	3 × 10 RM
Kettlebell	—	—	See description

June 2009. Surgical ACL reconstruction is performed using a semitendinosus-gracilis autograft.

April 2010. After 10 months of standardized rehabilitation (more details provided below), the player is deemed fully rehabilitated by medical professionals to return to preinjury sports activities, and the player returns to soccer at elite level.

May 2010. The player is involved in elite soccer at her preinjury level (Table 1). A second test for neuromuscular preactivity during a standardized sidecutting maneuver is performed. At this point in time, the player persists to display markedly reduced ST EMG preactivity during the sidecutting maneuver. Consequently, a 6-week training program involving kettlebell swing exercise is introduced to the player.

July 2010. A final third test involving neuromuscular preactivity assessment during a standardized sidecutting maneuver is performed in our lab after completion of the 6 weeks' kettlebell intervention.

In August 2011, the player sustained an ACL rerupture due to a traumatic contact situation during match play. The screening model used in the present study solely addresses the risk of noncontact ACL injury [5]. Thus, contact injuries are not accounted for in this model.

Written informed consent was obtained from the athlete prior to all testing and analyses.

3. Test Protocol

3.1. The Sidecutting Maneuver. The subject was screened for neuromuscular EMG preactivity while performing a standardized sidecutting maneuver in the laboratory. A previous study has demonstrated high test-retest reproducibility for magnitude and timing of the EMG activity during sidecutting [6] showing that this maneuver represents a consistent motor program in the CNS of trained players. In support of this notion, the sidecutting maneuver has been found to remain unchanged during a regular season with training and match play [6].

3.2. Neuromuscular Screening by EMG Recording. Surface EMG electrodes were placed on the preferred push-off leg (i.e., left leg) on vastus lateralis (VL), biceps femoris (BF), and semitendinosus (ST) muscles according to recommended standard procedures [7]. For detailed description of the laboratory setup see Zebis et al. (2009) [5].

During later offline analysis all EMG signals were high-pass filtered at a 5 Hz cutoff frequency (4th-order zero-lag Butterworth filter) and subsequently smoothed by a symmetrical moving RMS filter of 30 ms [8]. Mean RMS EMG amplitude was obtained for all muscles examined instantly before ground contact, defined as 0–10 ms prior to foot strike on the force plate, and subsequently normalized to the peak RMS EMG amplitude recorded during the sidecutting maneuver [6]. The average of 3 trials was calculated for each muscle in each test.

3.3. Countermovement Jump (CMJ). CMJ measurements were performed on a force plate (AMTI, Advanced Mechanical Technology, Inc.). Countermovement jumping was performed with the hands placed at the hip (akimbo), and maximal jump height was calculated by time-integration (0.001 time constant) of vertical ground reaction force as previously described by Caserotti et al. (2001) [9].

4. Rehabilitation after ACL Reconstruction

A standardized rehabilitation program, using generally accepted progression criteria was followed [10]. The rehabilitation protocol included specific goals for range of motion, muscle function, and functional performance, and these goals had to be met before the player could progress to the next level [10]. The player was supervised weekly during the entire postoperative rehabilitation phase by a trained physiotherapist.

In the first 12 weeks of rehabilitation, seated knee extension, squat on one leg, squat on two legs, heel raise, and standing on one leg were part of the training program, all exercises performed in a slow controlled manner. These exercises have previously been evaluated by EMG recording in ACL patients, 5 weeks after ACL reconstruction, demonstrating hamstring muscles activity levels corresponding to 19%–68% of MVC EMG [11]. The balance/coordination exercises during the first 12 weeks of rehabilitation included two-legged standing on wobble board and one-legged stance on balance mat, which previously has been reported to activate the hamstring muscles at low EMG activity levels [12].

A detailed description of the first 12 weeks of rehabilitation is presented in Table 2.

After 12 weeks of postoperative rehabilitation, strength training was progressively increased and open kinetic chain exercise, that is, loaded knee extension in machine, as well as free-weight barbell squat was included in the rehabilitation program. The majority of strength training exercises in the rehabilitation program were aimed at targeting the quadriceps muscles, with the hamstring muscles contracting actively as antagonists (knee extension) or synergists (hip extension). In a previous study, relatively low levels of ST EMG coactivation were observed during isolated knee extension exercise, free-weight squat, and seated leg press (9% to 22% of max EMG) in young healthy males [13]. Further, a preferential recruitment of the lateral hamstring muscle, biceps femoris (BF), over the medial hamstrings (ST) was noted during these exercises [13]. A single isolated strength training exercise for the hamstring muscles (prone leg curl exercise) was included in the rehabilitation protocol, which has been reported to involve high and comparable levels of ST and BF EMG muscle activities (>60% of max EMG) [13, 14]. After 4 months, higher level balance/coordination exercises on stable and unstable surface were included in the rehabilitation program. After 6 months, one-legged jump, landing, cutting, pivoting, and running drills were progressively included in the rehabilitation program [10]. However, a complete evidence-based neuromuscular training program was not followed by the player, for example, the program described by Myklebust et al., 2003 [15]. The ballistic balance/coordination exercises (i.e., one-legged jumps on different surfaces) have previously been evaluated in female elite athletes, where ST EMG activity levels were reported to range from 44% to 65% of MVC EMG [14]. After week 35, full soccer training was attended and at week 40 the player was engaged in full competition.

5. Return-to-Play

Upon completion of the postoperative rehabilitation phase, the player was tested according to the recommendations of return-to-play [16]. The player performed 3 single-legged hop tests: the single hop for distance, triple hop for distance, and single vertical hop. These tests have demonstrated good test-retest reliability in normal, young adults [17] and in patients after ACL reconstruction [18]. Finally, the player's self-reported knee function was scored by a validated questionnaire [19]. In April 2010, the player reached a level of the injured leg corresponding to ≥100% of the uninjured leg in all tests, and the player was cleared ready for return-to-play by the medical staff (PT, MD).

6. Kettlebell Swing Exercise Intervention

Since neuromuscular testing revealed that the players ST activation deficit persisted to exist during sidecutting after completion of the standard rehabilitation protocol, it was decided that the player should perform 6 weeks of additional training that was designed to preferentially target the medial hamstring muscle (more details given below). In this context, the kettlebell swing exercise has been reported to be particularly effective to targeting the ST muscle, demonstrating markedly higher EMG activity levels than ballistic one-legged balance/coordination exercises [14]. The kettlebell swing is a ballistic exercise performed standing on two legs where the highest external load is when the hamstring muscles are most stretched, that is, hip flexed and knee near straight. At this point, the knee joint position resembles the knee joint angle observed in a typical noncontact ACL injury situation

Table 2: Postoperative rehabilitation program.

Components	0–2 weeks	3–6 weeks	7–9 weeks	10–12 weeks
Soccer practice 90 min (/wk)	—	—	—	
Match play 90 min (/wk)	—	—	—	
Strength training (/wk)	—	—	—	3-4
Free-weight squat with barbell	—	—	—	—
Seated leg press (two-leg)	—	—	—	1 × 15 reps
Seated leg press (one-leg)	—	—	—	3 × 10 reps
Rotary calf	—	—	—	3 × 10 reps
Standing calf	—	—	—	3 × 10 reps
Knee extension	—	—	—	—
Prone leg curl	—			3 × 10 reps
Bicycling (/wk)	—	7	7	7
Exercises: unloaded (/wk)	7	7	7	7
Hip flexion/extension		3 × 10 reps	3 × 10 reps	3 × 10 reps
Knee flexion/extension		3 × 10 reps	3 × 10 reps	3 × 10 reps
Supine pelvic lifts (two-leg)		3 × 10 reps	3 × 10 reps	3 × 10 reps
Supine pelvic lifts (one-leg)		2 × 10 reps	2 × 10 reps	2 × 10 reps
Hip adduction (lying)		3 × 10 reps	3 × 10 reps	
Hip abduction (lying)		3 × 10 reps	3 × 10 reps	
Forward lunges		3 × 10 reps	3 × 10 reps	3 × 10 reps
Walking backwards		3 × 20 steps	3 × 20 steps	
Heel lifts		3 × 10 reps	3 × 10 reps	3 × 10 reps
Prone straight leg lift		3 × 10 reps	3 × 10 reps	
One-leg squat		—	3 × 10 reps	3 × 10 reps
Two-leg squat		—	3 × 10 reps	3 × 10 reps
Supine straight leg lift		—	3 × 10 reps	
One-leg standing		1 × 5 min	1 × 5 min	—
Exercises: equipment (/wk)	—	7	7	7
Hip abduction (elastics)		—	3 × 10 reps	3 × 10 reps
Prone knee flexion (elastics)		—	—	3 × 10 reps
Two-leg standing (wobble)		—	1 × 5 min	1 × 5 min
One-leg standing (mat)		—	—	3 × 10 reps
Step up (box)		—	2 × 10 reps	3 × 10 reps
Stretching exercises (/wk)		7	7	7
Quadriceps muscles		40 sec	40 sec	40 sec
Hamstring muscles		40 sec	40 sec	40 sec
Calf muscles		40 sec	40 sec	40 sec

[20]. Due to the stable two-legged position when swinging the kettlebell, the exercise is considered a safe exercise with respect to the knee joint. The kettlebell exercise intervention was initiated at the time when the player had returned to her preinjury activity level (May 2010, Table 1).

The player performed kettlebell swings using a 16 kg kettlebell according to the strength level of the subject and progressed later to 20 kg at the end of the intervention period. The kettlebell weight was chosen to match a weight where the subject was able to swing 20 times using proper technique. In this order, the kettlebell exercise has been shown to preferentially activate the medial hamstring muscle and at high EMG activity levels [14]. The player was supervised in proper technique by an educated kettlebell instructor. Kettlebell exercise was performed by forcefully swinging the kettlebell back between the legs by flexing the hips and keeping the knees slightly flexed (~10–15°) and to quickly reverse the direction with an explosive extension of the hips, swinging the kettlebell out to chest level where the hips and knees are extended and the subject is standing upright [14] (Figure 1).

In total, the player performed 10 training sessions during the 6-week period. Each training session consisted of 3–5 sets, with each single set corresponding to 20 swings and 20 seconds' pause in a 2-minute time interval. In sessions 1–4, kettlebell swings were performed using a 16 kg kettlebell. In

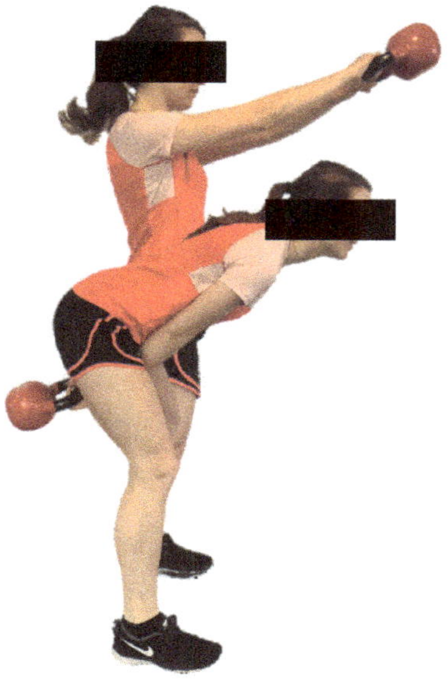

FIGURE 1: An illustration of the kettlebell swing exercise.

TABLE 3: Normalized EMG preactivity during sidecutting.

Preactivity	Test I: Before noncontact ACL injury	Test II: After surgery & rehabilitation	Test III: After kettlebell training
Semitendinosus (% of max EMG)	21%	23%	61%
Biceps femoris (% of max EMG)	23%	26%	17%

TABLE 4: Countermovement jump (CMJ) performance.

Height	Test I: Before noncontact ACL injury	Test II: After surgery & rehabilitation	Test III: After kettlebell training
CMJ (cm)	31.9	31.3	31.6

sessions 5–10, kettlebell swings were performed with a 20 kg kettlebell.

7. Results

7.1. Test I: Neuromuscular Coordination Assessment. Prior to ACL injury the player demonstrated a neuromuscular pattern during sidecutting known to increase the risk for noncontact ACL injury, that is, reduced EMG preactivity for the ST muscle (21% of max EMG, Table 3) and elevated EMG preactivity for the VL (i.e., VL-ST EMG preactivity difference ≥ 33%) [5].

7.2. Test II: Neuromuscular Coordination Assessment. Ten months after ACL reconstruction (including standardized postsurgical rehabilitation) the player was deemed ready to return to play by the medical staff (PT, MD). However, the player demonstrated a persisting pattern of high-risk neuromuscular activity during the sidecutting maneuver, characterized by reduced ST preactivity (23% of max EMG, Table 3). Six weeks of kettlebell training was therefore initiated, based on previous observation that kettlebell swing induces preferential high levels of semitendinosus EMG activity during execution [14].

7.3. Test III: Neuromuscular Coordination Assessment. After 6-week kettlebell training, the player increased ST preactivity during sidecutting from 23% to 61% of max EMG (Table 3), that is, increasing ST preactivity by 38 percentage points, consequently defined as a low-risk profile (VL-ST preactivity difference < 33%) [5]. In contrast, the lateral hamstring muscle (BF) displayed constancy in preactivity levels (17–26% of max EMG) across all time points examined (Table 3).

7.4. Countermovement Jump (CMJ). No change in functional performance, measured as maximal CMJ height, was observed throughout the study period (Table 4).

8. Discussion

In the present case study, a female elite soccer player was identified in retrospect with a high-risk neuromuscular profile [5] prior to sustaining a noncontact ACL rupture for the first time. Despite ACL reconstruction and subsequent period of standardized rehabilitation [10], the player continued to display a neuromuscular high-risk profile by the time of return-to-sport.

Although high quadriceps activity also seems to predispose for future ACL rupture, high knee extensor activity is essential to gain power and speed in explosive movements as the sidecutting maneuver. Thus, the main focus in the present case was to implement training that targeted an upregulation in medial hamstring (i.e., ST) muscle activity, for which reason the kettlebell exercise was chosen. Notably, six weeks of kettlebell training was effective for changing the neuromuscular profile during sidecutting from high- to low-risk behavior, due to an increased ST EMG preactivity during the sidecutting maneuver.

Excessive dynamic knee joint valgus moment during drop jumping has previously been identified to predispose for ACL injury [21]. The medial hamstring muscles are theoretically the only major muscles to actively counteract dynamic valgus [22]. In support of the medial ST muscle as the single most important ACL agonist, we have previously identified a "high-risk" zone for noncontact ACL injury comprised by low ST preactivity in concurrence with high VL preactivity during sidecutting [5]. In the present "high-risk" case, preventative efforts were not initiated prior to the athlete's first noncontact ACL injury because data from the screening study that established this risk profile had not been finally collected and analyzed. At the time of ACL injury and the subsequent rehabilitation, the neuromuscular screening method and ACL injury risk profile used in the present case study had been established and published [5]. Despite the fact that all standard procedures for ACL surgery, rehabilitation, and safe return-to-play were followed, the player persisted to display a high-risk profile characterized by low ST preactivity level during sidecutting. This finding indicates that standard rehabilitation did not sufficiently target the neuromuscular high-risk profile that the player displayed prior to the first-time ACL injury. In other words, the player appeared to remain at high-risk of noncontact ACL injury despite being discharged from rehabilitation and cleared to play.

We have previously reported that a multiexercise neuromuscular training program known to reduce the incidence of ACL injury among female elite athletes [15] may achieve this through a selective upregulation in ST preactivity during sidecutting [6]. In the present case report, various postural balance and intermuscular coordination exercises from the neuromuscular program [15] were introduced in the rehabilitation phase. Despite the implementation of such specific ACL injury prevention exercises, the player still demonstrated a high-risk profile at the time of "return-to-play." This indicates that a more aggressive training approach should be implemented when seeking to evoke a change in an established and consistent motor program. Thus, we focused exclusively on the ability to activate the semitendinosus and introduced an intervention with a single exercise, that is, kettlebell swing, known to preferentially activate the semitendinosus and at high activation levels [14].

The intervention strategy with six weeks of kettlebell training changed the neuromuscular profile from high- to low-risk [5]. Thus, the present case study indicates that a specific single exercise intervention targeting the ST muscle may be able to remodulate an existing motor program executed during a movement associated with noncontact ACL injury.

As seen in the present study participant, ACL ruptures typically are reconstructed by using the ST tendon as an autograft [23]. A follow-up MRI of the player in 2011 confirmed regeneration of the ST tendon. In line, a previous review reports that regeneration of the semitendinosus tendon may be confirmed in the majority of ACL patients reconstructed by harvesting of the ST tendon [24]. However, the volume of the semitendinosus muscle in the reconstructed limb has been reported to remain reduced compared to that of the uninjured limb [25]. Thus, in respect to dynamic knee joint control during sports activities involving cutting and pivoting tasks, it could be speculated whether ST graft harvesting actually leads to an elevated risk for sustaining secondary ACL injury (rerupture). In fact, recent data reveals that the revision rate after using hamstring tendon autograft reconstruction is higher compared with patella tendon autograft reconstruction, especially among the youngest patient group [26, 27]. Thus, introducing ballistic exercise modalities such as the kettlebell swing with preferentially high levels of medial hamstring activation seems essential, in both primary and secondary ACL injury preventative strategies.

In conclusion, this case describes an elite female soccer player who, after sustaining a noncontact ACL injury, having the ACL reconstructed and fulfilling 10 months of intensive ACL rehabilitation, still had a high-risk neuromuscular profile as she had preinjury. After only 6 weeks of kettlebell training, the neuromuscular pattern during sidecutting reversed from high- to low-risk. Thus, this exercise modality might be an important supplement to the standardized rehabilitation among patients aiming to return to sports activities. Future large-scale prospective studies should confirm whether the present findings can be used in the primary and secondary prevention of noncontact ACL injuries.

Competing Interests

The authors declare that there is no conflict of interests regarding the publication of this paper.

References

[1] P. Renstrom, A. Ljungqvist, E. Arendt et al., "Non-contact ACL injuries in female athletes: an International Olympic Committee current concepts statement," *British Journal of Sports Medicine*, vol. 42, no. 6, pp. 394–412, 2008.

[2] R. H. Brophy, S. A. Rodeo, R. P. Barnes, J. W. Powell, and R. F. Warren, "Knee articular cartilage injuries in the National Football League: epidemiology and treatment approach by team physicians," *Journal of Knee Surgery*, vol. 22, no. 4, pp. 331–338, 2009.

[3] S. M. Gianotti, S. W. Marshall, P. A. Hume, and L. Bunt, "Incidence of anterior cruciate ligament injury and other knee ligament injuries: a national population-based study," *Journal of Science and Medicine in Sport*, vol. 12, no. 6, pp. 622–627, 2009.

[4] J. Gilchrist, B. R. Mandelbaum, H. Melancon et al., "A randomized controlled trial to prevent noncontact anterior cruciate ligament injury in female collegiate soccer players," *American Journal of Sports Medicine*, vol. 36, no. 8, pp. 1476–1483, 2008.

[5] M. K. Zebis, L. L. Andersen, J. Bencke, M. Kjær, and P. Aagaard, "Identification of athletes at future risk of anterior cruciate ligament ruptures by neuromuscular screening," *The American Journal of Sports Medicine*, vol. 37, no. 10, pp. 1967–1973, 2009.

[6] M. K. Zebis, J. Bencke, L. L. Andersen et al., "The effects of neuromuscular training on knee joint motor control during sidecutting in female elite soccer and handball players," *Clinical Journal of Sport Medicine*, vol. 18, no. 4, pp. 329–337, 2008.

[7] H. J. Hermens, B. Freriks, C. Disselhorst-Klug, and G. Rau, "Development of recommendations for SEMG sensors and sensor placement procedures," *Journal of Electromyography and Kinesiology*, vol. 10, no. 5, pp. 361–374, 2000.

[8] P. Aagaard, E. B. Simonsen, J. L. Andersen, P. Magnusson, and P. Dyhre-Poulsen, "Increased rate of force development and neural drive of human skeletal muscle following resistance training," *Journal of Applied Physiology*, vol. 93, no. 4, pp. 1318–1326, 2002.

[9] P. Caserotti, P. Aagaard, E. B. Simonsen, and L. Puggaard, "Contraction-specific differences in maximal muscle power during stretch-shortening cycle movements in elderly males and females," *European Journal of Applied Physiology*, vol. 84, no. 3, pp. 206–212, 2001.

[10] R. B. Frobell, E. M. Roos, H. P. Roos, J. Ranstam, and L. S. Lohmander, "A randomized trial of treatment for acute anterior cruciate ligament tears," *New England Journal of Medicine*, vol. 363, no. 4, pp. 331–342, 2010.

[11] S. Tagesson, B. Öberg, and J. Kvist, "Tibial translation and muscle activation during rehabilitation exercises 5 weeks after anterior cruciate ligament reconstruction," *Scandinavian Journal of Medicine and Science in Sports*, vol. 20, no. 1, pp. 154–164, 2010.

[12] B. Juul-Kristensen, K. L. Johansen, P. Hendriksen, P. Melcher, J. Sandfeld, and B. R. Jensen, "Girls with generalized joint hypermobility display changed muscle activity and postural

sway during static balance tasks," *Scandinavian Journal of Rheumatology*, vol. 45, no. 1, pp. 57–65, 2016.

[13] L. L. Andersen, S. P. Magnusson, M. Nielsen, J. Haleem, K. Poulsen, and P. Aagaard, "Neuromuscular activation in conventional therapeutic exercises and heavy resistance exercises: implications for rehabilitation," *Physical Therapy*, vol. 86, no. 5, pp. 683–697, 2006.

[14] M. K. Zebis, J. Skotte, C. H. Andersen et al., "Kettlebell swing targets semitendinosus and supine leg curl targets biceps femoris: an EMG study with rehabilitation implications," *British Journal of Sports Medicine*, vol. 47, no. 18, pp. 1192–1198, 2013.

[15] G. Myklebust, L. Engebretsen, I. H. Brækken, A. Skjølberg, O.-E. Olsen, and R. Bahr, "Prevention of anterior cruciate ligament injuries in female team handball players: a prospective intervention study over three seasons," *Clinical Journal of Sport Medicine*, vol. 13, no. 2, pp. 71–78, 2003.

[16] D. Logerstedt, H. Grindem, A. Lynch et al., "Single-legged hop tests as predictors of self-reported knee function after anterior cruciate ligament reconstruction: the Delaware-Oslo ACL cohort study," *The American Journal of Sports Medicine*, vol. 40, no. 10, pp. 2348–2356, 2012.

[17] M. D. Ross, B. Langford, and P. J. Whelan, "Test-retest reliability of 4 single-leg horizontal hop tests," *Journal of Strength and Conditioning Research*, vol. 16, no. 4, pp. 617–622, 2002.

[18] A. Reid, T. B. Birmingham, P. W. Stratford, G. K. Alcock, and J. R. Giffin, "Hop testing provides a reliable and valid outcome measure during rehabilitation after anterior cruciate ligament reconstruction," *Physical Therapy*, vol. 87, no. 3, pp. 337–349, 2007.

[19] E. M. Roos, H. P. Roos, L. S. Lohmander, C. Ekdahl, and B. D. Beynnon, "Knee Injury and Osteoarthritis Outcome Score (KOOS)—development of a self-administered outcome measure," *Journal of Orthopaedic & Sports Physical Therapy*, vol. 28, no. 2, pp. 88–96, 1998.

[20] T. Krosshaug, A. Nakamae, B. P. Boden et al., "Mechanisms of anterior cruciate ligament injury in basketball: video analysis of 39 cases," *American Journal of Sports Medicine*, vol. 35, no. 3, pp. 359–367, 2007.

[21] T. E. Hewett, G. D. Myer, K. R. Ford et al., "Biomechanical measures of neuromuscular control and valgus loading of the knee predict anterior cruciate ligament injury risk in female athletes: a prospective study," *The American Journal of Sports Medicine*, vol. 33, no. 4, pp. 492–501, 2005.

[22] J. Bencke, D. Curtis, C. Krogshede, L. K. Jensen, T. Bandholm, and M. K. Zebis, "Biomechanical evaluation of the side-cutting manoeuvre associated with ACL injury in young female handball players," *Knee Surgery, Sports Traumatology, Arthroscopy*, vol. 21, no. 8, pp. 1876–1881, 2013.

[23] M. Lind, F. Menhert, and A. B. Pedersen, "The first results from the Danish ACL reconstruction registry: epidemiologic and 2 year follow-up results from 5,818 knee ligament reconstructions," *Knee Surgery, Sports Traumatology, Arthroscopy*, vol. 17, no. 2, pp. 117–124, 2009.

[24] R. Papalia, F. Franceschi, S. D'Adamio, L. Diaz Balzani, N. Maffulli, and V. Denaro, "Hamstring tendon regeneration after harvest for anterior cruciate ligament reconstruction: a systematic review," *Arthroscopy—Journal of Arthroscopic and Related Surgery*, vol. 31, no. 6, pp. 1169–1183, 2015.

[25] Y. Makihara, A. Nishino, T. Fukubayashi, and A. Kanamori, "Decrease of knee flexion torque in patients with ACL reconstruction: combined analysis of the architecture and function of the knee flexor muscles," *Knee Surgery, Sports Traumatology, Arthroscopy*, vol. 14, no. 4, pp. 310–317, 2006.

[26] A. Persson, K. Fjeldsgaard, J.-E. Gjertsen et al., "Increased risk of revision with hamstring tendon grafts compared with patellar tendon grafts after anterior cruciate ligament reconstruction: a study of 12,643 patients from the Norwegian Cruciate Ligament Registry, 2004–2012," *The American Journal of Sports Medicine*, vol. 42, no. 2, pp. 285–291, 2014.

[27] L. Rahr-Wagner, T. M. Thillemann, A. B. Pedersen, and M. Lind, "Comparison of hamstring tendon and patellar tendon grafts in anterior cruciate ligament reconstruction in a nationwide population-based Cohort study: results from the danish registry of knee ligament reconstruction," *The American Journal of Sports Medicine*, vol. 42, no. 2, pp. 278–284, 2014.

8

Superior Patellar Dislocation Misdiagnosed as Patellar Tendon Rupture: The Value of Ultrasonography

Artit Boonrod,[1] Sermsak Sumanont,[1] Manusak Boonard,[1] and Arunnit Boonrod[2]

[1]*Department of Orthopedics, Faculty of Medicine, Khon Kaen University, 123 Mittraphap Road, Khon Kaen 40002, Thailand*
[2]*Department of Radiology, Faculty of Medicine, Khon Kaen University, 123 Mittraphap Road, Khon Kaen 40002, Thailand*

Correspondence should be addressed to Artit Boonrod; artibo@kku.ac.th

Academic Editor: Johannes Mayr

Superior dislocation of the patella with intact patellar tendon is a rare condition. Most cases in literatures were diagnosed by clinical examination and plain radiography; however there are many cases that were misdiagnosed as patellar tendon rupture. In this case, we demonstrate the use of ultrasound for diagnosis of superior dislocation of the patella in the emergency department. We also include a literature review of similar cases and discuss the advantages of different types of imaging for diagnosis in this condition.

1. Introduction

Superior dislocation of the patella with intact patellar tendon is a rare condition [1]. The age group of the patient is between 45 and 80 years. Most of them had preexisting degenerative joint [1–23]. Most cases in literature review were usually diagnosed by clinical examination and plain radiography. The primary superior dislocation of the patella is easily treated with simple closed reduction under adequate anesthesia. However, there are many cases in which that treatment was delayed due to misdiagnose as patellar tendon rupture [3, 4, 10, 17]. In this report, we describe and provide discussion on the ultrasound used, as a helpful additional imaging, for diagnosis of superior dislocation of the patella in the emergency department.

2. Case Presentation

A 50-year-old man presented with right knee locked in hyperextension after falling with the knee extended. He had a severe knee pain and was unable to bend his knee. Initially, the patient was diagnosed as ruptured patellar tendon and was managed by immobilization with a long leg splint at a community hospital. The patient was referred to our hospital 5 hours after the injury. He had persistent anterior knee pain, inability to bend his knee, high-riding patella, anterior tilt of superior part of the patella, and skin dimple inferior to patella (Figure 1). The lateral radiograph of the right knee showed high-riding patella with inferior patellar osteophyte locked to osteophyte at the superior aspect of femoral condyle (Figures 2(a) and 2(b)). The physical examination and lateral radiographs of the knee represented superior patellar dislocation, but the patellar tendon integrity cannot be confirmed. Subsequently, the bedside ultrasonography, performed by an orthopedic surgeon, is used to evaluate the extensor mechanism of the knee. The patient was in supine position with his knee fixed in extension. Under high frequency transducer (GE healthcare, LOGIC Book, 8 MHz linear transducer), longitudinal ultrasound was performed through the entire length and width of the patellar tendon. Transverse scan was subsequently performed to complete the evaluation of patellar tendon in two perpendicular planes. The multiple, parallel echogenic lines of the patellar tendon were demonstrated between the lower pole of the patella and the tibial tuberosity (Figure 3). This ultrasound finding confirmed that the patellar tendon was intact. The dynamic study was not performed because the patient's knee was fixed in extension. The images were reviewed by a senior orthopedic surgeon and a radiologist, and the diagnosis of patellar dislocation with intact patellar tendon was agreed upon. After intravenous sedation, closed reduction was performed by using thumb and index finger to elevate the patella and gently

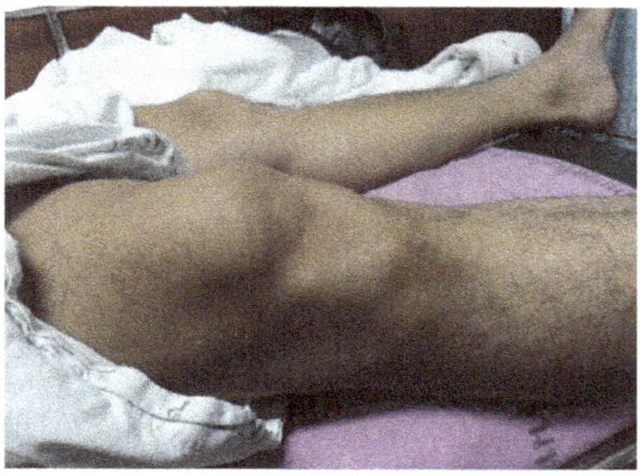

FIGURE 1: Clinical presentation with high-riding patella, anterior tilt of superior part of the patella, and skin dimple inferior to patella.

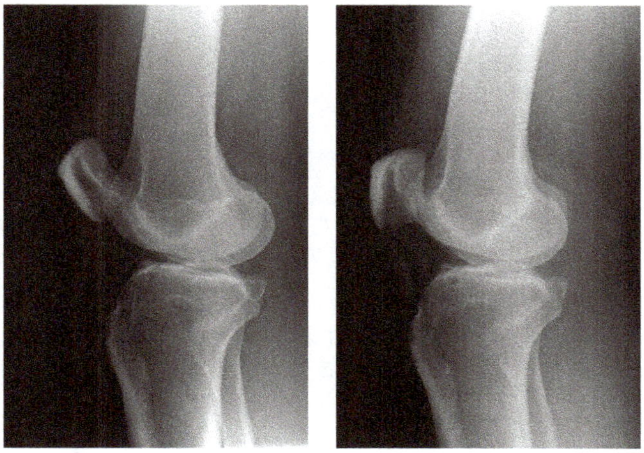

(a) (b)

FIGURE 2: Pre- and postreduction lateral radiographs show superior dislocation of the patella. (a) showed high-riding patella with inferior patellar osteophyte locked to osteophyte at the superior aspect of femoral condyle. (b) showed normal position of patella.

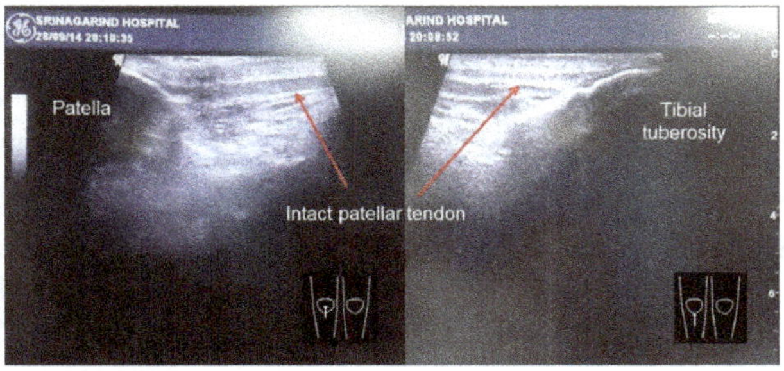

FIGURE 3: Under high frequency transducer (8 MHz linear transducer), the longitudinal scan showed multiple, parallel echogenic lines of the patellar tendon between the lower pole of the patella and the tibial tuberosity (arrowed). This ultrasound finding confirmed intact patellar tendon.

move the patella into superior and lateral directions. The patella was easily relocated. The patient was able to achieve full active range of motion immediately after reduction. A follow-up ultrasound evaluation and lateral radiograph of the knee confirmed the anatomic reduction without any complication. Compression dressing was applied and partial weight walking with axillary crutch was advocated for 2 weeks. At 18 months' follow-up he had no pain or recurrent dislocation.

3. Discussion

Superior dislocation of the patella with intact patellar tendon is a rare condition, only 20 of which have been reported in English medical literature [1]. The first case was reported by Watson-Jones in 1956 [22]. Most patients with this condition had preexisting degenerative joint [1–23]. Osteophytes at the inferior aspect of patella and at the anterior aspect of medial condyle of femur are the identified cause of the locked knee in extension [7, 8, 12, 18, 19, 23]. The usual mechanism of injury is forceful contraction of quadriceps tendon with or without a posteriorly directed force [9].

However to make the correct diagnosis on the first visit might be difficult because most physicians are more familiar with lateral dislocation of the patella and rupture of the patellar tendon [1]. Many of the cases in previous studies received delayed treatment due to being misdiagnosed as patellar tendon rupture [3, 4, 10, 17]. Diagnosis should be

Table 1: Additional imaging modalities.

Modality	Benefit
Ultrasound	(i) Evaluating the integrity of the patellar tendon [4, 10, 18]. (ii) Evaluating the medial structure injury such as vastus medialis tear [4]. (iii) Follow-up immediately after closed reduction [4, 18].
3D-computed tomography	(i) Evaluating the osteophytes at the inferior aspect of the patella and at the superior aspect of femoral condyle [1].
Magnetic resonance imaging	(i) Evaluating the integrity of the patellar tendon [4, 9, 13]. (ii) Evaluating the osteophytes at the inferior aspect of the patella and at the superior aspect of femoral condyle [4, 9, 13]. (iii) Evaluating any associated injury such as vastus medialis tear [4]. (iv) Evaluating the cartilage and other intra-articular pathologies.

differentiated from patellar tendon rupture because it is a surgical condition.

In most cases in literature, this condition is diagnosed by clinical examination and plain radiography. The presentations are anterior knee pain, locked knee in hyperextension, inability to bend knee, high-riding patella, anterior tilt of superior part of the patella, and skin dimple just inferior to the patella. Lateral radiograph shows superior dislocation of the patella and osteophytes at the inferior aspect of patella and at the anterior aspect of medial condyle of femur [4]. However, when the diagnosis is uncertain, additional imaging, such as ultrasound [4, 10], 3D-computed tomography [1], or magnetic resonance imaging [4, 9, 13], may be helpful (Table 1).

High-resolution ultrasonography has been recognized as an effective method of examining the extensor mechanism of the knee in both acute and chronic injuries. A key advantage of ultrasound over MRI is the ability to image tendons and bones dynamically and being useful for evaluating the reduction immediately in emergency department [4, 18]. Furthermore, in some cases, imaging is needed to look for any associated intra-articular damage such as osteophytes, osteochondral injury, or ligament tears. In this situation MRI provides a means of imaging of the intra-articular structures [4, 9, 13]. However, it is not recommended in the evaluation of most suspected extensor mechanism injuries because it is costly and usually unavailable in the emergency room. CT scan is useless imaging for diagnosis, because it is only shows the locked osteophytes [1], which can usually be clearly demonstrated by plain film.

In conclusion, although superior dislocation of the patella is a rare and non-life-threatening condition which may be unrecognized, a careful examination and investigation can lead to accurate diagnosis and appropriate management. At initial presentation, this condition may be confused with the rupture of the patellar tendon. Therefore, if physicians cannot exclude the rupture of the patellar tendon by clinical examination and plain radiograph, additional imaging studies such as ultrasound have an important role for correct diagnosis and confirmation of successful reduction immediately in the emergency department.

Competing Interests

The authors declare that there is no conflict of interests regarding the publication of this paper.

References

[1] H. Gakhar and A. Singhal, "Superior dislocation of the patella: case report and review of the literature," *Journal of Emergency Medicine*, vol. 44, no. 2, pp. 478–480, 2013.

[2] D. H. Bartlett, L. A. Gilula, and W. A. Murphy, "Superior dislocation of the patella fixed by interlocked osteophytes. A case report and review of the literature," *The Journal of Bone & Joint Surgery—American Volume*, vol. 58, no. 6, pp. 883–884, 1976.

[3] R. S. Bassi and B. A. Kumar, "Superior dislocation of the patella; a case report and review of the literature," *Emergency Medicine Journal*, vol. 20, no. 1, pp. 97–98, 2003.

[4] R. K. Clift and W. El-Alami, "Superior patellar dislocation: the value of clinical examination and radiological investigation," *BMJ Case Reports*, vol. 2012, 2012.

[5] X. Cusco, R. Seijas, O. Ares, J. R. Cugat, M. Garcia-Balletbo, and R. Cugat, "Superior dislocation of the patella: a case report," *Journal of Orthopaedic Surgery and Research*, vol. 4, article 29, 2009.

[6] T. Friden, "A case of superior dislocation of the patella," *Acta Orthopaedica Scandinavica*, vol. 58, no. 4, pp. 429–430, 2009.

[7] B. Hansen, C. Beck, and R. Townsley, "Arthroscopic removal of a loose body osteophyte fragment after superior patellar dislocation with locked osteophytes," *Arthroscopy*, vol. 19, no. 3, article E25, 2003.

[8] N. Harris, S. Hay, and D. Bickerstaff, "Recurrent traumatic superior dislocation of the patella with interlocking osteophytes," *The Knee*, vol. 2, no. 3, pp. 181–182, 1995.

[9] A. Iorwerth, R. Thomas, and D. J. Shewring, "Confirmation of an intact patellar tendon in superior dislocation of the patella using magnetic resonance imaging," *Injury*, vol. 32, no. 2, pp. 167–169, 2001.

[10] G. Joseph, K. Devalia, K. Kantam, and N. M. Shaath, "Superior dislocation of the patella. Case report and review of literature," *Acta Orthopaedica Belgica*, vol. 71, no. 3, pp. 369–371, 2005.

[11] R. Lai and Y. K. Lau, "Superior dislocation of the patella treated by closed reduction: a rare case report and review of the literature," *Hong Kong Journal of Emergency Medicine*, vol. 14, no. 4, pp. 225–227, 2007.

[12] T. G. McWilliams and M. S. Binns, "A locked knee in extension: a complication of a degenerate knee with patella alta," *Journal of Bone and Joint Surgery B*, vol. 82, article no. 890, 2000.

[13] O. Ofluoglu, D. Yasmin, R. Donthineni, and M. Yildiz, "Superior dislocation of the patella with early onset patellofemoral arthritis: a case report and literature review," *Knee Surgery, Sports Traumatology, Arthroscopy*, vol. 14, no. 4, pp. 350–355, 2006.

[14] J. P. Rao and M. A. Meese, "Irreducible superior dislocation of the patella requiring open reduction," *American Journal of Orthopedics*, vol. 26, no. 7, pp. 486–488, 1997.

[15] R. M. Roth and J. B. McCabe, "Nontraumatic superior dislocation of the patella," *Journal of Emergency Medicine*, vol. 3, no. 4, pp. 265–267, 1985.

[16] A. J. Saleemi, A. Hussain, M. J. Iqbal, M. G. Thuse, and A. A. George, "Superior dislocation of patella in a rugby player: an update on a extremely rare condition and review of literature," *Knee Surgery, Sports Traumatology, Arthroscopy*, vol. 15, no. 9, pp. 1112–1113, 2007.

[17] S. J. Scott, A. Molloy, and R. A. Harvey, "Superior dislocation of the patella—a rare but important differential diagnosis of acute knee pain—a case report and review of the literature," *Injury*, vol. 31, no. 7, pp. 543–545, 2000.

[18] M. A. Siddiqui and M. H. Tan, "Locked knee from superior dislocation of the patella-diagnosis and management of a rare injury," *Knee Surgery, Sports Traumatology, Arthroscopy*, vol. 19, no. 4, pp. 671–673, 2011.

[19] M. G. Siegel and S. S. Mac, "Superior dislocation of the patella with interlocking osteophytes," *Journal of Trauma*, vol. 22, no. 3, pp. 253–254, 1982.

[20] S. Takai, N. Yoshino, and Y. Hirasawa, "Arthroscopic treatment of voluntary superior dislocation of the patella," *Arthroscopy*, vol. 14, no. 7, pp. 753–756, 1998.

[21] D. D. Teuscher and T. H. Goletz, "Recurrent atraumatic superior dislocation of the patella: case report and review of the literature," *Arthroscopy*, vol. 8, no. 4, pp. 541–543, 1992.

[22] R. Watson-Jones, *Fractures and Joint Injuries*, Williams and Walkins, Baltimore, Md, USA, 5th edition, 1956.

[23] D. K. Yip, J. W. Wong, L. K. Sun, N. M. Wong, C. W. Chan, and P. Y. Lau, "The management of superior dislocation of the patella with interlocking osteophytes—an update on a rare problem," *Journal of orthopaedic surgery*, vol. 12, no. 2, pp. 253–257, 2004.

9

Giant Baker's Cyst Associated with Rheumatoid Arthritis

Levent Adiyeke,[1] Emre Bılgın,[2] Tahir Mutlu Duymus,[1]
İsmail Emre Ketencı,[1] and Meriç Ugurlar[3]

[1] *Haydarpasa Numune Training and Research Hospital, Department of Orthopaedics and Traumatology, İstanbul, Turkey*
[2] *Tepecik Education and Research Hospital, Department of Orthopaedics and Traumatology, Izmir, Turkey*
[3] *Şişli Etfal Training and Research Hospital, Department of Orthopaedics and Traumatology, İstanbul, Turkey*

Correspondence should be addressed to Levent Adiyeke; leventadiyeke@gmail.com

Academic Editor: John Nyland

We report a rare case of a "giant Baker's cyst-related rheumatoid arthritis (RA)" with 95 × 26 mm dimensions originating from the semimembranosus tendon. The patient presented with chronic pain and a palpable mass behind his left calf located between the posteriosuperior aspect of the popliteal fossa and the distal third of the calf. In MRI cystic lesion which was located in soft tissue at the posterior of gastrocnemius, extensive synovial pannus inside and degeneration of medial meniscus posterior horn were observed. Arthroscopic joint debridement and partial excision of the cyst via biomechanical valve excision were performed. The patient continued his follow-up visits at Rheumatology Department and there was no recurrence of cyst-related symptoms in 1-year follow-up. Similar cases were reported in the literature previously. However, as far as we know, a giant Baker's cyst-related RA, which was treated as described, has not yet been presented.

1. Introduction

Rheumatoid arthritis (RA) is a common chronic inflammatory autoimmune disease that affects 3% of females and 1% of males. This condition is characterized by neutrophil infiltration of soft tissues and hypertrophy of the joint capsule, synovia, tendon sheath, and bursa due to chronic inflammation [1]. Villi formation and intra-articular pannus formation develop as the amount of synovial fluid increases, leading to the proliferation of synovial tissue. Knee joints are the most commonly affected joints in 15% of RA patients [2, 3]. The joint capsule becomes tightened, which is associated with increasing amounts of synovial fluid. A palpable mass behind the knee joint, which typically expands the subcutaneous tissue, occurs between the semimembranosus and medial head of the gastrocnemius tendons [4, 5]. In this report, we present a giant Baker's cyst in a RA patient expanding to the middle of the calf.

2. Case

A 42-year-old male with left knee pain lasting for 9 months and swelling behind the knee was admitted to the orthopedics clinic. He stated that he had increased pain with standing and limited knee flexion. He had been receiving IV methotrexate (Metoject 20 mg/2 mL 1 × 1 per week) and oral sulfasalazine (Salazopyrin-en 500 Mg 2 × 2 per day) for 3 months for the RA. During physical examination, a large mass was observed behind the left knee, expanding to the proximal calf. The mass was immobile and soft when palpated. The range of motion (ROM) of the left knee was Fl/Ext 120/−10 degree. McMurray and Patellar Ballottement tests were positive. Neurovascular examination of the left lower extremity was normal. Laboratory studies showed the following: ESR, 18 mm/h; CRP, 5 mm/dL; and WBC, 10.000.

Minimal degenerative changes were observed at the medial plateau based on plain radiographs. Based on magnetic resonance imaging (MRI), a 95 mm × 26 mm cystic lesion had located in soft tissue at the posterior of the gastrocnemius, with extensive synovial pannus inside; degeneration of the medial meniscus posterior horn was observed (Figure 1). Diagnostic arthroscopy was performed and intense synovial hypertrophy signs and pannus formation were detected (Figure 2). Samples were obtained from synovial tissue for biopsy. Low-viscosity cyst material flowed into the

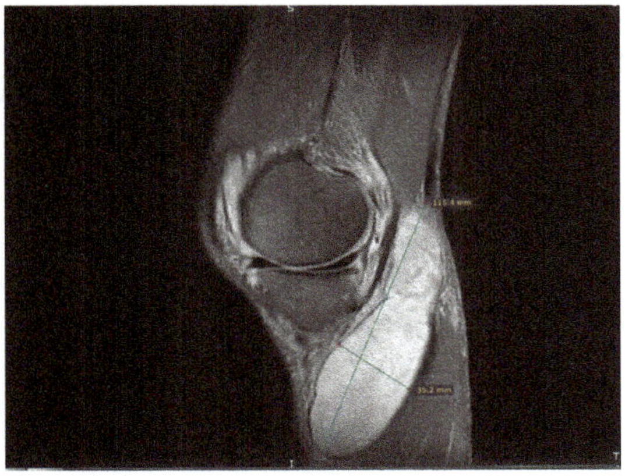

FIGURE 1: Magnetic resonance imaging sagittal plane view: cyst size.

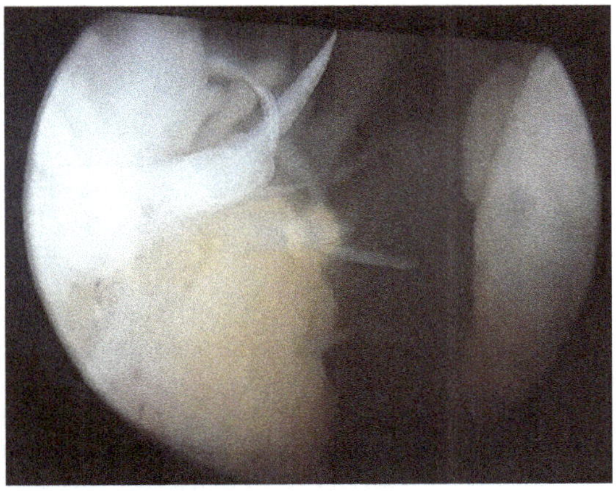

FIGURE 2: Arthroscopic view of pannus formation.

joint after controlling for the horizontal tear of the medial meniscus posterior horn with a probe (Figure 3). The canal from which the cyst content originated was expanded with a clamp, and the canal stoma was debrided using a shaver-blade. The cyst was reached by creating an approximately 9 cm posteromedial incision (Figure 4). The cyst was released from surrounding soft tissues, excised, and sent to pathology. Histopathological examination showed fibrohyalinized tissue covered with synovial epithelium. We also observed plasma cells due to active chronic inflammation, as well as fibrovascular tissue fragments compatible with the cyst wall. Analysis of synovial fluid showed the following: WBC, 27200; PMN (%), 75; glucose, 67; and culture negative. Pain and swelling decreased after discharge, and full ROM of the left knee was observed at follow-up visits.

3. Discussion

RA is a chronic immune system-induced disease that leads to increased production of synovial fluid depending on inflammation in the knee joint. In this disease in which synovial tissue has a strong effect on the knee joint, chondral damage and connective tissue involvement may be present [1, 6, 7]. This disease is associated with increased synovial fluid in the knee and can lead to the formation of a Baker's cyst, with a one-way valve mechanism formed in the knee joint. Baker's cyst, which is generally palpated with asymptomatic swelling in the popliteal fossa, may occur depending on meniscal tears and arthrosis [8, 9]. In a study by Fielding et al., which was performed with MRI, they stated that Baker's cyst was seen in adult populations at a rate of 4%; this rate was higher in the elderly population [10] and is even higher in diseases such as RA and gout. In situations involving pain, swelling in the popliteal fossa and severe limitation of knee ROM, further evaluation is required. Deep vein thrombosis, popliteal artery aneurysm and cyst rupture should be considered in the differential diagnosis [9, 11–14]. The differential diagnosis should also include malignant tumors, which can settle in the popliteal region and have cystic characteristics (synovial sarcoma, fibrosarcoma, and malignant fibrous histiocytoma). To evaluate Baker's cyst, MRI and ultrasound (US) are the most important diagnostic tools in terms of the exclusion of

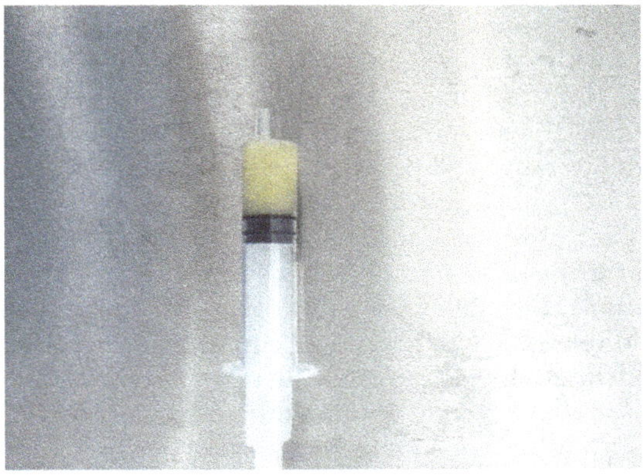

FIGURE 3: Cyst aspiration material compatible with subacute inflammatory period.

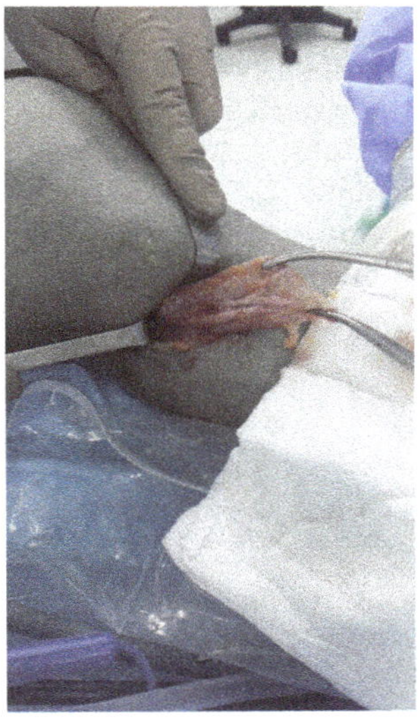

FIGURE 4: Excision of the Baker's cyst by posteromedial incision.

different diagnoses and characterizing the relationship of cyst content with the joint [8, 10, 15, 16].

For the treatment of Baker's cyst, various conservative and surgical treatments were applied depending on the underlying cause and accompanying pathology. Within the conservative applications, successful results were reported with joint aspiration and corticosteroid (KS) injection in osteoarthritis related cases [6, 17–19]. Acebes et al. reported successful results following aspiration of cyst contents and KS injection in osteoarthritis related cases [17]. In similar cases, Bandinelli et al. also reported successful results using US-guided steroid injection directly into the cyst and intraarticular steroid injection; both methods were considered effective [18]. In the treatment of Baker's cyst accompanied with RA, Hofman-González et al. stated that methotrexate application to the cyst may be an alternative method for patients with surgical risk factors [20]. In our case, active complaints of the patient were present, despite ongoing IV methotrexate treatment.

Although successful results were obtained in Baker's cyst treatment with conservative methods, surgical interventions may be required. Cyst excision is one of the options for surgical interventions, although extensive exposure is required. However, arthroscopic methods have become more popular. By performing arthroscopy, intra-articular pathology leading to cyst formation can be intervened, and biomechanical valve mechanisms thought to be responsible for cyst formation can be treated [21, 22]. Rupp et al. indicated that Baker's cyst is often accompanied by a medial meniscal tear and chondral lesions. It was reported that regression of the cyst was observed after performing arthroscopic debridement, partial meniscectomy, and microfracture for low-grade chondral lesions. However, formation of an effusion was not adequately controlled and treatment success was limited in grades 3 and 4 chondral lesions [23].

In a previous study, Sansone and De Ponti obtained good results following arthroscopic treatment of biomechanical valves and accompanying intra-articular disorders in a series of 30 patients with a two-year follow-up. Moreover, 95% of patients benefited from this method [22]. In a similar study, Calvisi et al. stated that, after suturing the canal valve using the all-inside arthroscopic technique with anterolateral and posteromedial portals and treatment of the intra-articular conditions, Baker's cyst disappeared in 64% of cases after two-year follow-up. Regression of the cyst was observed at a rate of 27%, and the cyst progressed in 9% of cases [24].

Intervention of intra-articular disorders and expansion of canal diameter with excision of the canal valve by performing arthroscopy is a recently accepted method. Ahn et al. stated that they achieved 94% success in a three-year follow-up period using this method [25]. In a study by Cho, using a similar method, good clinical results were obtained in a two-year follow-up with no recurrence [26]. In our case, the canal diameter of the cyst was expanded and intra-articular pathology was treated by shaving the medial meniscus posterior horn through arthroscopy. Symptoms related to the Baker's cyst, which extended to the posteromedial calf, were eliminated by partial cyst excision. The patient continued their follow-up visits at the Rheumatology Department, and there was no recurrence of cyst-related symptoms during a 1-year follow-up.

Successful results can be obtained by performing arthroscopic debridement and biomechanical valve excision in cases with Baker's cyst accompanied by intra-articular damage. Additionally, open cyst excision should be considered in symptomatic and recurrent cases.

Competing Interests

No competing interests were declared by the authors.

References

[1] M. H. Ozsoy, L. Altınel, K. Basarır, A. Cavuoğlu, and V. Dincel, "Romatoid artritte eklem hastalığının patogenezi," *TOTBID Dergisi*, vol. 5, no. 3-4, pp. 101–110, 2006.

[2] P. N. Chalmers, S. L. Sherman, B. S. Raphael, and E. P. Su, "Rheumatoid synovectomy: does the surgical approach matter?" *Clinical Orthopaedics and Related Research*, vol. 469, no. 7, pp. 2062–2071, 2011.

[3] P. Triolo, R. Rossi, F. Rosso, D. Blonna, F. Castoldi, and D. E. Bonasia, "Arthroscopic synovectomy of the knee in rheumatoid arthritis defined by the 2010 ACR/EULAR criteria," *The Knee*, vol. 23, no. 5, pp. 862–866, 2016.

[4] D. Fritschy, J. Fasel, J.-C. Imbert, S. Bianchi, R. Verdonk, and C. J. Wirth, "The popliteal cyst," *Knee Surgery, Sports Traumatology, Arthroscopy*, vol. 14, no. 7, pp. 623–628, 2006.

[5] L. Martí-Bonmatí, E. Mollá, R. Dosdá, C. Casillas, and P. Ferrer, "MR imaging of Baker cysts—prevalence and relation to internal derangements of the knee," *Magnetic Resonance Materials in Physics, Biology and Medicine*, vol. 10, no. 3, pp. 205–210, 2000.

[6] M. Köroğlu, M. Callıoğlu, H. N. Eriş et al., "Ultrasound guided percutaneous treatment and follow-up of Baker's cyst in knee osteoarthritis," *European Journal of Radiology*, vol. 81, no. 11, pp. 3466–3471, 2012.

[7] E. Nogueira, A. Gomes, A. Preto, and A. Cavaco-Paulo, "Update on therapeutic approaches for rheumatoid arthritis," *Current Medicinal Chemistry*, vol. 23, no. 21, pp. 2190–2203, 2016.

[8] S.-T. Liao, C.-S. Chiou, and C.-C. Chang, "Pathology associated to the Baker's cysts: A Musculoskeletal Ultrasound Study," *Clinical Rheumatology*, vol. 29, no. 9, pp. 1043–1047, 2010.

[9] S. Artul, H. Jabaly-Habib, F. Artoul, and G. Habib, "The association between Baker's cyst and medial meniscal tear in patients with symptomatic knee using ultrasonography," *Clinical Imaging*, vol. 39, no. 4, pp. 659–661, 2015.

[10] J. R. Fielding, P. D. Franklin, and J. Kustan, "Popliteal cysts: a reassessment using magnetic resonance imaging," *Skeletal Radiology*, vol. 20, no. 6, pp. 433–435, 1991.

[11] P. F. DeLuca and A. R. Bartolozzi, "Tibial neuroma presenting as a Baker cyst. A case report," *The Journal of Bone & Joint Surgery—American Volume*, vol. 81, no. 6, pp. 856–858, 1999.

[12] A. Gombert, H. Jalaie, M. J. Jacobs, and J. Grommes, "Popliteal artery aneurysma as an important differential diagnosis," *Sportverletzung-Sportschaden*, vol. 29, no. 1, pp. 51–52, 2015.

[13] J. S. Kim, S. H. Lim, B. Y. Hong, and S. Y. Park, "Ruptured popliteal cyst diagnosed by ultrasound before evaluation for deep vein thrombosis," *Annals of Rehabilitation Medicine*, vol. 38, no. 6, pp. 843–846, 2014.

[14] N. Alonso-Gómez, A. Pérez-Piqueras, A. Martínez-Izquierdo, and F. Sáinz-González, "Giant baker' cyst. Differential diagnosis of deep vein thrombosis," *Reumatologia Clinica*, vol. 11, no. 3, pp. 179–181, 2015.

[15] L. Riente, A. Delle Sedie, E. Filippucci et al., "Ultrasound imaging for the rheumatologist XXVII. Sonographic assessment of the knee in patients with rheumatoid arthritis," *Clinical and Experimental Rheumatology*, vol. 28, no. 3, pp. 300–303, 2010.

[16] V. J. De de Beer, E. R. Bogoch, and H. A. Smythe, "Lymphoma presenting as a popliteal mass in a patient with rheumatoid arthritis," *Journal of Rheumatology*, vol. 17, no. 9, pp. 1242–1243, 1990.

[17] J. C. Acebes, O. Sánchez-Pernaute, A. Díaz-Oca, and G. Herrero-Beaumont, "Ultrasonographic assessment of Baker's cysts after intra-articular corticosteroid injection in knee osteoarthritis," *Journal of Clinical Ultrasound*, vol. 34, no. 3, pp. 113–117, 2006.

[18] F. Bandinelli, R. Fedi, S. Generini et al., "Longitudinal ultrasound and clinical follow-up of Baker's cysts injection with steroids in knee osteoarthritis," *Clinical Rheumatology*, vol. 31, no. 4, pp. 727–731, 2012.

[19] M. K. Smith, B. Lesniak, M. G. Baraga, L. Kaplan, and J. Jose, "Treatment of popliteal (baker) cysts with ultrasound-guided aspiration, fenestration, and injection: long-term follow-up," *Sports Health*, vol. 7, no. 5, pp. 409–414, 2015.

[20] F. Hofman-González, C. Hernández-Díaz, C. Solano-Ávila, A. G. López-Reyes, A. Peña-Ayala, and C. Pineda-Villaseñor, "Giant Baker's cyst treated with intralesional methotrexate," *Cirugia y Cirujanos*, vol. 81, no. 1, pp. 64–68, 2013.

[21] A. Pankaj, D. Chahar, and D. Pathrot, "Arthroscopic management of popliteal cysts," *Indian Journal of Orthopaedics*, vol. 50, no. 2, pp. 154–158, 2016.

[22] V. Sansone and A. De Ponti, "Arthroscopic treatment of popliteal cyst and associated intra-articular knee disorders in adults," *Arthroscopy*, vol. 15, no. 4, pp. 368–372, 1999.

[23] S. Rupp, R. Seil, P. Jochum, and D. Kohn, "Popliteal cysts in adults: prevalence, associated intraarticular lesions, and results after arthroscopic treatment," *American Journal of Sports Medicine*, vol. 30, no. 1, pp. 112–115, 2002.

[24] V. Calvisi, S. Lupparelli, and P. Giuliani, "Arthroscopic all-inside suture of symptomatic Baker's cysts: a technical option for surgical treatment in adults," *Knee Surgery, Sports Traumatology, Arthroscopy*, vol. 15, no. 12, pp. 1452–1460, 2007.

[25] J. H. Ahn, S. H. Lee, J. C. Yoo, M. J. Chang, and Y. S. Park, "Arthroscopic treatment of popliteal cysts: clinical and magnetic resonance imaging results," *Arthroscopy - Journal of Arthroscopic and Related Surgery*, vol. 26, no. 10, pp. 1340–1347, 2010.

[26] J. H. Cho, "Clinical results of direct arthroscopic excision of popliteal cyst using a posteromedial portal," *Knee Surgery & Related Research*, vol. 24, no. 4, pp. 235–240, 2012.

Multiple Giant Cell Tumors of Tendon Sheath Found within a Single Digit of a 9-Year-Old

John S. Hwang,[1] Valerie A. Fitzhugh,[2] Peter D. Gibson,[1] Jacob Didesch,[1] and Irfan Ahmed[1]

[1]*Department of Orthopaedic Surgery, Rutgers, The State University of New Jersey, New Jersey Medical School, Newark, NJ 07103, USA*
[2]*Department of Pathology and Laboratory Medicine, Rutgers, The State University of New Jersey, New Jersey Medical School, Newark, NJ 07103, USA*

Correspondence should be addressed to John S. Hwang; hwangjo@njms.rutgers.edu

Academic Editor: Narender Kumar Magu

Giant cell tumor of tendon sheath is one of the most common soft tissue tumors of the hand. These tumors typically occur in the third or fourth decade of life and present as solitary nodules on a single digit. Currently, the greatest reported number of lesions found within a single digit is five. Although uncommon, giant cell tumor of tendon sheath does occur in the pediatric population. Herein we present a report of a rare case of GCTTS in a child in which seven lesions were identified within a single digit—the greatest number of lesions within a single digit reported to date.

1. Introduction

Giant cell tumor of tendon sheath (GCTTS) is the second most common soft tissue tumor of the hand, second to ganglion cyst [1–3]. This tumor is also known as localized tenosynovial giant cell tumor. These tumors were previously described as localized nodular synovitis, fibrous xanthoma, or pigmented villonodular tenosynovitis. Furthermore, GCTTS is histologically identical to pigmented villonodular synovitis (PVNS), with the only distinction being the location of the masses; GCTTS is located within a tendon, while PVNS is an intraarticular lesion. Typically, GCTTS occurs within the ages of 30–50 and affects women twice as often as men [3].

Though uncommon, GCTTS has been seen in the pediatric population. A case series performed by Gholve et al. demonstrated that GCTTS in the pediatric population behaves similarly to the adult lesion [4]. These lesions are often solitary within a single digit, but cases have been reported in which multiple lesions were identified within a single digit. Currently, the greatest number of lesions reported in a single digit was five [5]. Herein we present a report of a rare case of GCTTS in a child where seven lesions were identified within a single digit, the most reported to date.

Informed consent was obtained from the patient's guardian for print and electronic publication.

2. Case Presentation

A 9-year-old female, right hand dominant, presented to our institution with a one-year history of left middle finger pain and palpable growing masses. The patient was first evaluated by her pediatrician. Plain radiographs were performed by her pediatrician and the report stated no significant findings. Her past medical history is significant for hypothyroidism which is being treated with levothyroxine. Magnetic resonance imaging (MRI) was performed to further evaluate the masses. The study demonstrated multiple hypodense masses and seven identifiable masses, on the volar aspect of the proximal, middle, and distal phalanx of the left middle finger (Figures 1(a) and 1(b)).

Three months after obtaining the MRI, the patient was seen in the clinic for evaluation by the orthopaedic hand service. Physical examination revealed mild swelling and tenderness throughout her left middle finger; however, no sensory deficits were noted, and brisk capillary refills were present.

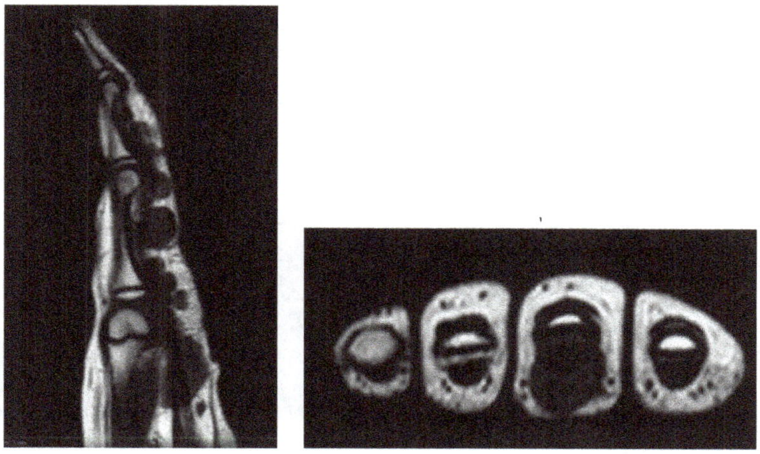

(a) (b)

FIGURE 1: (a) MRI T1 sagittal image demonstrating hypodense masses on the volar aspect of the middle finger. (b) MRI T1 axial image demonstrating hypodense masses on the volar aspect of the middle finger.

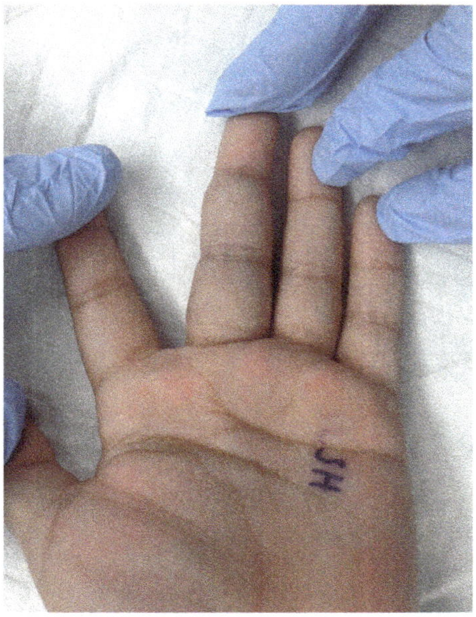

FIGURE 2: Preoperative image of left hand demonstrating fullness of the middle finger with bluish discoloration.

Three palpable small masses could be felt throughout the volar aspect of her finger. Bluish discoloration could be seen over some of these masses (Figure 2). The range of motion of her finger was significantly limited due to pain and swelling: 0–10 degrees in proximal interphalangeal joint, 0–15 degrees in distal interphalangeal joint, and 0–30 degrees in metacarpophalangeal joint. There were no enlarged lymph nodes found on physical examination. The patient denied recent weight loss, fevers, chills, fatigue, or trauma. A decision was made to perform an excisional biopsy to identify the masses through histological examination.

The patient initially underwent excisional biopsy of two of the masses that were abutting each other. Definitive diagnosis was not obtainable from the initial frozen section. The third mass was located more proximal and a decision was made to not excise this lesion until a definitive diagnosis could be made. Tissue was submitted for further histological examination. Standard sections revealed a cellular process including giant cells and mononuclear stromal cells within a collagenous matrix (Figure 3(a)). Hemosiderin deposition and clusters of xanthomatous cells were also identified (Figures 3(b) and 3(c)). These findings were consistent with GCTTS. Two months after the initial surgery, a decision was made to excise the remaining masses. Five additional lobular masses were identified intraoperatively and resected (Figures 4(a) and 4(b)). Permanent sections from the remaining masses were consistent with GCTTS and histologically analogous to the previous biopsy.

At this time, the patient is two years from her second surgery. She denies any pain and has full range of motion of her left middle finger. Her incisions are well healed and no foci of recurrence are noted at this time (Figure 5).

3. Discussion

GCTTS is a common benign soft tissue tumor found in the hand which originates in the synovium of the flexor sheath. They typically go through stages of dormancy and increased activity making these lesions suddenly symptomatic or noticeable. Although they most often occur in the hand and fingers, these tumors can also occur in larger joints like the feet, ankles, knees, and elbow. In the hand, they typically occur adjacent to the distal interphalangeal joint of the index or long finger.

With recurrence rates reported up to 45% [6], careful attention must be paid when excising these tumors. A systematic review study performed by Fotiadis et al. examined possible risk factors for recurrence [7]. They stated that poor surgical technique with incomplete excision increased the risk of recurrence. The authors found that careful dissection and excision with magnification equipment resulted in the lowest

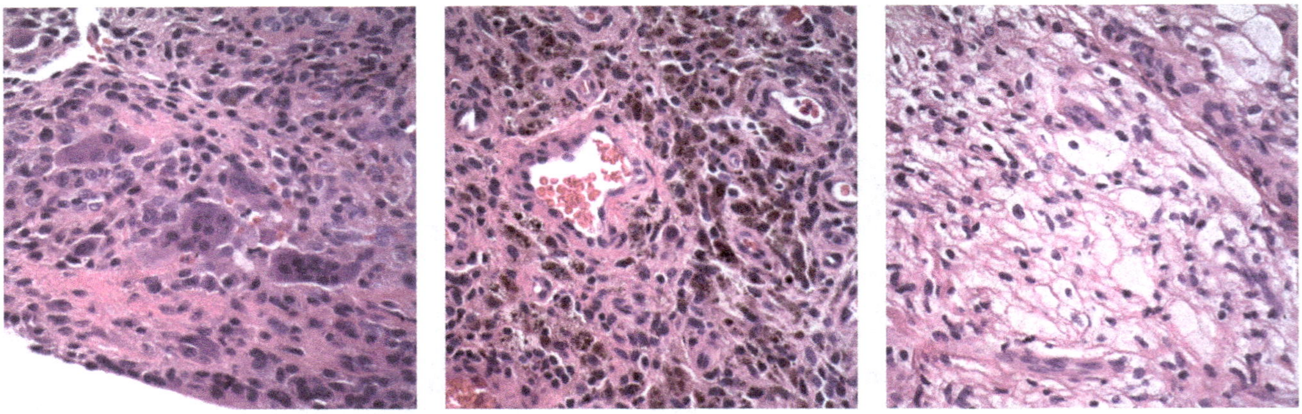

(a) (b) (c)

FIGURE 3: (a) Hematoxylin and eosin stained section demonstrating giant cells and mononuclear cells embedded within a collagenous matrix (600x). (b) Hematoxylin and eosin stained section demonstrating hemosiderin laden cells (600x). (c) Hematoxylin and eosin stained section demonstrating clusters of xanthomatous cells (600x).

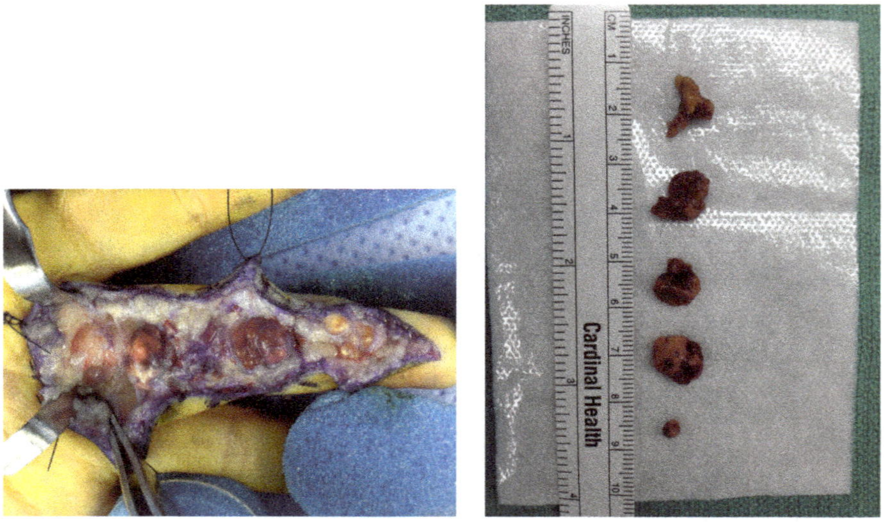

(a) (b)

FIGURE 4: (a) Intraoperative image demonstrating five masses within the flexor tendon sheath of the middle finger. (b) Gross pathology demonstrated five resected masses found within the flexor tendon sheath of the middle finger.

recurrence rate. Additional risk factors for recurrence included location at distal interphalangeal joint of finger, osseous pressure erosion, mitotic activity on histology, proximity to arthritic joint, gene nm 23, and Al-Qattan type II tumors.

In 2001, Al-Qattan described a classification system for GCTTS. The classification systems were macroscopically divided into two main types, tumor with or without a single pseudocapsule [2]. The patient in this study had seven discrete lesions within one digit. According to this study, our patient is classified as having a Type IIC tumor, which is multicentric type with separate discrete lesions in the same digit. Type II tumors, ones which are not surrounded by one pseudocapsule, were found to have a recurrence rate of 38%. In our case, our patient currently has not had a recurrence with one-year follow-up.

Our case also represents the largest number documented discrete GCTTS lesions in a single digit in current literature. Singh et al. reported a case in an adult with five lesions within a single digit [5]. That patient had complete excision of the lesion and no recurrences. In the study by Al-Qattan, one patient was found to have Type IIC classification with a history of recurrence.

In 2007, Gholve et al. published the largest case series of GCTTS in the pediatric population [4]. The researchers found the rate recurrence in their retrospective review of 29 children to be 0%. Although the mean follow-up was four years, they state that meticulous dissection with

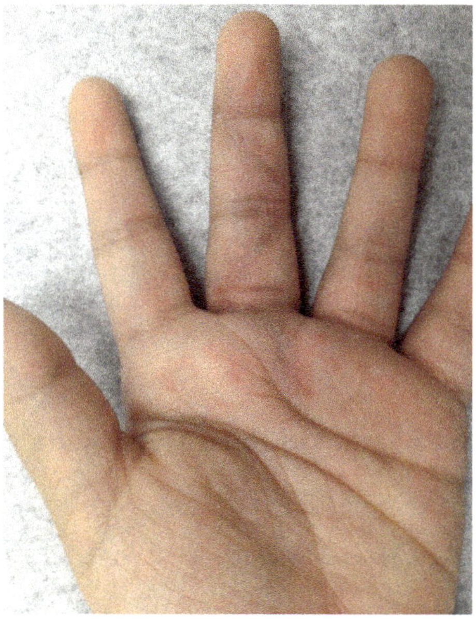

FIGURE 5: Healed incision of the left hand.

magnification equipment may assist in decreasing the rate of recurrence. Other studies have also made similar recommendations in preventing recurrences of GCTTS [1].

In conclusion, our case represents a rare case of GCTTS in a child with seven lesions found within a single digit. To our knowledge, this is the first case where more than five solitary lesions were found within a single digit. In addition, these lesions were found in a child which is even less typical. Due to the relatively high rate of recurrence found with these tumors, especially those with multiple solitary lesions, complete and meticulous resection of these tumors with magnification equipment is recommended.

Competing Interests

The authors declare that they have no competing interests.

References

[1] S. S. Suresh and H. Zaki, "Giant cell tumor of tendon sheath: case series and review of literature," *Journal of Hand and Microsurgery*, vol. 2, no. 2, pp. 67–71, 2010.

[2] M. M. Al-Qattan, "Giant cell tumours of tendon sheath: classification and recurrence rate," *Journal of Hand Surgery*, vol. 26, no. 1, pp. 72–75, 2001.

[3] D. P. Green, *Green's Operative Hand Surgery*, Elsevier/Churchill Livingstone, Philadelphia, Pa, USA, 2005.

[4] P. A. Gholve, H. S. Hosalkar, P. A. Kreiger, and J. P. Dormans, "Giant cell tumor of tendon sheath: largest single series in children," *Journal of Pediatric Orthopaedics*, vol. 27, no. 1, pp. 67–74, 2007.

[5] T. Singh, S. Noor, and A. W. Simons, "Multiple localized giant cell tumor of the tendon sheath (GCTTS) affecting a single tendon: a very rare case report and review of recent cases," *Hand Surgery*, vol. 16, no. 3, pp. 367–369, 2011.

[6] P. P. Kotwal, V. Gupta, and R. Malhotra, "Giant-cell tumour of the tendon sheath. Is radiotherapy indicated to prevent recurrence after surgery?" *The Journal of Bone & Joint Surgery—British Volume*, vol. 82, no. 4, pp. 571–573, 2000.

[7] E. Fotiadis, A. Papadopoulos, T. Svarnas, P. Akritopoulos, N. P. Sachinis, and B. E. Chalidis, "Giant cell tumour of tendon sheath of the digits. A systematic review," *Hand*, vol. 6, no. 3, pp. 244–249, 2011.

11

Unusual Presentation of Popliteal Cyst on Magnetic Resonance Imaging

Tsuyoshi Ohishi,[1] Masaaki Takahashi,[2] Daisuke Suzuki,[1] and Yukihiro Matsuyama[3]

[1]*Department of Orthopaedic Surgery, Enshu Hospital, Hamamatsu, Shizuoka 430-0929, Japan*
[2]*Joint Center, Jyuzen Memorial Hospital, Hamamatsu, Shizuoka 434-0042, Japan*
[3]*Department of Orthopaedic Surgery, Hamamatsu University School of Medicine, Hamamatsu, Shizuoka 431-3192, Japan*

Correspondence should be addressed to Tsuyoshi Ohishi; t-ohishi@ken.ja-shizuoka.or.jp

Academic Editor: Zbigniew Gugala

Popliteal cyst commonly presents as an ellipsoid mass with uniform low signal intensity on T1-weighted magnetic resonance images and high signal intensity on T2-weighted images. Here, we describe a popliteal cyst with unusual appearance on magnetic resonance imaging, including heterogeneous intermediate signal intensity on T2-weighted images. Arthroscopic cyst decompression revealed that the cyst was filled with necrotic synovial villi, indicative of rheumatoid arthritis. Arthroscopic enlargement of unidirectional valvular slits with synovectomy was useful for the final diagnosis and treatment.

1. Introduction

Popliteal cyst, or Baker's cyst, is commonly seen in patients with rheumatoid arthritis [1]. It is easily differentiated from other cystic or solid tumours according to its appearance on magnetic resonance imaging (MRI) [2]. Here, we present a case of popliteal cyst in a patient with rheumatoid arthritis that had an unusual appearance on MRI. Arthroscopic enlargement of unidirectional valvular slits was useful for the final diagnosis and treatment.

2. Case Report

A 74-year-old man was referred to our hospital with a 2-month history of a painful mass in the popliteal fossa of the right knee. The patient had undergone conservative treatment for a diagnosis of osteoarthritis of the right knee for the previous 4 months at a nearby clinic. The patient was 158 cm tall and weighed 58 kg and demonstrated a limp due to right knee pain. He had emphysema and carcinoma of the stomach, both of which were well controlled.

On physical examination of the right knee, an elastic soft mass measuring 5 cm × 3 cm with a smooth surface was palpable in the popliteal fossa. The mass was tender on palpation without redness or warmth. Range of motion was −10° of extension and 120° of flexion due to contracture. Tenderness was elicited on the medial joint line. McMurray's test was positive with pain on the medial joint line, but a clicking sound was not elicited. Patellar ballottement also was positive. No anteroposterior or lateral instability was observed. Laboratory data revealed a C-reactive protein level of 1.26 mg/dL and a haemoglobin level of 12.9 mg/dL but were otherwise within normal range. Blood examinations pertaining to rheumatoid arthritis were not performed at the initial visit. Plain radiographs of the right knee showed grade 2 medial compartment osteoarthritis. MRI revealed a well-defined popliteal mass with low signal intensity on T1-weighted images and heterogeneous intermediate signal intensity on T2-weighted images (Figures 1(a) and 1(b)). The cyst connected to the subgastrocnemius bursa through a path between the medial head of the gastrocnemius muscle and the semimembranosus tendon (Figure 1(c)). The provisional diagnosis was popliteal cyst with some solid contents inside the cyst in an osteoarthritic knee.

Arthroscopic surgery under general anaesthesia was performed. Synovial proliferation was observed in the suprapatellar pouch and gutters of both sides, which were excised. To access the popliteal cyst, a transseptal portal was made after creating posteromedial and posterolateral portals using

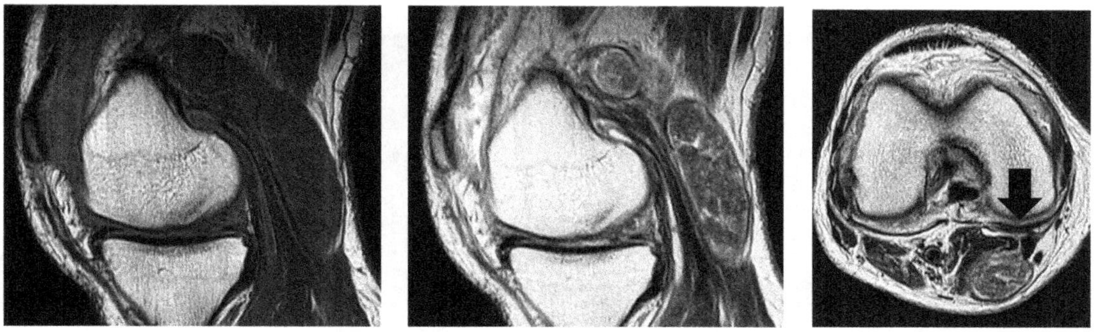

(a) (b) (c)

FIGURE 1: Preoperative sagittal T1-weighted (a) and T2-weighted (b) and axial T2-weighted (c) magnetic resonance images. A cyst was detected with low signal intensity on T1-weighted images and heterogeneous intermediate signal intensity on T2-weighted images. A connecting path was seen between the cyst and the subgastrocnemius bursa (arrow), compatible with the characteristics of popliteal cyst.

our technique [3]. Synovial proliferation also was observed in the posteromedial and posterolateral compartments. Arthroscopic cyst decompression was performed using our procedure [4]. First, the synovial fold was identified (Figure 2(a)) and removed using a motorized shaver from the posteromedial portal while viewing from the posterolateral portal via the transseptal portal. A vertical slit between the medial head of the gastrocnemius muscle and the semimembranosus tendon was identified (Figure 2(b)) and enlarged by destructing the unidirectional valvular slit (Figure 2(c)). Once the orifice of the cyst was enlarged, abundant yellowish synovia-like fragments were pushed out manually from behind until the popliteal mass was not palpable on the back (Figure 2(d)). Pathologic examination revealed that the synovial villi in the suprapatellar pouch were thickened with inflammatory cells, blood vessels, and fibrinoid-degenerated connective tissue, compatible with rheumatoid arthritis. The material inside the cyst included fragments of necrotic synovial villi with fibrinoid degeneration (Figure 3).

Range of motion of the right knee and weight-bearing gait were allowed from 2 days postoperatively. Postoperative blood examinations revealed positive results for rheumatoid factor and an anticyclic citrullinated peptide antibody level of 78.1 U/mL. The final diagnosis was popliteal cyst filled with necrotic synovia accompanied by rheumatoid arthritis. No swelling, deformity, or tenderness was found in other joints, including the contralateral knee, fingers, elbows, or shoulders. Administration of methotrexate 6 mg/week was started after surgery. MRI performed 1 year postoperatively showed no evidence of the popliteal cyst (Figure 4). At 2 years postoperatively, recurrence of the cyst was not observed and the patient had no difficulty in performing activities of daily living.

3. Discussion

Popliteal cyst, or Baker's cyst, is caused by a one-way valvular mechanism of the slits between the medial head of the gastrocnemius muscle and the semimembranosus muscle [5]. On MRI, popliteal cyst commonly presents as an ellipsoid mass with uniform low signal intensity on T1-weighted images and high signal intensity on T2-weighted images [2]. The connection between the cyst and the subgastrocnemius bursa also can be detected on axial MRI. In our case, the ellipsoid shape with connection between the cyst and the subgastrocnemius bursa was compatible with popliteal cyst, but the signal intensities inside the cyst were unusual. The popliteal cyst in this case showed low signal intensity on T1-weighted images and heterogeneous intermediate signal intensity on T2-weighted images. Thus far, pigmented villonodular synovitis, hematoma, and infection have been reported in cases of popliteal cyst with unusual appearance on MRI [6, 7]. Unless the connection between the cyst and the subgastrocnemius bursa can be identified on MRI, malignant tumour, aneurysm, or benign solid tumour should be considered [8]. In all previous cases with unusual signal intensities inside the popliteal cyst, open resection was performed for diagnosis and treatment [6, 7]. The unusual presentation of the popliteal cyst on preoperative MRI was due to necrotic synovial villi inside the cyst. A one-way valvular mechanism between the cyst and the joint could have been responsible for the accumulation and concentration of synovial villi in the cyst, with proliferation in the joint due to rheumatoid arthritis.

In addition to rheumatoid arthritis, popliteal cysts can be caused by many other underlying pathologies [9]. Anatomically, a popliteal cyst can be divided into two categories. Primary cysts have no communication between joint and cyst and are predominantly found in children without joint disorders. In contrast, secondary cysts have a communication between joint and cyst through a one-way valve mechanism and are mostly observed in adolescents [10]. The majority of popliteal cysts are classified as secondary cysts. All pathologies that cause joint effusion may also cause a secondary popliteal cyst. Meniscal tears, ligament insufficiency, cartilage lesions, osteoarthritis, infectious arthritis, villonodular synovitis, and rheumatoid arthritis can cause a popliteal cyst [9]. Among these, rheumatoid arthritis is a well-known cause of popliteal cysts, since inflammation and synovial proliferation can destroy the unidirectional valve mechanism between the medial head of the gastrocnemius muscle and semimembranosus muscle [11].

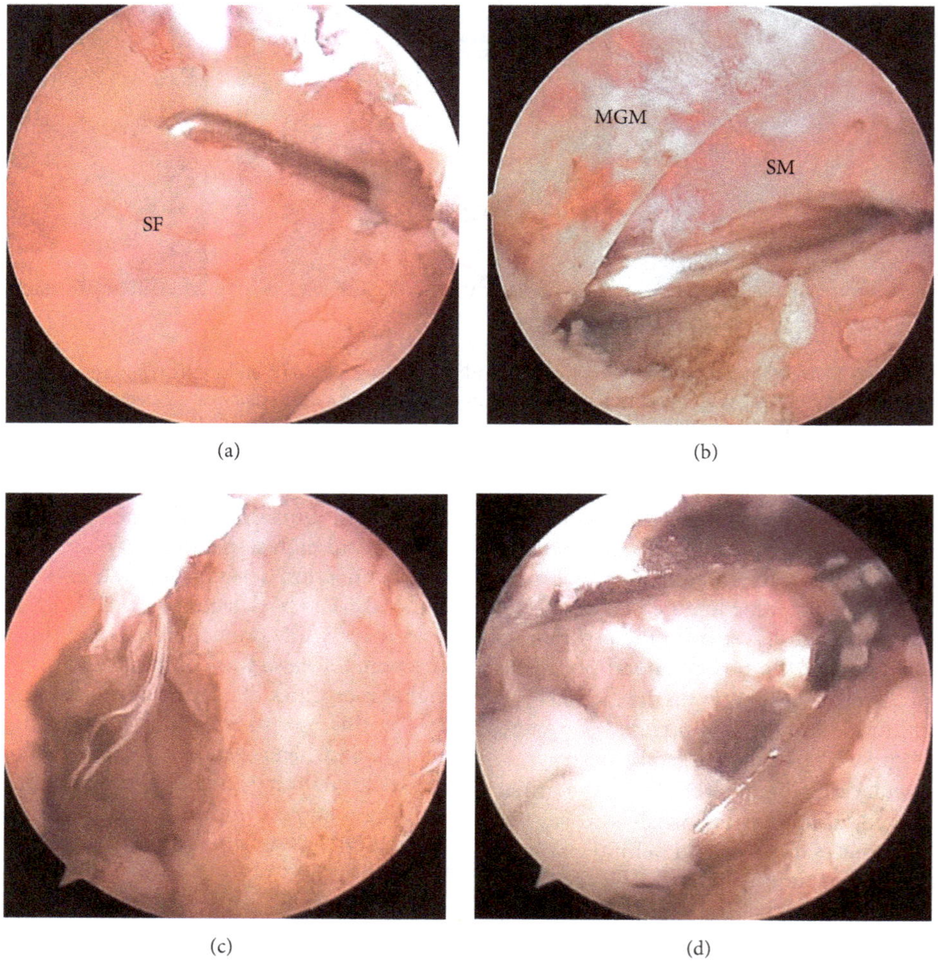

FIGURE 2: Arthroscopic views from the posterolateral portal through the transseptal portal. (a) The synovial fold (SF) was identified using a probe introduced from the posteromedial portal. (b) After removing the synovial fold, a switching rod was inserted between the medial head of the gastrocnemius muscle (MGM) and the semimembranosus muscle (SM), which was the orifice of the popliteal cyst. (c) The orifice of the popliteal cyst was enlarged by resecting the limited parts of the medial head of the gastrocnemius muscle and the semimembranosus muscle. (d) The material inside the cyst was pushed out from behind and removed using forceps.

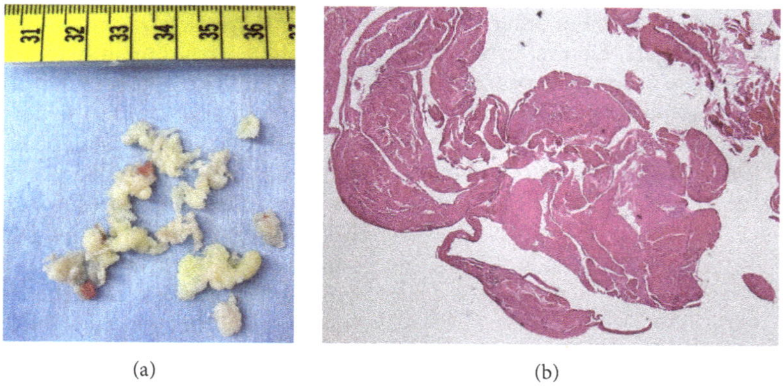

FIGURE 3: Photographs of gross (a) and histologic (magnification ×40) (b) findings of the material inside the cyst. Fragments of necrotic synovial villi with fibrinoid degeneration are observed.

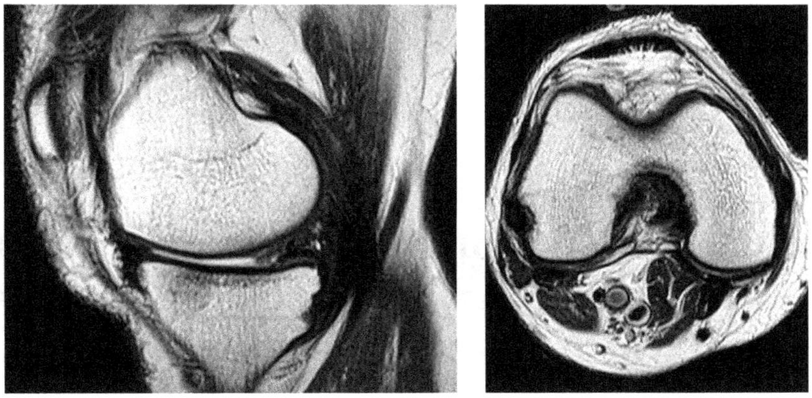

(a) (b)

FIGURE 4: T2-weighted sagittal (a) and axial (b) magnetic resonance images taken 1 year postoperatively. No evidence of the popliteal cyst is observed.

Conservative therapy including antirheumatic drugs is the first choice of treatment for popliteal cyst with rheumatoid arthritis. However, we could not diagnose this patient with rheumatoid arthritis preoperatively. According to previous reports, open excision of popliteal cyst results in a high rate of recurrence [12]. Arthroscopic enlargement of the unidirectional valvular slit with or without cystectomy, which recently has become widely accepted, is less invasive and has a low rate of recurrence [4, 13]. In this case, arthroscopic surgery followed by administration of antirheumatic drugs was effective for the final diagnosis and treatment.

Competing Interests

The authors confirm that there are no known competing interests associated with this publication, and no significant financial support was provided for this work that could have influenced the outcome.

References

[1] H. W. Meyerding and R. E. van Demark, "Posterior hernia of the knee (Baker's cyst, popliteal cyst, semimembranosus bursitis, medial gastrocnemius bursitis and popliteal bursitis)," *The Journal of the American Medical Association*, vol. 122, no. 13, pp. 858–861, 1943.

[2] G. Hermann, I. F. Abdelwahab, T. T. Miller, M. J. Klein, and M. M. Lewis, "Tumour and tumour-like conditions of the soft tissue: magnetic resonance imaging features differentiating benign from malignant masses," *British Journal of Radiology*, vol. 65, no. 769, pp. 14–20, 1992.

[3] T. Ohishi, E. Torikai, D. Suzuki, T. Banno, and Y. Honda, "Arthroscopic treatment of a medial meniscal cyst using a posterior trans-septal approach: a case report," *Sports Medicine, Arthroscopy, Rehabilitation, Therapy & Technology*, vol. 2, no. 1, article 25, 2010.

[4] T. Ohishi, M. Takahashi, D. Suzuki et al., "Treatment of popliteal cysts via arthroscopic enlargement of unidirectional valvular slits," *Modern Rheumatology*, vol. 25, no. 5, pp. 772–778, 2015.

[5] W. Rauschning and P. G. Lindgren, "The clinical significance of the valve mechanism in communicating popliteal cysts," *Archives of Orthopaedic and Traumatic Surgery*, vol. 95, no. 4, pp. 251–256, 1979.

[6] H. Tatari, O. Baran, B. Lebe, S. Kiliç, M. Manisali, and H. Havitçioglu, "Pigmented villonodular synovitis of the knee presenting as a popliteal cyst," *Arthroscopy*, vol. 16, no. 6, p. 13, 2000.

[7] M. J. Yoo, J. S. Yoo, H. S. Jang, and C. H. Hwang, "Baker's cyst filled with hematoma at the lower calf," *Knee Surgery & Related Research*, vol. 26, no. 4, pp. 253–256, 2014.

[8] M. G. Butler, K. D. Fuchigami, and A. Chako, "MRI of posterior knee masses," *Skeletal Radiology*, vol. 25, no. 4, pp. 309–317, 1996.

[9] D. Fritschy, J. Fasel, J.-C. Imbert, S. Bianchi, R. Verdonk, and C. J. Wirth, "The popliteal cyst," *Knee Surgery, Sports Traumatology, Arthroscopy*, vol. 14, no. 7, pp. 623–628, 2006.

[10] D. Stein, M. Cantlon, B. MacKay, and C. Hoelscher, "Cysts about the knee: evaluation and management," *Journal of the American Academy of Orthopaedic Surgeons*, vol. 21, no. 8, pp. 469–479, 2013.

[11] I. M. Pinder, "Treatment of the popliteal cyst in the rheumatoid knee," *The Journal of Bone & Joint Surgery—British Volume*, vol. 55, no. 1, pp. 119–125, 1973.

[12] W. Rauschning and P. G. Lindgren, "Popliteal cysts (Baker's cysts) in adults. I. Clinical and roentgenological results of operative excision," *Acta Orthopaedica Scandinavica*, vol. 50, no. 5, pp. 583–591, 1979.

[13] J. H. Ahn, S. H. Lee, J. C. Yoo, M. J. Chang, and Y. S. Park, "Arthroscopic treatment of popliteal cysts: clinical and magnetic resonance imaging results," *Arthroscopy*, vol. 26, no. 10, pp. 1340–1347, 2010.

12

Fabella Syndrome as an Uncommon Cause of Posterolateral Knee Pain after Total Knee Arthroplasty: A Case Report and Review of the Literature

Eriko Okano,[1] Tomokazu Yoshioka,[1,2] Takaji Yanai,[3] Sho Kohyama,[3] Akihiro Kanamori,[1] Masashi Yamazaki,[1] and Toshikazu Tanaka[3]

[1]*Department of Orthopedic Surgery, Faculty of Medicine, University of Tsukuba, 1-1-1 Tennodai, Tsukuba, Ibaraki 305-8575, Japan*
[2]*Division of Regenerative Medicine for Musculoskeletal System, Faculty of Medicine, University of Tsukuba, 1-1-1 Tennodai, Tsukuba, Ibaraki 305-8575, Japan*
[3]*Department of Orthopaedic Surgery, Kikkoman General Hospital, 100 Miyazaki, Noda, Chiba 278-0005, Japan*

Correspondence should be addressed to Tomokazu Yoshioka; yoshioka@md.tsukuba.ac.jp

Academic Editor: Werner Kolb

The fabella is a sesamoid bone that is located in the lateral head of the gastrocnemius muscle and has been identified on magnetic resonance imaging in 31% of Japanese people. In the present case, a 65-year-old woman experienced posterolateral knee pain, accompanied by a clicking "sound" during active knee flexion, after undergoing total knee arthroplasty for knee osteoarthritis. Eight months of conservative therapy failed to produce an improvement, with progressive osteoarthritic change of the fabella identified on plain radiography. Based on this evidence, a diagnosis of fabella syndrome was made and the patient underwent a fabellectomy. Fabellectomy provided immediate resolution of posterolateral knee pain and the clicking sound with knee flexion, with the patient remaining symptom-free 18 months after fabellectomy and with no limitations in knee function. Fabellectomy eliminated symptoms in all of five case reports that have been previously published and is regarded as an effective first choice for treating fabella syndrome after total knee arthroplasty.

1. Introduction

Pain after total knee arthroplasty (TKA) can result from multiple factors [1, 2]. Fabella syndrome has been identified as an uncommon, but relevant, cause of pain post-TKA due to mechanical irritation of the posterolateral tissues of the knee. The symptoms of fabella syndrome are posterolateral pain and a catching sensation (or clicking sound) with knee flexion [3, 4]. We report the case of a patient presenting with fabella syndrome after routine TKA and include a brief review of literature.

2. Case Report

A 66-year-old woman was referred to our specialty clinic for assessment of persistent right knee pain, 8 months after undergoing a TKA for knee osteoarthritis. The patient had undergone right cemented TKA, using a LEGION cruciate-retaining total knee system (Smith & Nephew, Memphis, TN, USA), without patella resurfacing. Range of motion, standing, and walking exercises under full weight bearing were started from the first postoperative day. The pain in her right knee developed one week after her TKA and was localized to the popliteal fossa and was associated with catching/clicking with active knee flexion. The patient had undergone successful left TKA at age of 58, and her medical history was otherwise unremarkable. The patient reported her main occupation as being a housewife.

The physical assessment at the first visit identified the following. Upon visual examination, no redness or swelling was observed, and scarring of the surgical incision, along the midline of the patella, was confirmed. On palpation, no heat or hydrarthrosis was identified. However, deep palpation between the iliotibial tract, on the proximal head of the fibula,

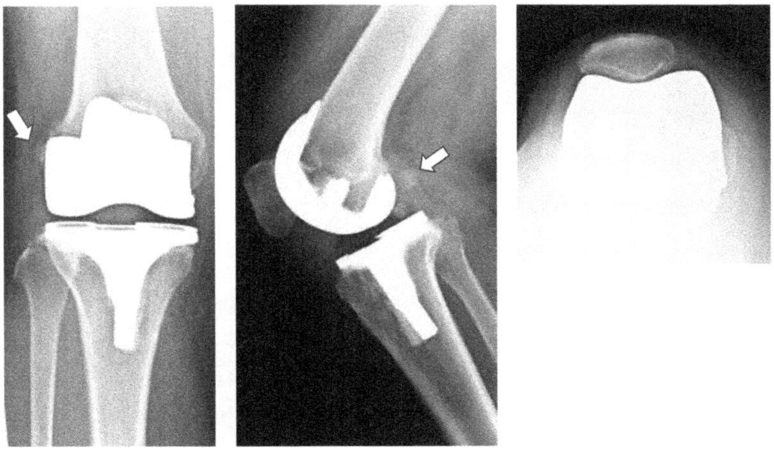

FIGURE 1: Plain radiographs on first visit; the white arrow identifies the fabella.

and the biceps femoris elicited mild tenderness. A snapping was palpated over the same region during active knee flexion, in the range of 80°–90°, accompanied by pain, identified at an intensity of 91 mm on a 100 mm visual analogue scale (VAS). The snapping was not reproducible on passive knee extension and flexion. Total range of motion of the right knee was 10°–120°, with no obvious instability. Neurological examination and blood work were unremarkable. The Japanese Orthopedic Association (JOA) score was administered. The JOA is as a patient-derived knee scoring system to evaluate physical impairment and disability in patients with knee osteoarthritis that is commonly used in Japanese clinical practice. The JOA score evaluates four domains: pain on walking, pain on ascending or descending stairs, range of motion, and joint effusion [5]. The patient reported a total JOA score of 65, with the following domain-specific scores: pain on walking, 25; pain on ascending or descending stairs, 5; range of motion, 25; and joint effusion, 10. Plain radiographs of the right knee were obtained on the first visit (Figure 1). While standing, the femorotibial angle (FTA) was 174°, and the femoral and tibial component angles were within the normal range: 97° for α angle; 88° for β angle; 6° for γ angle; and 89° for δ angle [6]. The posterior condyle offset was 29 mm, with a 1° tibial posterior declining angle [7]. A fabella was identified at the posterior femoral condyle, 11 mm along the major axis of the fabella (Figure 1). Comparison of plain radiographs of the right knee joint at several points in time confirmed presence of a fabella prior to surgery and progressive osteoarthrosis, with osteophyte formation, over the posterior femoral condyle over the 5- to 7-month post-TKA period (Figure 2).

Review of computed tomography (CT) images obtained at 7 months post-TKA (Figure 3) identified a fabella, 11 × 10 mm in size, over the posterior femoral condyle. The femoral component was fixed in 2° of internal rotation, with respect to the clinical epicondylar axis, and the anterior-posterior axis of the tibial component was aligned with the medial edge of the tibial tuberosity and the PCL attachment. Therefore, there were no abnormal findings in the position of the femoral or tibial components.

Considering that (1) the symptom started one week after TKA surgery, (2) the pain was localized in the posterolateral aspect of the knee, and (3) the pain and snapping were caused by active knee flexion, fabella syndrome was identified as the primary diagnosis. The following were considered as differential diagnoses: (1) impairment associated with remaining cement or resected bone fragments; (2) soft tissue impingement; and (3) popliteal tendinitis.

Based on our information, we determined excision of the fabella (fabellectomy), through a separate posterolateral incision, to be the treatment of choice. We first performed an arthroscopic examination to diagnostically rule out the potential differential diagnoses. Arthroscopic examination confirmed absence of damage or abrasion to the polyethylene components, with unremarkable findings on visualization of the remaining cement or bone fragments, the popliteal tendon and posterior cruciate ligament, and absence of soft tissue impingement. The extirpation of the fabella was performed using a posterolateral approach between the iliotibial tract and the biceps femoris, confirming the presence of snapping between the femoral component and fabella during knee flexion. The size of the fabella was 20 mm along the major axis, with osteophyte and deformation of the articular cartilage confirmed (Figure 4).

Subjective symptoms resolved immediately after the surgery, and, at 1 month after surgery, range of motion was 0°–120° and the VAS score improved to 10 mm. At 18 months after the surgery, the JOA score had improved to a total score of 85: pain on walking, 30; pain on ascending or descending stairs, 20; range of motion, 25; and joint effusion, 10. There was no recurrence of snapping or pain over the posterolateral aspect of the knee.

3. Discussion

Sources of knee pain after TKA can be divided into 4 categories: originating from mechanical or biological factors, with location of the lesion either inside or outside of the knee joint [2]. We based our primary diagnosis of fabella syndrome on the following information: radiographs confirming

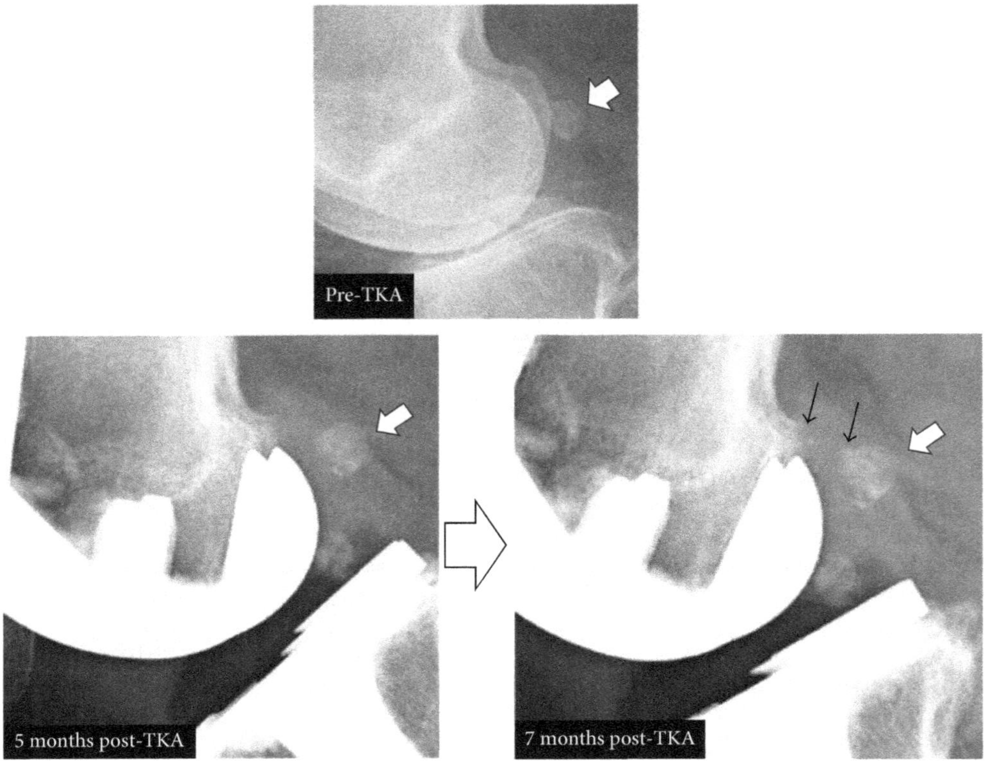

FIGURE 2: Plain, lateral view radiographs of the knee at several time points; the white arrow identifies the fabella and the black arrow onset and progression of osteoarthrosis.

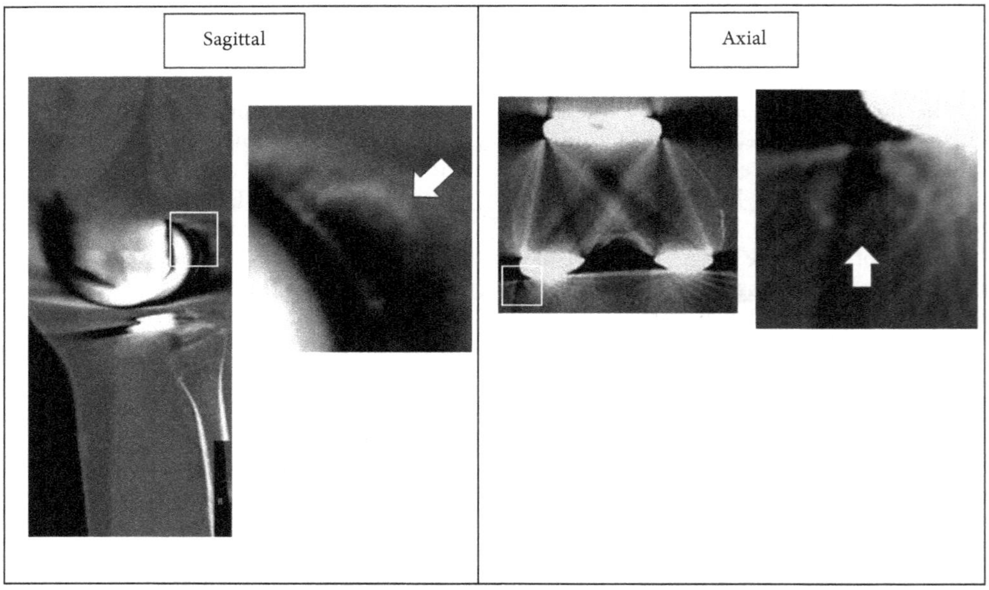

FIGURE 3: Position of the femoral component and the fabella; the white arrow identifies the fabella.

absence of abnormalities in the positioning of the artificial components; appearance of symptoms 1 week post-TKA; pain localized to the posterolateral area of the knee, specific to the location of the fabella; and a chief complaint of snapping and pain with active knee flexion, which is specific of fabella syndrome.

A summary of the causes and presentation of fabella symptom identified in our review of the literature is provided in Table 1. The major symptoms of fabella syndrome are pain due to a mechanical irritation of local soft tissues during knee extension, causing tension, by pressure from the fabella, on the lateral femoral condyle, regardless of the history of knee

Table 1: Previous reports on fabella syndrome after TKA.

Previous report (published year)	Age/sex M: male F: female	Onset time after TKA	Symptoms	Movement that causes symptoms	Etiology	Treatment
Jaffe et al. 1988 [3]	63 F	6 days	Pain located in the posterolateral part of the knee & snapping & clicking	Knee flexion at 90°	The posterior edge of the polyethylene component	Fabellectomy
Laird 1991 [9]	68 M	3 months	Pain behind the knee & hard lump	During knee flexion & extension	Posterior condyle of the prosthesis	Fabellectomy
Larson and Becker 1993 [10]	67 F	3 months	Pain localized to the posterolateral aspect of the knee & catching	During knee motion	Moderate mediolateral laxity & polyethylene insert	Changed to a thicker polyethylene & fabellectomy
Erichsen 1997 [11]	64 F	1 year	Pain in the lateral part of popliteal fossa & clicking	When the knee was extended from full flexion	The edge of the femoral component	Fabellectomy
Segal et al. 2004 [12]	53 F	8 weeks	Pain at the posterolateral aspect of the popliteal fossa & crepitus	Knee flexion & extension	Lateral edge of the prosthetic femoral condyle	Fabellectomy
Present study	66 F	1 week	Posterolateral knee pain & snapping	Active knee flexion at 80–90°	Lateral edge of the femoral component and femoral condyle	Fabellectomy

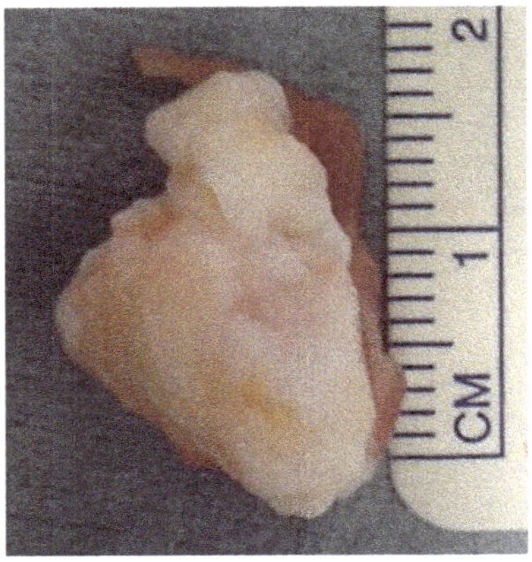

FIGURE 4: Gross pathology of the excised fabella, confirming significant osteoarthrosis.

surgery [4, 8]. There are five case reports of fabella syndrome that have been documented post-TKA [3, 9–12]. The average age of the patients presenting with fabella syndrome, 1 man and 5 women, was 63, and the time to onset of symptoms after surgery varied between 6 days and 1 year, with an early postoperative occurrence being more common. The major symptoms resulted from mechanical irritation and stress symptoms, such as pain, catching, clicking, and crepitus, in the posterolateral region of the knee with active knee flexion and extension. Two mechanical causes have been reported in the literature, 2 cases resulting from "catching" of the fabella on the polyethylene insert [3, 10], and 3 cases resulting from the fabella being pressed onto the lateral femoral condyle [9, 11, 12]. With regard to fabella syndrome appearing after TKA, the following characteristics have been reported: (1) size of the fabella was ≥1.0 cm along its major axis [3], (2) anatomically exceptional fabella in the lateral head of the gastrocnemius, (3) abnormal placement or mismatch of prosthetic components resulting in impingement of the fabella, and (4) ligament instability possibly caused by an unbalanced distribution of soft tissue [12]. Fabellectomy was the treatment of choice in all reported cases, with immediate resolution of symptoms. Therefore, we believe fabellectomy should be the first choice of treatment in the absence of abnormal positioning and/or size of the TKA components.

In conclusion, we reported the case of one patient presenting with fabella syndrome after TKA. Fabella syndrome should be included as one of the differential diagnoses of post-TKA knee pain, with fabellectomy providing an optimal treatment option.

Ethical Approval

The study was carried out in accordance with the Declaration of Helsinki and within the appropriate ethical framework.

Consent

Written informed consent was obtained from the patient for publication of this case report and any accompanying images.

Competing Interests

The authors declare that they have no competing interests.

Acknowledgments

The authors would like to thank Editage (http://www.editage.jp/) for English language editing.

References

[1] S. Hofmann, G. Seitlinger, O. Djahani, and M. Pietsch, "The painful knee after TKA: a diagnostic algorithm for failure analysis," *Knee Surgery, Sports Traumatology, Arthroscopy*, vol. 19, no. 9, pp. 1442–1452, 2011.

[2] R. Seil and D. Pape, "Causes of failure and etiology of painful primary total knee arthroplasty," *Knee Surgery, Sports Traumatology, Arthroscopy*, vol. 19, no. 9, pp. 1418–1432, 2011.

[3] F. F. Jaffe, S. Kuschner, and M. Klein, "Fabellar impingement: a cause of pain after total knee replacement. A case report," *The Journal of Bone and Joint Surgery—American Volume*, vol. 70, no. 4, pp. 613–616, 1988.

[4] A. Driessen, M. Balke, C. Offerhaus et al., "The fabella syndrome-a rare cause of posterolateral knee pain: a review of the literature and two case reports," *BMC Musculoskeletal Disorders*, vol. 15, no. 1, article 100, 2014.

[5] M. Okuda, S. Omokawa, K. Okahashi, M. Akahane, and Y. Tanaka, "Validity and reliability of the Japanese Orthopaedic Association score for osteoarthritic knees," *Journal of Orthopaedic Science*, vol. 17, no. 6, pp. 750–756, 2012.

[6] F. C. Ewald, "The Knee Society total knee arthroplasty roentgenographic evaluation and scoring system," *Clinical Orthopaedics and Related Research*, no. 248, pp. 9–12, 1989.

[7] P. Massin and A. Gournay, "Optimization of the posterior condylar offset, tibial slope, and condylar roll-back in total knee arthroplasty," *Journal of Arthroplasty*, vol. 21, no. 6, pp. 889–896, 2006.

[8] S. Ehara, "Potentially symptomatic fabella: MR imaging review," *Japanese Journal of Radiology*, vol. 32, no. 1, pp. 1–5, 2014.

[9] L. Laird, "Fabellar joint causing pain after total knee replacement," *The Journal of Bone & Joint Surgery*, vol. 73, no. 6, pp. 1007–1008, 1991.

[10] J. E. Larson and D. A. Becker, "Fabellar impingement in total knee arthroplasty. a case report," *Journal of Arthroplasty*, vol. 8, no. 1, pp. 95–97, 1993.

[11] H. Erichsen, "Bilateral fabellar impingement after knee replacement—a case report," *Acta Orthopaedica Scandinavica*, vol. 68, no. 4, p. 403, 1997.

[12] A. Segal, T. T. Miller, and E. S. Krauss, "Fabellar snapping as a cause of knee pain after total knee replacement: assessment using dynamic sonography," *American Journal of Roentgenology*, vol. 183, no. 2, pp. 352–354, 2004.

13

Sacral Emphysematous Osteomyelitis Caused by *Escherichia coli* after Arthroscopy of the Knee

Mirko Velickovic and Thomas Hockertz

Department of Orthopedic Surgery and Traumatology, Städtisches Klinikum Wolfenbüttel, Alter Weg 80, 38302 Wolfenbüttel, Germany

Correspondence should be addressed to Mirko Velickovic; mirko.velickovic@klinikum-wolfenbuettel.de

Academic Editor: Nikolaos K. Kanakaris

Emphysematous osteomyelitis is a rare but serious condition which is often associated with a fatal outcome. The typical appearances of emphysematous osteomyelitis are clusters of small gas bubbles within the medullary cavity. We report a case of a 62-year-old male who presented with emphysematous osteomyelitis due to hematogenous spread of *Escherichia coli* from the knee after arthroscopy.

1. Case Report

A 62-year-old man presented to our emergency center with severe lower back pain. His complaint started a month ago and the pain in the lower spine was now increasing. Oral painkillers did not produce significant pain relief. The patient denied any history of trauma. On admission to hospital, the patient suffered from lower back pain radiating to the left buttock but not to the leg. There was no numbness or any neurologic deficit. The rest of the physical examination was without any pathologic findings. The patient was febrile (38.4°), blood pressure was 142/88 mmHg, heart rate was 103/minute, and SaO_2 was 98%. Routine laboratory investigations revealed raised CRP 132,7 mg/L, and the leukocytes were normal. Glucose blood levels were slightly raised up to 206 mg/dL. Lumbar spine radiographs showed degenerative changes but no fracture (Figure 1). The medical history revealed that the patient had an arthroscopy of the right knee two months ago with total synovectomy, chondroshaving, and partial meniscectomy of the medial meniscus as well as lateral release. The physical examination of the knee was unspecific except for slight effusion in the knee with very few symptoms. There was no redness, swelling, atrophy, or any deformity. The scars were healed. The patient walked normally without any limping and with no gait disturbances. There was no need for imaging the knee in the emergency center. The patient was admitted to the ward. Control laboratory examination on the next day showed a marked increase of CRP 164,7 (mg/L—Normal < 5 mg/L) as well as leukocytes ($16,2 \times 10^3/\mu L$—Normal 4–11 $\times 10^3/\mu L$). Procalcitonin was however markedly increased (1,70 ng/mL—Normal 0,05–0,5 ng/mL), and HBA1C was normal. We started an antibiotic treatment with Amoxiclav (Amoxicillin and Clavulanic Acid) intravenously. The first blood cultures (aerobe and anaerobe) verified the presence of a multisensible *Escherichia coli* strain. Transthoracic and transesophageal echocardiography excluded endocarditis. A sonography of the abdomen was inconspicuous.

Stool analysis excluded the presence of pathologic germs. Due to the strong pain in the lower back, we assumed spondylodiscitis but this was excluded by MRI. But the MRI demonstrated the presence of osteomyelitis of the massa lateralis of the sacrum (Figure 2). The additional CT scan of the abdomen and pelvis showed edema of the iliacus and lumbricales muscles of the left side as well as splenomegaly and nephritis and multiple free air bubbles in the massa lateralis of the sacrum (Figure 3). In the follow-up CT scan of the pelvis 12 days later, there was no free air any more detectible but there was an abscess formation around the piriformis muscle and beginning osteomyelitis of the ilium bone (Figure 4). There were also no more signs of nephritis detectible. Surgery was strongly recommended but the patient refused any kind of surgical interventions including open surgical debridement of the sacrum as well as

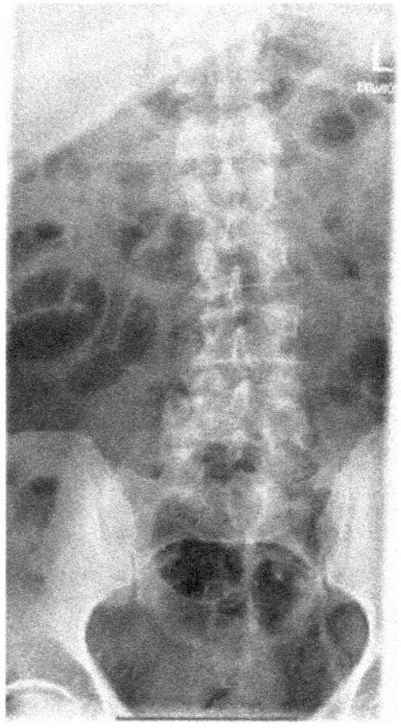

FIGURE 1: Lumbar spine radiographs on admission showed degenerative changes.

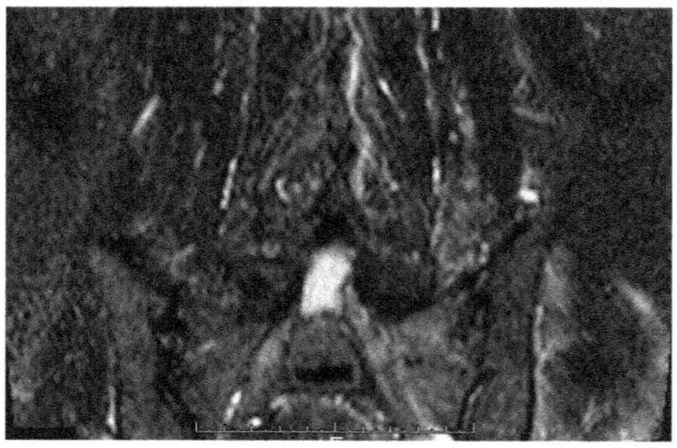

FIGURE 2: MRI with osteomyelitis of the sacrum as well as free air bubbles in the sacrum.

drainage of the abscess by interventional radiologic methods such as percutaneous catheterization. We continued the high dose antibiotic treatment and performed regular laboratory examinations. The patient clinically improved, and the symptoms markedly declined. There was no fever any more. On discharge after 31 days in hospital, leucocytes were normal and CRP was 17,3 mg/L. There were 4 follow-up examinations in our outpatient clinic in 2 months. As part of the control, we performed a CT scan and an MRI of the pelvis one month after discharge from hospital which showed marked osteolytic destruction of the massa lateralis of the sacrum but there was a decline of the abscess formation along the piriformis muscle (Figures 5(a) and 5(b)). In one of the outpatient follow-up examinations, the patient complained of pain and gait disturbances in the knee so an MRI of the knee was done. This demonstrated extensive effusion of the knee with contrast accumulation compatible with a synovitis as a sign of the inflammatory changes and zones of subchondral edema at the medial tibia and the medial femur (Figure 6). The patient again refused any surgical intervention and did not apply for follow-up examinations. In total, Amoxiclav (Amoxicillin and Clavulanic Acid) was administered intravenously for 3 weeks and orally for 9 weeks.

2. X-Rays

See Figures 1, 2, 3, 4, 5, and 6.

3. Discussion

Emphysematous osteomyelitis is a rare but serious condition and may result in a fatal outcome. It was first described by Ram and colleagues in 1981 [1]. There are less than 30 cases of emphysematous osteomyelitis reported in English literature. Most cases are associated with immunosuppression due to diabetes mellitus or malignancies [2–4]. However, our patient was negatively tested to have diabetes mellitus. A malignancy was not known previously and there were no signs of malignancy in the CT or MRI imaging so we considered a malignancy as the origin to be unlikely. Nevertheless, additional diagnostic procedures such as oncologic examinations or colonoscopy can be useful especially in cases of a positive family history for malignancies. Blood cultures revealed the presence of *Escherichia coli* which was treated according to the resistogram. Most cases of emphysematous osteomyelitis are monomicrobial and are caused either by an anaerobe or as in our case by a member of the Enterobacteriaceae family although causative organisms include the whole spectrum of aerobic and anaerobic bacteria. Monomicrobial infections are most commonly due to hematogenous spread and polymicrobial infections due to contiguous spread. Nearly every bone can be affected but most cases occur in the vertebrae, sacrum, and lower extremities [2].

We cannot prove that the development of the osteomyelitis of the sacrum was unequivocally based on the arthroscopy of the knee, but we consider hematogenous spread from the knee to be very likely. Another source for the infection could not be found. Cases of spontaneous of emphysematous osteomyelitis are described in literature but in our case the patient underwent surgery of the knee and complained about constant symptoms with slight pain during the in-patient stay. Although the physical examination of the knee was still unremarkable, the MRI of the knee demonstrated signs of inflammatory changes with marked effusion, synovitis, and subchondral edema at the medial tibia and the medial femur. The presence of intraosseous gas is not always pathologic. Degenerative joint diseases as well as vacuum phenomena, ischemic necrosis, malignancies, and cysts may lead to accumulation of gas. However, intraosseous gas together with systematic symptoms such as fever has to be considered as a serious condition and may be caused by gas-forming organisms. Emphysematous osteomyelitis is associated with high mortality (32%); therefore, immediate diagnosis and treatment are crucial for the outcome. Ordinary X-rays showed intraosseous gas so we performed a CT scan not only to confirm the X-ray findings but also to show the extent and exact location of the gas formation. To reveal the presence of an additional abscess or soft tissue process, an MRI is recommended. In most cases, early surgical treatment is essential. In our case, surgery was recommended but the patient refused any surgical intervention. Due to extensive antibiotic therapy, the patient survived. On discharge, there

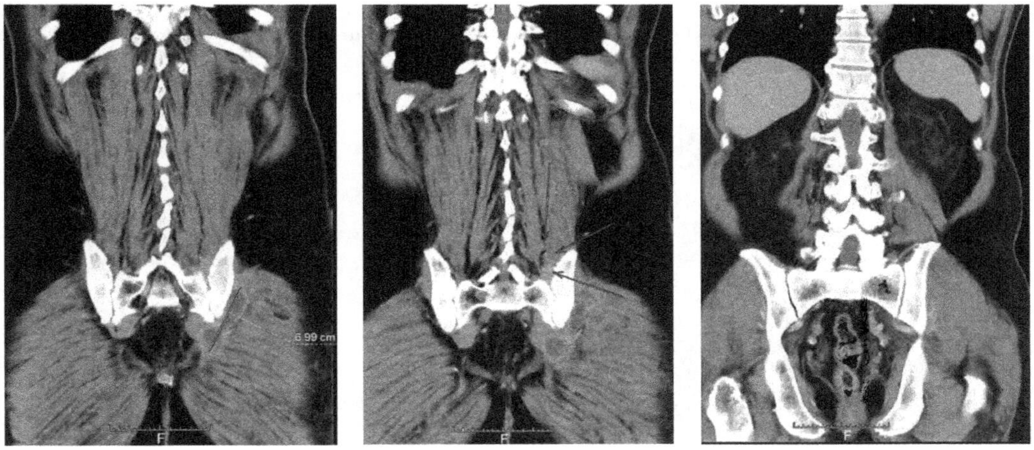

FIGURE 3: CT scan with multiple free air bubbles in the massa lateralis of the sacrum as well as edema of the iliacus and lumbricales muscles of the left side.

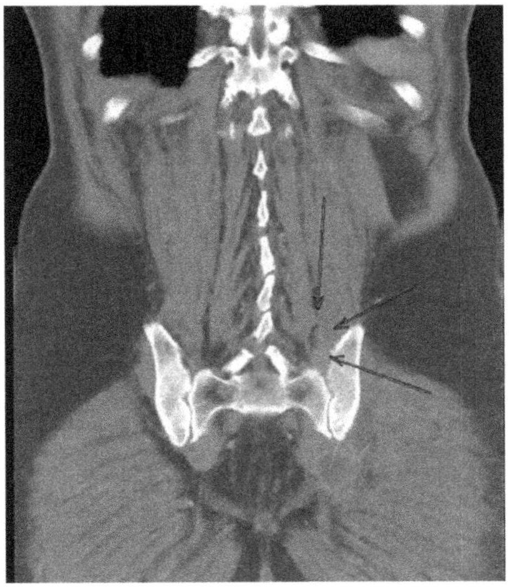

FIGURE 4: Abscess formation around the piriformis muscle and beginning osteolytic destruction of the ilium bone.

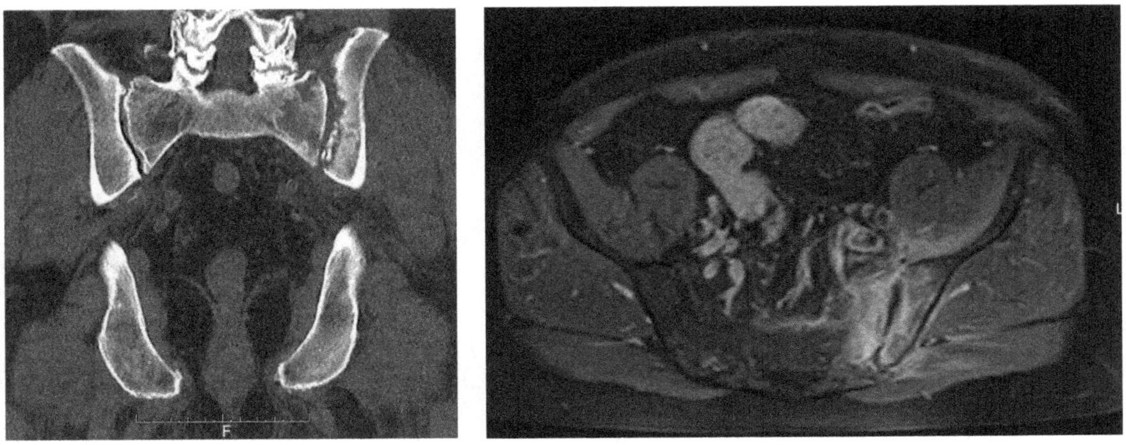

(a) (b)

FIGURE 5: Control CT and MRI of the pelvis 2 months later: osteolytic destruction of the massa lateralis with fluid around the piriformis muscle and the ilium bone.

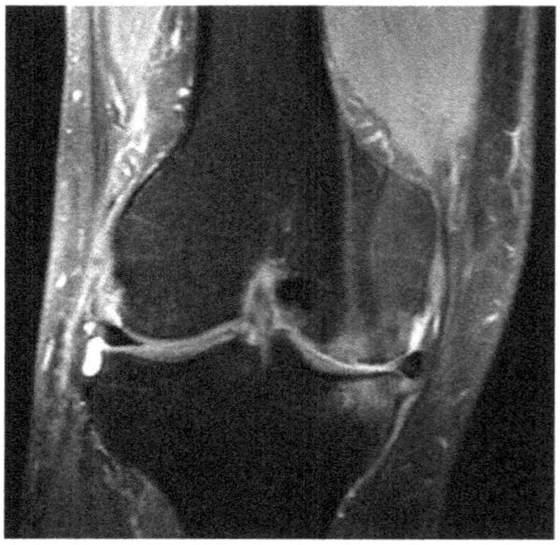

Figure 6: MRI of the knee: inflammatory changes with marked effusion and synovitis as well as subchondral edema at the medial tibia and the medial femur.

were no signs of fever anymore detectible and the laboratory control examination showed nearly normal values.

4. Conclusion

Emphysematous osteomyelitis is a rare but potentially fatal condition. It should always be considered whenever intraosseous gas is identified on imaging. Most reported cases are secondary to an intra-abdominal infection or surgery or are associated with immunosuppression like in malignancies or diabetes mellitus so taking history is crucial. Diagnostic procedures should include X-rays, CT, and MRI laboratory examinations and exclude or include comorbidities such as diabetes mellitus and malignancies. In general, early and extensive treatment is crucial for an adequate outcome.

Consent

Written informed consent was obtained from the patient for publication of this case report and accompanying images.

Competing Interests

The authors declare that they have no competing interests.

References

[1] P. C. Ram, S. Martinez, M. Korobkin, R. S. Breiman, H. R. Gallis, and J. M. Harrelson, "CT detection of intraosseous gas: a new sign of osteomyelitis," *American Journal of Roentgenology*, vol. 137, no. 4, pp. 721–723, 1981.

[2] C. Luey, D. Tooley, and S. Briggs, "Emphysematous osteomyelitis: a case report and review of the literature," *International Journal of Infectious Diseases*, vol. 16, no. 3, pp. e216–e220, 2012.

[3] S. K. Aiyappan, U. Ranga, and S. Veeraiyan, "Spontaneous emphysematous osteomyelitis of spine detected by computed tomography: report of two cases," *Journal of Craniovertebral Junction and Spine*, vol. 5, no. 2, pp. 90–92, 2014.

[4] O. McDonnell and Z. Khaleel, "Emphysematous osteomyelitis," *JAMA Neurology*, vol. 71, no. 4, 2014.

14

Metastatic Prostate Cancer of Hand

Akihito Nagano,[1] Takatoshi Ohno,[2] Koji Oshima,[3] Daichi Ishimaru,[1] Yutaka Nishimoto,[4] Yoshiyuki Ohno,[5] Akihiro Hirakawa,[1] Tatsuhiko Miyazaki,[6] and Haruhiko Akiyama[1]

[1] *The Department of Orthopaedic Surgery, Gifu University School of Medicine, 1-1 Yanagido, Gifu 501-1193, Japan*
[2] *The Department of Orthopaedic Surgery, Japanese Red Cross Gifu Hospital, 3-36 Iwakuracho, Gifu 502-0844, Japan*
[3] *The Department of Orthopaedic Surgery, Ibi Kousei Hospital, 2547-4 Miwa, Ibigawa-cho, Gifu 501-0691, Japan*
[4] *The Department of Nursing Course, Gifu University School of Medicine, 1-1 Yanagido, Gifu 501-1193, Japan*
[5] *The Department of Orthopaedic Surgery, Gifu Municipal Hospital, 7-1 Kashima-cho, Gifu 500-8323, Japan*
[6] *The Division of Pathology, Gifu University Hospital, 1-1 Yanagido, Gifu 501-1193, Japan*

Correspondence should be addressed to Akihito Nagano; a-nagano@lucky.odn.ne.jp

Academic Editor: Kaan Erler

Soft tissue metastases of prostate cancer to other sites are extremely rare, and, to our best knowledge, there have been no reports of metastasis to soft tissue of the hand. A 63-year-old man was diagnosed with prostatic cancer. During treatment, bone and soft tissue metastases to the right hand, appearing in the first web space, were observed. The tumor was resected, along with both the first and second metacarpal bones. The thumb was reconstructed by pollicization of the remaining index finger, enabling the patient to use the pollicized thumb for activities of daily living. This is the first case report of prostate cancer metastasizing to the soft tissue in hand. After wide resection, pollicization was able to reconstruct a functional hand and thumb.

1. Introduction

Prostate cancer has been found to metastasize to the bones, regional lymph nodes, and lungs, with several previous reports describing metastases to other sites. Here, we present the first case of a prostate cancer that metastasized to the soft tissue of the hand.

2. Case Presentation

During a routine check-up a 63-year-old man was found to have a high prostate specific antigen (PSA) concentration (7.9 ng/mL). Transrectal fine needle aspiration (FNA) of the prostate provided a definitive diagnosis of poorly differentiated adenocarcinoma (cT3a, Gleason score 8 (4 + 4), 8/8 cores affected). No metastases were detected, and treatment with both the nonsteroidal antiandrogen bicalutamide (Casodex) and goserelin (Zoladex) reduced his PSA level to 0.2 ng/mL within three months. Five years later, however, despite his PSA level remaining low, local extension to the bladder and metastasis to the S1 vertebra were detected. Furthermore, he developed a gradually enlarging painless mass in the first web space of his right hand, adversely affecting his activities of daily living. Therefore he was referred to our department.

Physical examination showed a well-circumscribed, elastic soft mass located between the right thumb and index finger. This mass, which was palpable but not mobile, measured $5 \times 4 \times 3$ cm in size. The skin over the mass was discolored, suggesting that the tumor had invaded the skin. Daily living was impaired due to restricted range of motion (ROM) of the thumb. Although no pain was associated with the mass, the patient experienced sensory disturbance of the right thumb (Figure 1).

Laboratory tests showed elevation of alkaline phosphatase but low PSA level (0.036 ng/mL).

2.1. Radiographic Findings. A roentgenogram of the right hand showed enlargement of first metacarpal interspace, indicating noncalcification of the soft tissue mass. The metacarpal bones adjacent to the mass were normal without any bony destruction.

Magnetic resonance imaging (MRI) of the right hand revealed a well-defined, clearly circumscribed mass, with iso-

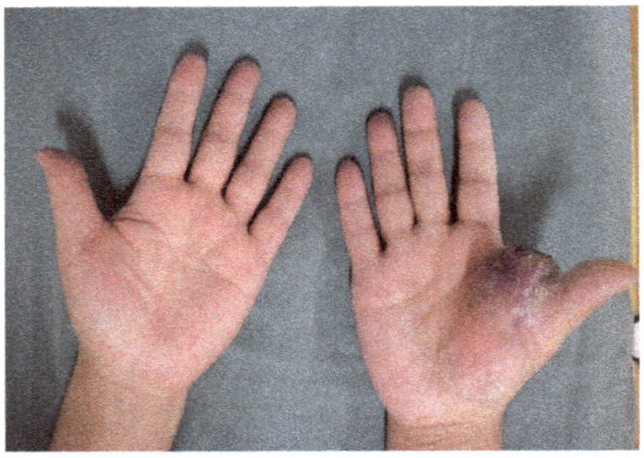

FIGURE 1: Soft tissue mass in the right hand. The mass was located in the first intercarpal space, with the overlying skin showing discoloration.

to low intensity on T1 weighted images and heterogeneously high intensity on T2 weighted images. After intravenous administration of gadolinium-based contrast agent, the mass was well enhanced peripherally, but the central region was poorly enhanced, suggesting necrosis. The mass was adjacent to the first metacarpal bone (Figure 2).

Thallium scintigraphy showed marked accumulation in the right hand but no accumulation in other parts of the body.

Computed tomography (CT) of the entire body revealed a lytic and sclerotic lesion of the sacrum, which was considered metastatic.

Based on these findings, the patient was differentially diagnosed with a primary malignant soft tissue tumor, such as a myxoid liposarcoma or myxofibrosarcoma, or with a metastatic lesion of the adenocarcinoma of the prostate.

2.2. Histological Examination. An open biopsy of the mass in the right hand and a CT-guided biopsy of the lesion of the S1 vertebra were obtained to make a definitive diagnosis. Pathological examination of both lesions showed multinodular growth of small-sized but pleomorphic anaplastic tumor cells with numerous mitotic figures. Some tumor cells were plump with eosinophilic cytoplasm. A focal sheet-like arrangement was observed, with no distinct organoid structure. Immunohistochemical evaluation showed that the tumor cells were positive for cytokeratin AE1/AE3, CAM5.2, vimentin, prostate specific acid phosphatase, and androgen receptor and negative for PSA, S-100, CD34, CD68, and smooth muscle actin. Reticulin silver impregnation showed an epithelioid-like structure. These findings indicated that the tumor was an anaplastic carcinoma rather than a mesenchymal malignancy. The patient was therefore diagnosed with metastatic prostate cancer (Figure 3).

2.3. Treatment. The treatment of patient with cancer should be performed on a case-by-case basis, depending on the patient's prognosis and functional capabilities especially in patients with multiple metastasis. Generally, palliative treatment, such as radiation therapy, is chosen because of the dismal prognosis of patients with metastasis. In the present case, the prognosis was thought to be relatively better than the other cancer; in fact, the prognosis of prostate cancer with bone metastasis is reported as 3.0–3.5 years [1]. Furthermore, an amputation would bring about unacceptable degree of functional disability, because the affected hand was dominant. Incomplete resection might lead to local recurrence.

After discussion of treatment options with the patient and his family, he agreed to wide resection of the hand tumor and systemic chemotherapy.

The tumor, along with the surrounding tissues, was resected *en bloc*. Wide resection of the tumor was accompanied by disarticulation of the carpometacarpal (CMC) joint, osteotomy of the proximal second metacarpal bone, disarticulation of the second metacarpophalangeal (MCP) joint, resection of the tendons and neurovascular bundles of the thumb and index finger, and resection of both the first dorsal interosseous and lumbrical muscles. Concurrently, the thumb was reconstructed by pollicization of the remaining index finger, and the skin defect was covered with a skin graft. The pathological findings of the tumor were the same as the specimen at the time of biopsy, and microscopically free margin (R0 resection) was achieved. After surgery, the patient underwent chemotherapy with docetaxel (DTX) and estramustine. The patient was able to use the pollicized thumb for activities of daily living, such as writing, six months after the operation (Figure 4). Chemotherapy was continued, with no local recurrence in the hand. However, because of multiple metastases to the lungs and spine, the patient died four years after surgery.

3. Discussion

The most common locations of prostate cancer metastases are the pelvic lymph nodes and bone, followed by the lungs, bladder, and liver [2]. Soft tissue metastases of prostate cancer to other sites are extremely rare, and, to our knowledge, there have been no reports of metastasis to soft tissue of the hand. Of 47 patients with soft tissue or nonregional lymphatic metastases of prostate carcinoma, 16 had soft tissue metastasis to the lungs, liver, kidneys, bladder, penile glans, subcutaneous tissue of the scalp, thoracic wall, and thigh [3]. Autopsies of 1885 patients with prostate cancer showed metastases in 1367. Sites of metastasis included the lymph nodes, bones, and other visceral organs, but none of these patients had metastases to the hand.

As described previously, a prostate cancer tends to metastasize to the bone. However, acrometastasis, that is, bone metastasis distal to the elbow and the knee, are rare,

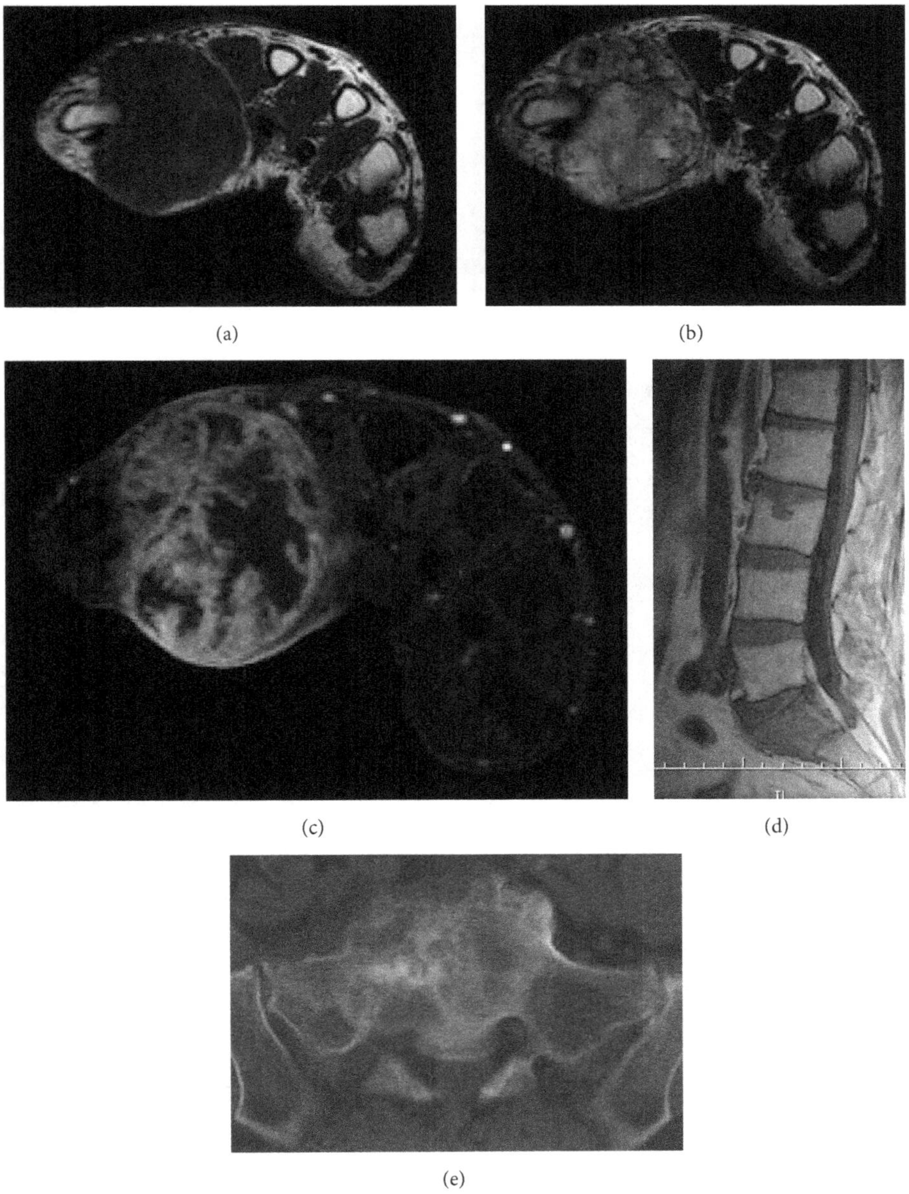

FIGURE 2: (a) T1 weighted, (b) T2 weighted, and (c) enhanced MRI images of the right hand suggested a malignant neoplasm. (d) MRI and (e) CT of the sacrum showed a lytic and sclerotic lesion, which was regarded as a prostate cancer metastasis.

accounting for approximately 0.1% of all cases with skeletal metastasis. Men were almost twice as likely to acrometastasis as women. The most prevalent primary diagnosis is lung, followed by colon, breast, and genitourinary tract [4, 5]. In the present case, the metastatic tumor was attached to the first metacarpal bone but not invasive, suggesting that metastasis occurred in the soft tissue, not in the bone.

Metastases of well-differentiated prostatic adenocarcinoma show typical pathological features and are not difficult to diagnose. In contrast, metastases of poorly differentiated prostatic adenocarcinoma may present a diagnostic challenge. Immunohistochemical staining, especially for PSA, is useful in assessing the prostatic origin of these less latter tumors. However, higher-grade poorly differentiated adenocarcinoma may lack both pathological features and diagnostic antigenicity, including for PSA [6]. Our patient had an anaplastic carcinoma negative for PSA, making a definitive diagnosis of metastatic prostatic carcinoma quite difficult. The findings that tumor cells were partially positive for both cytokeratin and vimentin and that both the sacral and hand lesions showed similar pathological features and are positive for prostate specific acid phosphatase and androgen receptor strongly suggested that the tumor was metastatic rather than a primary soft tissue sarcoma.

Treatment of patients with advanced prostate cancer must strike a balance between efficacy and acceptable side effects.

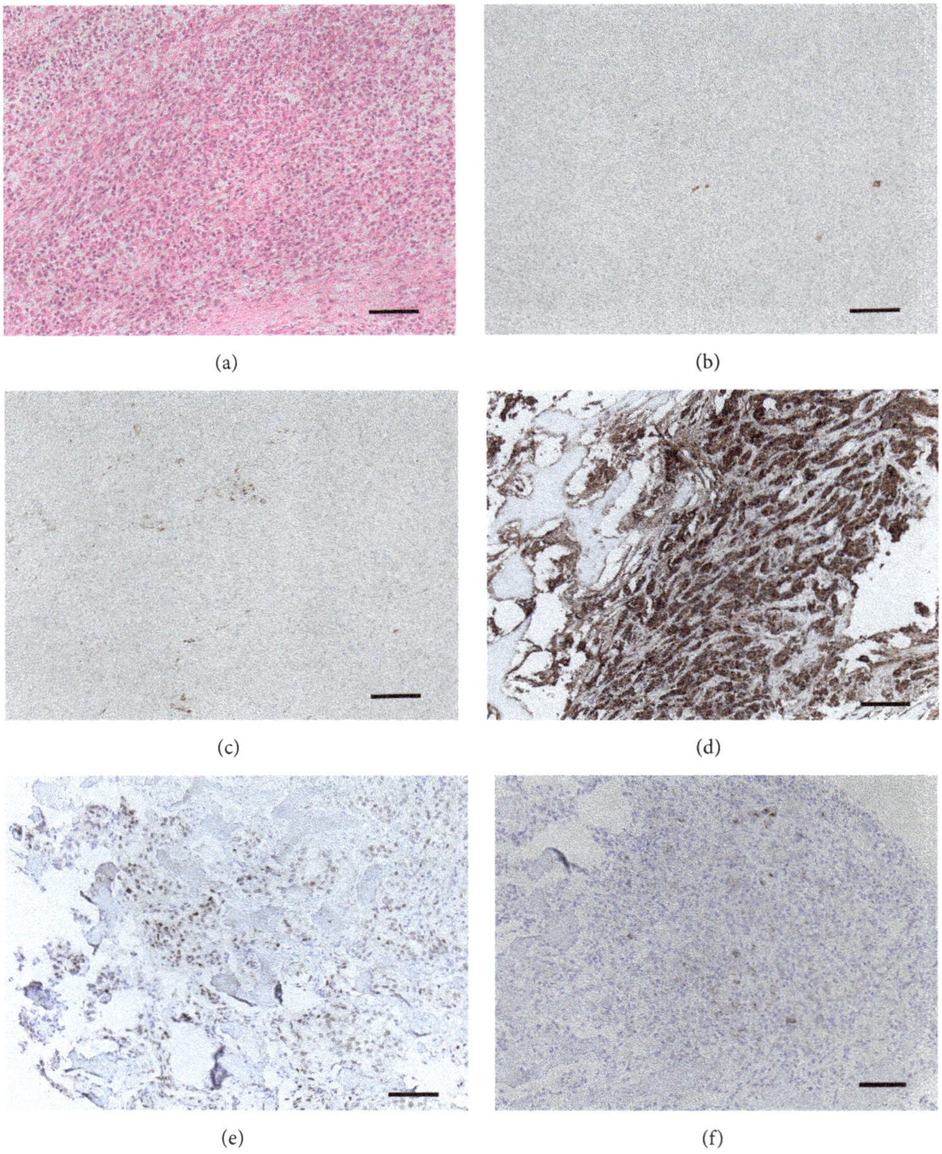

FIGURE 3: Staining with (a) hematoxylin and eosin (×20), (b) CAM5.2, (c) vimentin, (d) prostate specific acid phosphatase, and (e) androgen receptor showed small-sized but pleomorphic anaplastic tumor cells. (f) Reticulin silver impregnation showed epithelioid-like structures, indicative of carcinoma (bar: 100 μm).

After assessment of disease risk, patients should be informed about the benefits and side effects of all options [1]. In addition, the presence of bone metastases reduces median survival to about 3.0–3.5 years [1]. The patient in this study was informed of the risks of surgery and prognosis of the disease and chose wide resection in combination with reconstruction of the thumb by pollicization of the index finger, allowing the affected thumb to retain its function. No major complications occurred during or after the operation, and the patient was satisfied with the functional results of the operation.

4. Conclusion

We have reported the first case of metastatic prostate adenocarcinoma to the hand. Wide resection of the metastatic tumor and reconstruction of the thumb by pollicization of the index finger resulted in satisfactory clinical and functional outcomes.

Consent

Written informed consent was obtained from the wife of the patient for publication of this case report and any accompanying images.

Competing Interests

The authors declare that there is no conflict of interests regarding the publication of this paper.

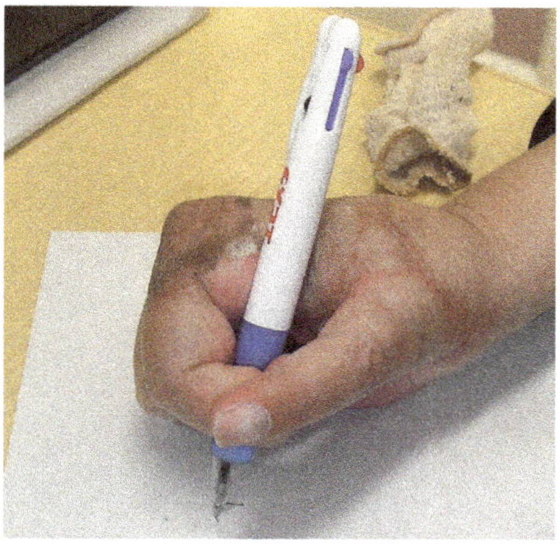

FIGURE 4: Postoperative appearance of the right hand. The patient used the pollicized thumb for activities of daily living, such as writing.

Acknowledgments

The authors wish to thank the family for their cooperation in this study. And they are deeply grateful to Mr. Yasuo Katagiri for his brilliant technical support in immunohistochemical study.

References

[1] R. Kirby, "Case study: management of advanced prostate cancer with soft tissue metastases," *Prostate Cancer and Prostatic Diseases*, vol. 8, no. 3, pp. 290–292, 2005.

[2] H. Saitoh, M. Hida, T. Shimbo, K. Nakamura, J. Yamagata, and T. Satoh, "Metastatic patterns of prostatic cancer. Correlation between sites and number of organs involved," *Cancer*, vol. 54, no. 12, pp. 3078–3084, 1984.

[3] G. Saeter, S. D. Fossa, S. Ous, G. P. Blom, and O. Kaalhus, "Carcinoma of the prostate with soft tissue or non-regional lymphatic metastases at the time of diagnosis: a review of 47 cases," *British Journal of Urology*, vol. 56, no. 4, pp. 385–390, 1984.

[4] C. J. Flynn, C. Danjoux, J. Wong et al., "Two cases of acrometastasis to the hands and review of the literature," *Current Oncology*, vol. 15, no. 5, pp. 51–58, 2008.

[5] A. F. Mavrogenis, G. Mimidis, Z. T. Kokkalis et al., "Acrometastases," *European Journal of Orthopaedic Surgery and Traumatology*, vol. 24, no. 3, pp. 279–283, 2014.

[6] A. V. Parwani and S. Z. Ali, "Prostatic adenocarcinoma metastases mimicking small cell carcinoma on fine-needle aspiration," *Diagnostic Cytopathology*, vol. 27, no. 2, pp. 75–79, 2002.

15

An Unusual and Complicated Course of a Giant Cell Tumor of the Capitate Bone

Ingo Schmidt

SRH Poliklinik Gera GmbH, Straße des Friedens 122, 07548 Gera, Germany

Correspondence should be addressed to Ingo Schmidt; schmidtingo62@googlemail.com

Academic Editor: Kaan Erler

A 51-year-old female patient presented with a carpal giant cell tumor (GCT) of the right capitate bone. The lesion was initially misdiagnosed as having an osteomyelitis. First, the diagnosis of a benign GCT was confirmed by histological examination. Second, an intralesional curettage and packing of the cavity with cancellous iliac crest bone grafts combined with a fusion of the third carpometacarpal (CMC III) joint were carried out. Third, due to a secondary midcarpal osteoarthritis and a secondary scaphoid nonunion, the CMC III joint fusion plate was removed and the midcarpal joint completely excised. Fourth, in the absence of recurrence of GCT, a four-corner fusion (4CF) with a corticocancellous iliac crest bone graft and complete excision of the scaphoid bone had to be performed. Fifth, a total wrist arthroplasty (TWA) was performed due to hardware failure of 4CF with migration of a headless compression screw into radiocarpal joint which led to erosion of articular surface of the distal radius. At the 3-year follow-up that includes a 1-year follow-up after TWA, there was no recurrence of GCT, and the TWA was not failed. The patient reported that she would have the motion-preserving TWA again.

1. Introduction

Giant cell tumor (GCT) of the bone is a rare, benign, and locally aggressive tumor, constituting 4-5% of all primary bone tumors and 18–20% of all benign bone tumors. Two malignant variants are known—first, the primary malignant GCT that was found in up to 10% of cases; and second, the rare sarcomatous proliferation appears inside the lesion previously documented as a benign GCT. Usually, GCT occurs in skeletally mature individuals, the patient's age ranges from 20 to 50 years, and the peak age incidence is in the third and fourth decade of life with slight female predominance. Typically, the tumor site is subchondral at the long bone metaepiphysis, especially the distal radius and femur, and proximal humerus and tibia [1–3].

GCT of the carpal bones is a very rare entity, only few case reports have described unifocal or multifocal appearance involving the proximal and/or distal row [4, 5]. We present an unusual and complicated course of GCT of the capitate bone which required five surgical procedures within two years. To our knowledge, such a case finally resulting in a total wrist arthroplasty (TWA) has not been reported thus far.

2. Case Report

The posteroanterior (PA) radiograph of a 51-year-old female patient showed an intraosseous lytic lesion of the right capitate bone (Figure 1(a)) that was associated with a marked radionuclide uptake in all carpal bones using bone-granulocyte scintigraphy (Figure 1(b)) and magnetic resonance imaging (MRI) demonstrated low to intermediate signal intensity of the lesion without soft-tissue extension (Figure 1(c)). Due to these findings, an osteomyelitis of the capitate bone was suggested by the radiologist. At first, free intraosseous sample was taken that revealed a benign GCT in histological examination. The chest radiograph did not show pulmonal pathology. Second, intralesional curettage and packing of the cavity with cancellous iliac crest bone grafts combined with a fusion of the third carpometacarpal (CMC III) joint using a 2,0 mm titanium plate (Medartis, Basel, Switzerland) were performed.

One year after, the PA and lateral radiographs showed union of the CMC III joint fusion without hardware failure, but there was pronounced destruction at the proximal pole of the reconstructed capitate bone and at the distal facet of

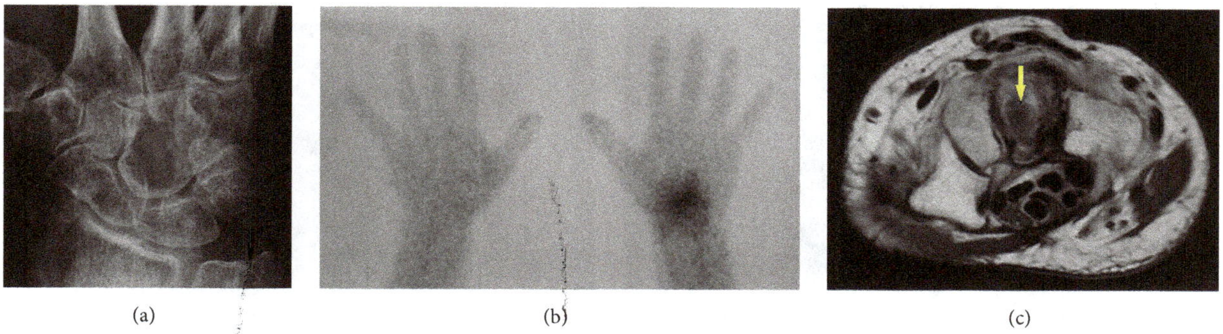

FIGURE 1: Case report (preoperative diagnostic findings): (a) PA radiograph showing lytic lesion in capitate bone with cortical thinning and cortical destruction distally; (b) bone-granulocyte scintigraphy of both hands showing increased radionuclide uptake in the region of right carpal bones 45 minutes after application; (c) axial MRI sequence showing low to intermediate signal intensity in capitate bone and no soft-tissue extension *(arrow)*.

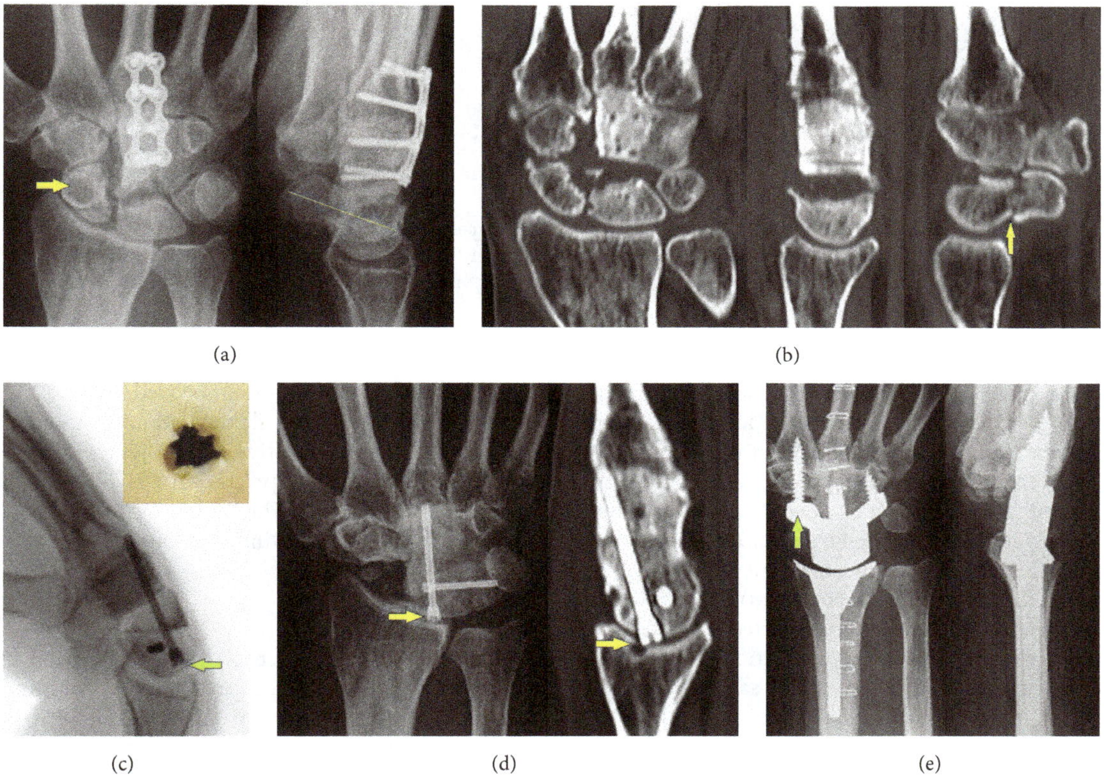

FIGURE 2: Case report (course): (a) PA and lateral radiographs showing union of CMC III joint fusion, severe destruction of midcarpal joint, positive ring sign *(arrow)*, and distinctive volar tilt of capitate bone *(line)*; (b) coronar and sagittal CT scans showing removal of CMC III joint fusion plate, solid bony structure of reconstructed capitate bone, no recurrence of GCT, complete union of CMC III joint fusion, complete resection of midcarpal joint for histological examination, and humpback deformity due to a nonunion at the waist of scaphoid bone *(arrow)*; (c) intraoperative clinical photograph and lateral fluoroscopy demonstrating safe subchondral placement of the longitudinally inserted 4CF headless compression screw at the lunate bone *(arrow)*; (d) PA radiograph and sagittal CT scan showing loosening and migration of longitudinally inserted compression screw into radiocarpal joint with erosion of articular surface at the distal radius *(arrows)*; (e) postoperative AP and lateral radiographs demonstrating correct alignment of TWA, note the scaphoid augment of carpal component *(arrow)*.

lunate bone, and a positive ring sign associated with distinctive volar tilt of scaphoid bone in the absence of an injury after the second procedure (Figure 2(a)). Third, the CMC III joint fusion plate was removed and the midcarpal joint completely excised. The histological examination did not show recurrence of GCT but revealed pronounced midcarpal osteoarthritis (OA). Intraoperatively, a nonunion at the waist of scaphoid bone was seen. Postoperatively, computed tomography (CT) scans showed complete union of CMC III joint fusion associated with sufficient osseointegration of

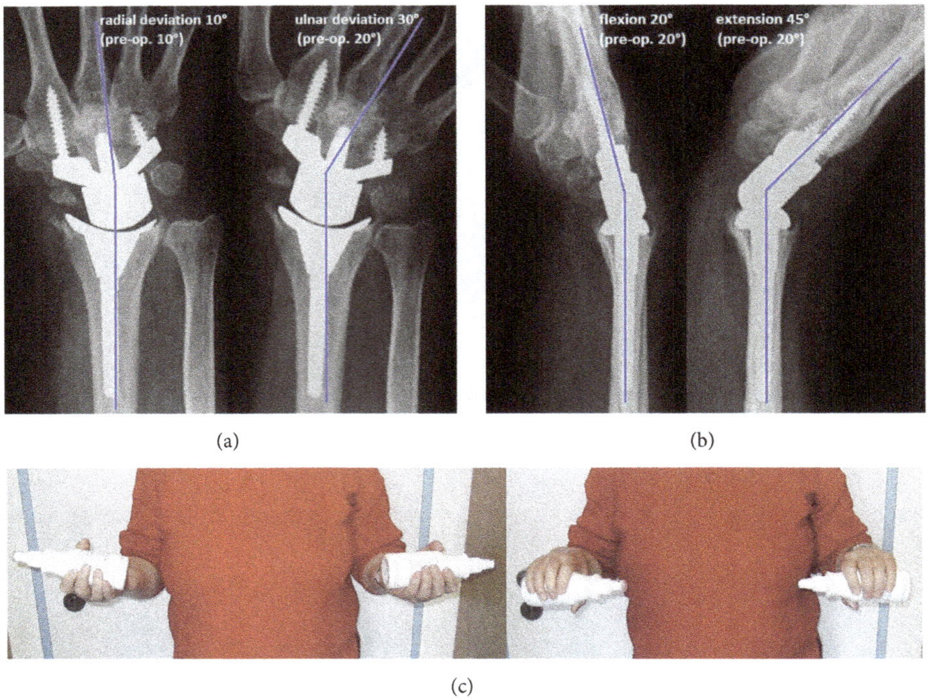

Figure 3: Case report (3-year follow-up): (a) PA radiographs showing no recurrence of GCT, unchanged correct alignment of TWA without any signs of loosening, and no impingement with terminal ranges of motion; (b) lateral PA radiographs with terminal ranges of motion showing no instability of TWA; (c) clinical photographs demonstrating 90° supination and 90° pronation of both forearms.

cancellous bone grafts at the capitate bone and additionally the humpback deformity due to a nonunion at the waist of scaphoid bone (Figure 2(b)). Fourth, an open 4CF with excision of the entire scaphoid bone using a corticocancellous iliac crest bone graft and two cannulated headless titanium compression screws (Medartis, Basel, Switzerland) was performed. One 2,2 mm screw was transversely inserted into triquetrum bone, and the second 3.0 mm screw was longitudinally inserted into the reconstructed capitate bone in an antegrade manner breaching the articular surface of lunate bone. Intraoperatively, there was a safe subchondral placement of the longitudinally inserted compression screw at the lunate bone (Figure 2(c)).

One year after 4CF, a migration of the longitudinally inserted compression screw into radiocarpal joint with erosion of the articular surface at the distal radius was present (Figure 2(d)). The patient declined a total wrist fusion (TWF), and a TWA using the relatively new angle-stable Maestro™ Wrist Reconstructive System (WRS, Biomet, Warsaw, Indiana/USA) with the use of a scaphoid augment distally was performed (Figure 2(e)). After that, the course was uncomplicated.

At the 3-year follow-up (including 1-year follow-up after TWA), the radiographs did not show recurrence of GCT, the TWA was not loosened, and there were no signs of impingement nor instability with terminal ranges of motion (Figures 3(a)-3(b)). Pain improved from 8 to 2 in visual analog score (0–10 points). Patient-rated wrist evaluation (0–100 points) improved from 88 to 37. Wrist extension and wrist ulnar deviation improved from 20° to 45° and from 20° to 30°. Wrist flexion and wrist radial deviation were equal to preoperative. The forearm motion arc with 90° supination and 90° pronation was 100% to the opposite forearm (Figure 3(c)). The patient reported that she would have the motion-preserving TWA again.

3. Discussion

GCTs of bone rarely occur in the hand. When they do, the metacarpals and phalanges are the most commonly affected bones. Based on a review of 1228 cases of GCT of all bones, Averill et al. [5] found that only 3% of cases occurred in the hand and extremely rare with 0,32% in carpal bones, patients are often younger than patients with appearance in other locations, recurrence is more rapidly than in other locations, the incidence of multifocal appearance of GCT of bones in the hand is 18%, and 87% of GCTs in the hand treated by curettage recurred. GCT of carpal bones affected in 31% the hamate, in 24% the capitate, in 14% the scaphoid, in 10% the lunate, in 7% the triquetrum, in 7% the trapezium, in 7% the trapezoid, and multifocal appearance was found in 14% of all cases [4]. Multifocal GCT of carpal bones and multicentric occurrence involving nine sites of both upper extremities including the lunate bone in a course over 16 years were also described in two skeletally immature male patients with age of 14 and starting with age of 13 years [6, 7].

In a review of literature including hand published articles from 1935 to 2005, only 29 cases of GCT of carpal bones (averaged age of patients 32,6 years ranging from 16 to 80 years, data from three publications not available) could be found by Shigematsu et al. [4], and the high incidence of local recurrence with 24% of all cases was associated only with performed intralesional procedures and recurrence occurred between three months and four years, whereas in cases treated with an excisional procedure recurrence did not occur. Why the marked midcarpal OA and humpback deformity of the scaphoid due to a nonunion after the secondary procedure (curettage/cancellous bone grafting/CMC III joint fusion) occurred in our case is unclear.

Radiographically, GCT of carpal bones resembles other lytic lesions. As with other musculoskeletal neoplasm, CT and MRI are superior to conventional radiographs [8]. On the other hand, benign GCT of bone can also initially misdiagnosed on MRI as a malignancy [9]. Bone scintigraphy demonstrates increased radionuclide uptake in the vast majority of GCTs; however, bone scintigraphy is nonspecific, does not aid in the detection of GCT, does not differentiate benign from malignant GCT, and is most likely secondary to other bony abnormalities or local and/or regional hyperemia [10]. For detection of benign GCT of bone, histological examination of free intralesional samples is absolutely necessary.

Treatment strategy for GCT of bone has been evolved over the years with different surgical options, which can be summarized under two main categories: first, intralesional curettage and/or chemical treatment (hydrogen peroxide, phenol, and alcohol) and/or cryosurgery (instillation of liquid nitrogen), followed by packing of the cavity with bone grafts, bone graft substitutes, and/or polymethylmethacrylate (PMMA); and, second, en bloc resection of the entire tumor followed by reconstruction in the form of arthroplasty or arthrodesis using nonvascularized or vascularized bone grafts. When using an intralesional procedure, meticulous high-speed burring is recommended to improve the quality of curettage, but the use of autologous bone grafts is likely unable to prevent recurrence sufficiently [11, 12]. In contrast to autologous bone grafting, it has been reported that combined treatment of selective GCT in the hand with curettage, cryosurgery, and additional cementation (PMMA) appears to be safe and effective [13]. In a review of literature, it has been reported that some types of GCT of bones still have the ability to metastasize in the presence of a recurrence rate up to 45% [14]. Approximately, up to 3% of GCTs metastasizes to lung at certain time points after the confirmed diagnosis [15], and for patients who experienced local recurrence it has been estimated that they can have a six-fold higher risk of lung metastasis [16].

For treatment of GCT of carpal bones, care must be taken when using an intralesional curettage with or without bone grafting, and an excisional procedure is recommended to prevent recurrence [17–19]. If the scaphoid, lunate, or triquetrum is affected, proximal row carpectomy (PRC) or complete excision of the involved bone combined with an intercarpal fusion is the method of choice [20–22]. The use of retrograde or, such as in our case, antegrade inserted headless compression screws for 4CF has proven to be a suitable and reliable option with an union rate up to 94% [23–26], but hardware migration into radiocarpal joint despite complete union of 4CF, such as in our case, is a concern. Richards et al. [25] reported on proximal backing out of the screws in 14% of 21 treated patients; and it was also observed in all of four treated patients who underwent the insertion of headless compression screws in antegrade manner after averaged six months (4–8 months) despite union of all 4CFs [27]. If the distal row is affected, complete excision of the involved bone combined with an intercarpal fusion is the method of choice as well [28]; however, complete excision of the capitate without reconstruction of distal row or distal row carpectomy also can be surgical option [18, 29]. Vergara-Fernández et al. [30] reported on complex replacement of excised carpal bones using a long corticocancellous bone graft from the third metacarpal bone which was distracted by an external fixateur in a 15-year-old male patient. Averill et al. [5] reported on one case with multifocal carpal, metacarpal, and phalangeal appearance in an 18-year-old male patient that required a ray amputation. For recurrence of GCT after a primary excisional procedure or failed intercarpal fusion, total wrist fusion (TWF) with the use of large corticocancellous iliac crest bone grafts is to be considered as one salvage option. The overall complication rate of 4CF is 29% versus 14% for PRC, respectively [31]; main complications of 4CF are delayed or nonunion and/or, such as in our case, hardware failure [32], and the reported conversion rate to a TWF after a failed 4CF or PRC (including conversion to TWA) ranges from 8,7 to 14,8% [33–36].

TWA is the motion-preserving alternative to TWF, and it has proven to be successful after failed 4CF or PRC in single cases [35–40]. For this purpose in our case, the essential prerequisite was that the bone stock of the primary reconstructed capitate bone demonstrated a solid bony structure for safe fixation of the carpal TWA monoblock component with its central peg into the reconstructed capitate in the absence of local recurrence of GCT or local postoperative osteitis. The Maestro total wrist, developed by *Strickland/Palmer/Graham* in 2002 and available since January 2005, is a biaxial-anatomical third-generation type that is current in use, and first encouraging short-term results were published in 2009 [41]. In a single-center study, published in 2015, the cumulative implant survival after eight years ($N = 68$) is reported to be 95%, and at the 5-year follow-up radiographic loosening was present only in 2% of all cases [42]. Currently, the Maestro total wrist achieves the most favorable functional outcome as compared to other third-generation types (Remotion, Universal 2), and it may be justified in preserving resection-related carpal height due to its three various carpal heads in combination with its design of ellipsoid surface articulation [43]. Such as in our case, the design of implant allows the excision of the entire scaphoid bone accompanied with its replacement utilizing a carpal component that incorporates various scaphoid augments; therefore, it is not always necessary to attempt fusion of the distal pole of the scaphoid to the surrounding carpal bones ([41], Figures 4(a)-4(b)).

However, patients undergoing treatment with TWA must be prepared that it might end with TWF; therefore, limited bone resection is a common feature of all contemporary wrist replacements [44, 45]. The Maestro total wrist has

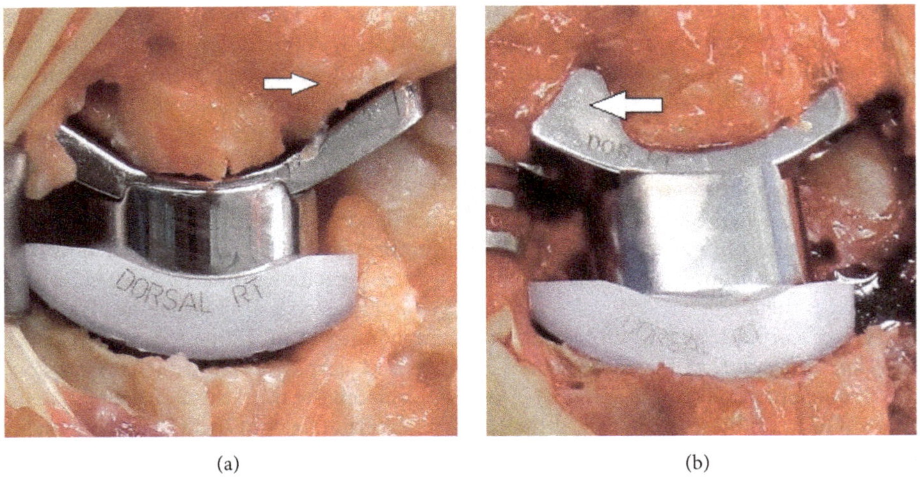

FIGURE 4: Technical note (Maestro WRS): (a) Clinical photograph demonstrating the use of carpal component without scaphoid augment, the distal pole of scaphoid bone is not excised *(arrow)*; (b) clinical photograph demonstrating the use of carpal component with scaphoid augment *(arrow)*, the entire scaphoid bone is excised.

demonstrated uncomplicated conversion to TWF [40, 42, 43, 46].

Competing Interests

The author declares that he has no conflict of interests concerning this article.

Acknowledgments

The author would like to thank Dr. Torsten Doenicke and Dr. Reinhard Friedel (both from the University Hospital Jena, Germany) and Professor Dr. Reiner Oberbeck (SRH Waldklinikum Gera GmbH, Germany) for her support in the treatment of this patient.

References

[1] D. C. Dahlin, "Giant cell tumor of bone: highlights of 407 cases," *American Journal of Roentgenology*, vol. 144, no. 5, pp. 955–960, 1985.

[2] M. Campanacci, N. Baldini, S. Boriani, and A. Sudanese, "Giant-cell tumor of bone," *The Journal of Bone & Joint Surgery—American Volume*, vol. 69, no. 1, pp. 106–114, 1987.

[3] M. Werner, "Giant cell tumour of bone: morphological, biological and histogenetical aspects," *International Orthopaedics*, vol. 30, no. 6, pp. 484–489, 2006.

[4] K. Shigematsu, Y. Kobata, H. Yajima, K. Kawamura, N. Maegawa, and Y. Takakura, "Giant-cell tumors of the carpus," *Journal of Hand Surgery*, vol. 31, no. 7, pp. 1214–1219, 2006.

[5] R. M. Averill, R. J. Smith, and C. J. Campbell, "Giant-cell tumors of the bones of the hand," *Journal of Hand Surgery*, vol. 5, no. 1, pp. 39–50, 1980.

[6] M. T. Ansari, P. K. Prakash, and M. V. Machhindra, "Wrist preserving surgery for multifocal giant cell tumor of carpal bones in a skeletally immature patient: a case report," *Orthopaedic Surgery*, vol. 6, no. 4, pp. 322–325, 2014.

[7] E. N. Novais, A. Y. Shin, A. T. Bishop, and T. C. Shives, "Multicentric giant cell tumor of the upper extremities: 16 years of ongoing disease," *Journal of Hand Surgery*, vol. 36, no. 10, pp. 1610–1613, 2011.

[8] M. D. Murphey, G. C. Nomikos, D. J. Flemming, F. H. Gannon, H. T. Temple, and M. J. Kransdorf, "From the archives of AFIP. Imaging of giant cell tumor and giant cell reparative granuloma of bone: radiologic-pathologic correlation," *Radiographics*, vol. 21, no. 5, pp. 1283–1309, 2001.

[9] M. Pujani, S. Bahadur, Z. S. Jairajpuri, S. Jetley, and J. Jameel, "Giant cell tumor bone in an elderly male- an unusual case misdiagnosed on MRI as a malignant sarcoma," *Indian Journal of Surgical Oncology*, vol. 6, no. 3, pp. 285–287, 2015.

[10] D. Van Nostrand, J. E. Madewell, L. M. McNiesh, R. W. Kyle, and D. Sweet, "Radionuclide bone scanning in giant cell tumor," *Journal of Nuclear Medicine*, vol. 27, no. 3, pp. 329–338, 1986.

[11] F. Gouin, V. Dumaine, and French Sarcoma and Bone Tumor Study Groups GSF-GETO, "Local recurrence after curettage treatment of giant cell tumors in peripheral bones: retrospective study by the GSF-GETO (French Sarcoma and Bone Tumor Study Groups)," *Orthopaedics & Traumatology: Surgery & Research*, vol. 99, supplement 6, pp. S313–S318, 2013.

[12] H. Algawahmed, R. Turcotte, F. Farrokhyar, and M. Ghert, "High-speed burring with and without the use of surgical adjuvants in the intralesional management of giant cell tumor of bone: a systematic review and meta-analysis," *Sarcoma*, vol. 2010, Article ID 586090, 5 pages, 2010.

[13] J. C. Wittig, B. M. Simpson, J. Bickels, K. L. Kellar-Graney, and M. M. Malawer, "Giant cell tumor of the hand: superior results with curettage, cryosurgery, and cementation," *Journal of Hand Surgery*, vol. 26, no. 3, pp. 546–555, 2001.

[14] D. Li, J. Zhang, Y. Li et al., "Surgery methods and soft tissue extension are the potential risk factors of local recurrence in giant cell tumor of bone," *World Journal of Surgical Oncology*, vol. 14, no. 1, article 114, 2016.

[15] A. Muheremu and X. Niu, "Pulmonary metastasis of giant cell tumor of bones," *World Journal of Surgical Oncology*, vol. 12, article 261, 2014.

[16] M. G. Rock, "Curettage of giant cell tumor of bone. Factors influencing local recurrences and metastasis," *La Chirurgia degli organi di Movimento*, vol. 75, no. 1, supplement 1, pp. 204–205, 1990.

[17] P. Moreel and D. Le Viet, "Failure of initial surgical treatment of a giant cell tumor of the capitate and its salvage: a case report," *Chirurgie de la Main*, vol. 25, no. 6, pp. 315–318, 2006.

[18] D. J. McDonald and F. Schajowicz, "Giant cell tumor of the capitate. A case report," *Clinical Orthopaedics and Related Research*, no. 279, pp. 264–268, 1992.

[19] A. Angelini, A. F. Mavrogenis, and P. Ruggieri, "Giant cell tumor of the capitate," *Musculoskeletal Surgery*, vol. 95, no. 1, pp. 45–48, 2011.

[20] W. A. Abdu, J. M. Murphy, and V. A. Memoli, "Giant cell tumor of the scaphoid: a case report and review of the literature," *Journal of Hand Surgery*, vol. 19, no. 6, pp. 1003–1005, 1994.

[21] D. J. FitzPatrick and P. G. Bullough, "Giant cell tumor of the lunate bone: a case report," *Journal of Hand Surgery*, vol. 2, no. 4, pp. 269–270, 1977.

[22] D. S. Louis, F. M. Hankin, and E. M. Braunstein, "Giant cell tumour of the triquetrum," *Journal of Hand Surgery. British Volume*, vol. 11, no. 2, pp. 279–280, 1986.

[23] M. Henry, "Internal headless compression screw method for 4-corner fusion," *Journal of Hand and Microsurgery*, vol. 1, no. 1, pp. 45–49, 2016.

[24] B. Ball and J. W. Bergman, "Scaphoid excision and 4-corner fusion using retrograde headless compression screws," *Techniques in Hand and Upper Extremity Surgery*, vol. 16, no. 4, pp. 204–209, 2012.

[25] A. A. Richards, A. M. Afifi, and M. S. Moneim, "Four-corner fusion and scaphoid excision using headless compression screws for SLAC and SNAC wrist deformities," *Techniques in Hand & Upper Extremity Surgery*, vol. 15, no. 2, pp. 99–103, 2011.

[26] T. Ozyurekoglu and T. Turker, "Results of a method of 4-corner arthrodesis using headless compression screws," *Journal of Hand Surgery*, vol. 37, no. 3, pp. 486–492, 2012.

[27] G. D. Shifflett, E. A. Athanasian, S. K. Lee, A. J. Weiland, and S. W. Wolfe, "Proximal migration of hardware in patients undergoing midcarpal fusion with headless compression screws," *Journal of Wrist Surgery*, vol. 3, no. 4, pp. 250–261, 2014.

[28] S. Duman, H. Sofu, Y. Camurcu, S. Gursu, and R. Oke, "Giant cell tumor of the capitate: an unusual case with 10 years follow-up," *SICOT Journal*, vol. 1, article 18, 2015.

[29] G. G. Gupta, G. L. Lucas, and M. Pirela-Cruz, "Multifocal giant cell tumor of the capitate, hamate, and triquetrum: a case report," *Journal of Hand Surgery*, vol. 20, no. 6, pp. 1003–1006, 1995.

[30] H. J. Vergara-Fernández, D. Ortiz-Arellano, B. Martínez-Hernández, R. M. Mosiñoz, and J. A. Arellano, "Hand reconstructive surgery secondary to giant cell tumor," *Acta Ortopédica Mexicana*, vol. 24, no. 5, pp. 343–348, 2010.

[31] B. M. Saltzman, J. M. Frank, W. Slikker, J. J. Fernandez, M. S. Cohen, and R. W. Wysocki, "Clinical outcomes of proximal row carpectomy versus four-corner arthrodesis for post-traumatic wrist arthropathy: a systematic review," *Journal of Hand Surgery. European Volume*, vol. 40, no. 5, pp. 450–457, 2015.

[32] R. W. Wysocki and M. S. Cohen, "Complications of limited and total wrist arthrodesis," *Hand Clinics*, vol. 26, no. 2, pp. 221–228, 2010.

[33] J. D. Krakauer, A. T. Bishop, and W. P. Cooney, "Surgical treatment of scapholunate advanced collapse," *Journal of Hand Surgery*, vol. 19, no. 5, pp. 751–759, 1994.

[34] A. K. Dacho, S. Baumeister, G. Germann, and M. Sauerbier, "Comparison of proximal row carpectomy and midcarpal arthrodesis for the treatment of scaphoid nonunion advanced collapse (SNAC-wrist) and scapholunate advanced collapse (SLAC-wrist) in stage II," *Journal of Plastic, Reconstructive & Aesthetic Surgery*, vol. 61, no. 10, pp. 1210–1218, 2008.

[35] H. Chim and S. L. Moran, "Long-term outcomes of proximal row carpectomy: a systematic review of the literature," *Journal of Wrist Surgery*, vol. 1, no. 2, pp. 141–148, 2012.

[36] M. H. Ali, M. Rizzo, A. Y. Shin, and S. L. Moran, "Long-term outcomes of proximal row carpectomy: a minimum of 15-year follow-up," *Hand*, vol. 7, no. 1, pp. 72–78, 2012.

[37] G. Herzberg, "Prospective study of a new total wrist arthroplasty: short term results," *Chirurgie de la Main*, vol. 30, no. 1, pp. 20–25, 2011.

[38] W. Cooney, J. Manuel, J. Froelich, and M. Rizzo, "Total wrist replacement: a retrospective comparative study," *Journal of Wrist Surgery*, vol. 1, no. 2, pp. 165–172, 2012.

[39] M. Nicoloff, "Total wrist arthroplasty—indications and state of the art," *Zeitschrift für Orthopädie und Unfallchirurgie*, vol. 153, no. 1, pp. 38–45, 2015.

[40] M. P. Gaspar, J. Lou, P. M. Kane, S. M. Jacoby, A. L. Osterman, and R. W. Culp, "Complications following partial and total wrist arthroplasty: a single-center retrospective review," *Journal of Hand Surgery*, vol. 41, no. 1, pp. 47–53.e4, 2016.

[41] D. Dellacqua, "Total wrist arthroplasty," *Techniques in Orthopaedics*, vol. 24, no. 1, pp. 49–57, 2009.

[42] M. Sagerfors, A. Gupta, O. Brus, and K. Pettersson, "Total wrist arthroplasty: a single-center study of 219 cases with 5-year follow-up," *Journal of Hand Surgery*, vol. 40, no. 12, pp. 2380–2387, 2015.

[43] M. Sagerfors, A. Gupta, O. Brus, M. Rizzo, and K. Pettersson, "Patient related functional outcome after total wrist arthroplasty: a single center study of 206 cases," *Hand Surgery*, vol. 20, no. 1, pp. 81–87, 2015.

[44] O. Reigstad and M. Røkkum, "Wrist arthroplasty: where do we stand today? A review of historic and contemporary designs," *Hand Surgery*, vol. 19, no. 2, pp. 311–322, 2014.

[45] B. D. Adams, B. P. Kleinhenz, and J. J. Guan, "Wrist arthrodesis for failed total wrist arthroplasty," *Journal of Hand Surgery*, vol. 41, no. 6, pp. 673–679, 2016.

[46] J. A. Nydick, S. M. Greenberg, J. D. Stone, B. Williams, J. A. Polikandriotis, and A. V. Hess, "Clinical outcomes of total wrist arthroplasty," *Journal of Hand Surgery*, vol. 37, no. 8, pp. 1580–1584, 2012.

Solitary Spinal Epidural Metastasis from Gastric Cancer

Taisei Sako,[1] Yasuaki Iida,[1] Yuichirou Yokoyama,[1] Shintaro Tsuge,[1] Keiji Hasegawa,[1] Akihito Wada,[1] Tetsuo Mikami,[2] and Hiroshi Takahashi[1]

[1]*Department of Orthopaedic Surgery, Toho University School of Medicine, Tokyo, Japan*
[2]*Department of Pathology, Toho University School of Medicine, Tokyo, Japan*

Correspondence should be addressed to Hiroshi Takahashi; drkan@med.toho-u.ac.jp

Academic Editor: Eyal Itshayek

Solitary epidural space metastasis of a malignant tumor is rare. We encountered a 79-year-old male patient with solitary metastatic epidural tumor who developed paraplegia and dysuria. The patient had undergone total gastrectomy for gastric cancer followed by chemotherapy 8 months priorly. The whole body was examined for suspected metastatic spinal tumor, but no metastases of the spine or important organs were observed, and a solitary mass was present in the thoracic spinal epidural space. The mass was excised for diagnosis and treatment and was histopathologically diagnosed as metastasis from gastric cancer. No solitary metastatic epidural tumor from gastric cancer has been reported in English. Among the Japanese, 3 cases have been reported, in which the outcome was poor in all cases and no definite diagnosis could be made before surgery in any case. Our patient developed concomitant pneumonia after surgery and died shortly after the surgery. When a patient has a past medical history of malignant tumor, the possibility of a solitary metastatic tumor in the epidural space should be considered.

1. Introduction

In most cases of metastatic epidural tumor the tumor expanding from a vertebral metastasis grows into the spinal canal, and solitary epidural metastasis of a malignant tumor is rare. We encountered a patient with a solitary metastatic epidural tumor from gastric cancer and with no vertebral metastasis.

2. Case Report

The patient was a 79-year-old man with the chief complaints of paraplegia and dysuria.

Bilateral muscle weakness of the lower limbs developed with no known cause in October 20××. The symptoms gradually became aggravated, and it became difficult for the patient to stand up from November. Dysuria appeared after several days and activities of daily living also became difficult. Thus, the patient was urgently admitted for close examination and treatment.

The patient had a past medical history of gastric cancer and had undergone total gastrectomy in March, followed by postoperative chemotherapy (combination of oral 5FU preparation S-1 + cisplatin) from April to July.

The muscle strength of the lower limbs on admission was MMT3 in all of the bilateral iliopsoas, quadriceps, tibialis anterior, extensor hallucis longus, and flexor hallucis longus muscles, showing complete bilateral muscle weakness of the lower limbs. Regarding sensation, 1/10 hypaesthesia was noted in the T4 or lower regions. The bilateral patellar tendon and Achilles tendon reflexes were normal, and Babinski and Chaddock reflexes were negative. Since difficulty in urination and abdominal distension were noted, urethral catheterization was performed, and 1400 mL of urine was drained.

On blood testing, WBC was 4,200/μL and CRP was 0.6 mg/dL, showing a mild inflammatory response, Hgb was 9.9 g/dL, and Plt was $10.9 \times 10^4 \mu$L, showing pancytopenia. LDH was 275 IU/L, AST was 33 IU/L, and ALT was 59 IU/L, indicating elevation of liver enzymes. ALP was 355 IU/L, and Ca was 8.0 mg/dL. With respect to tumor markers, CEA, CA19-9, and AFP were increased to 15.2 ng/mL, 1,420 U/mL, and 1,034 ng/mL, respectively.

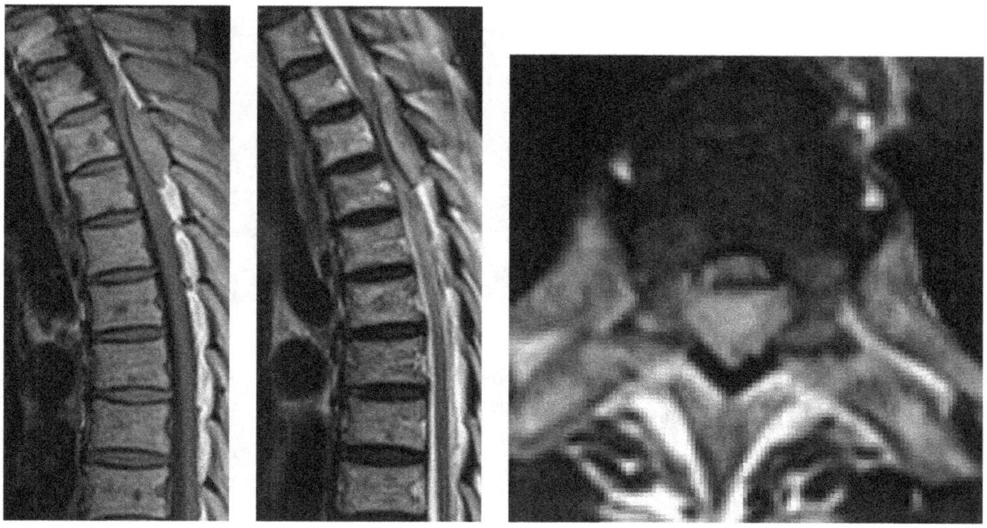

(a) Sagittal T1 WI (b) Sagittal T2 WI (c) Axial T2 WI

FIGURE 1: Thoracic spine MRI before operation. A thoracic epidural mass lesion was evident showing low intensity on the T1 weighted image and iso-high intensity on the T2 weighted image.

On cerebrospinal fluid testing, the fluid was transparent, and the cell count was elevated to 32/μL (polymorphonuclear leukocyte: 81%, mononuclear cell: 19%). The glucose and protein levels were increased to 104 mg/dL and 181 mg/dL, respectively. CEA was <0.50 ng/dL, which was within the normal range. No malignant findings were noted on cerebrospinal fluid cytology, which was judged as Class I.

On thoracic spinal plain radiography, no apparent abnormal findings, that is, osteolytic findings of the vertebrae and pedicle sign, were noted. On thoracic spinal MRI, a low-isointensity region was observed in the dorsal dura mater on T1-weighted imaging and an iso-high intensity mass lesion was observed on T2-weighted imaging at the T2–4 level; the lesion excluded the dural canal from the dorsal side (Figure 1). On head, chest, and abdominal CT, head and spinal MRI, and PET, no apparent mass lesions other than the thoracic spinal epidural mass were observed (Figure 2).

Paralysis progressed from Frankel C to A at 4 days after admission, and emergency surgery was performed to treat the epidural occupying lesion of the thoracic spine. Laminectomy and tumor excision were applied at the T2–5 level. A grayish white tumorous lesion was present in the dorsal dura mater and markedly obstructed the dural canal from the posterior side. The tumor parenchymal tissue was fragile and hemorrhagic. Since adhesion between the dura mater and tumor was marked, en bloc excision was attempted but was difficult, and the lesion was resected piece by piece as much as possible, and sufficient decompression of the dural canal was achieved.

On pathological examination, outgrowth of cells containing swollen nuclei to a solid tumor was observed, with a few gland duct-like structures. Alcian-blue staining-positive mucus production was observed, suggesting poorly differentiated adenocarcinoma (Figure 3). The histology of the lesion was similar to that of lymph node metastasis, which is observed in gastric cancer surgery, suggesting metastasis from gastric cancer.

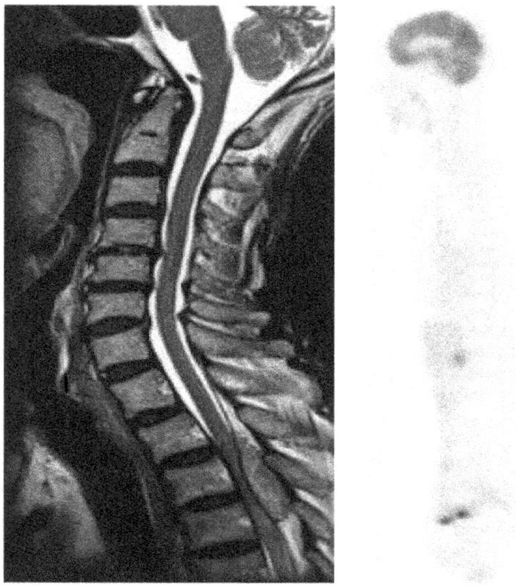

(a) Cervical spine MRI (b) PET-CT

FIGURE 2: No apparent mass lesions other than the thoracic spinal epidural mass were observed.

The neurologic manifestation did not improve after surgery. The lesion was clinically diagnosed as metastatic tumor of gastric cancer, and treatment with irradiation and chemotherapy were suggested; however, best supportive care was selected because the general condition was poor due to the complication with pneumonia. Ultimately, pneumonia-aggravated, disseminated intravascular coagulation (DIC) occurred, and the patient died 27 days after admission.

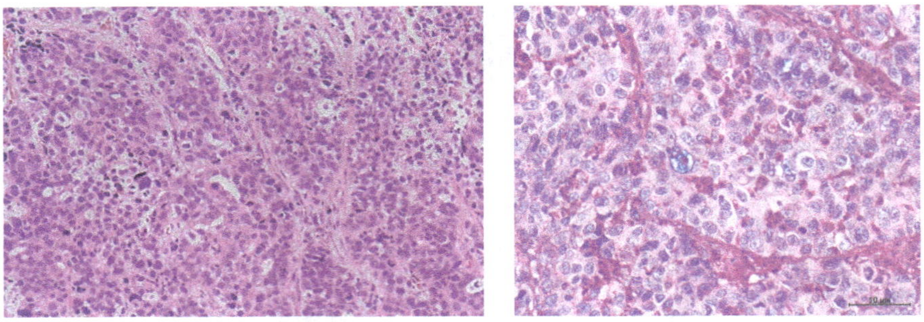

(a) (b)

FIGURE 3: (a) Hematoxylin and eosin (HE) staining showed outgrowth of cells containing swollen nuclei to a solid tumor which was observed, with a few gland duct-like structures (×400). (b) Alcian-blue staining-positive mucus production was observed, suggesting poorly differentiated adenocarcinoma (×400).

3. Discussion

When a patient with a past medical history of a malignant tumor develops spinal paralysis during the course of treatment, metastatic spinal tumor-associated paralysis should be the primary suspected etiology.

Since our patient had a past medical history of malignant tumor, head, chest, and abdominal CT, head and spinal MRI, and PET were performed in consideration of spinal metastasis. However, no apparent mass lesion, other than the thoracic spinal epidural mass, was noted. The sensitivities and specificities of MRI and PET for metastatic bone tumor screening are high, and those of MRI have been reported to be 91 and 95%, respectively, compared with 90 and 97%, respectively, for PET [1, 2]. Furthermore, the cerebrospinal fluid cytology finding was Class 1, indicating that this case was not a metastatic vertebral tumor but that it was likely to be a hematoma, abscess, or an epidural lesion. After admission, the paralysis worsened rapidly, and surgery was performed to local regions or via the cerebrospinal fluid. The pathological findings of the excised specimen did not contradict the features of metastasis from gastric cancer, and it was diagnosed as a solitary metastatic epidural tumor from gastric cancer.

Regarding the route of metastasis to the spine, Batson [3] proposed that an epidural internal vertebral venous plexus and a vertebral venous plexus distributing in the vertebra communicate closely and that slow blood flow transports cancer cells allowing them to implant in the spine. In other local metastatic routes, tumor cells infiltrate directly from local regions or reach via the cerebrospinal fluid; although this is not common [4]. In our patient, the route was not infiltration through spinal metastasis, but it was assumed to be solitary metastasis to the epidural space via the Batson venous plexus.

While there have been no English language reports on solitary metastatic epidural tumor from gastric cancer in PubMed, 3 cases, excluding the current case, have been reported in Japan [5–7].

No definite diagnosis was made before surgery in any of these reported cases, and laminectomy and tumor resection were performed without radiotherapy. The survival time was short (from < one month to about 5 months) (Table 1).

Metastatic epidural spinal cord compression (MESCC) was first reported by Spiller in 1925 [8]. Metastatic cancer lesions typically develop in the vertebra or epidural space and induce secondary spinal cord compression. Regarding the mechanism of the pathogenesis, tumor cells cause vertebral metastasis through the circulation in the early phase and reach the spinal cord via an indirect route in about 85% of cases [9, 10], and the paravertebral tumor grows into the spinal canal through the intervertebral foramen leading to direct compression of the spinal cord in about 15% of all cases [9, 11]. Our case exhibited spinal cord paralysis, which was induced by solitary epidural metastasis, and its development did not occur through either mechanism of MESCC. MESCC has been reported to be a common complication that develops in 2.5–5% of terminal cancer patients within 2 years before death [12–14] and the annual incidence has been reported to be 3.4% among hospitalized patients [15]. Gastric cancer patients accounted for 1-2% of patients who developed MESCC [1, 16, 17], thus, a relatively low rate. In our patient, MESCC was due to the solitary metastatic epidural tumor from gastric cancer, which could be considered very rare.

Rades et al. [17] scored the survival rate of 29 gastric cancer-associated MESCC patients, based on clinical factors, and established an index to predict outcome. Specifically, Rades et al. investigated vertebral body metastasis-induced spinal cord compression. The four cases reported in Japan, including our patient, exhibited spinal cord paralysis induced by solitary metastatic epidural tumor, and the pathogenetic mechanism was different from that of MESCC. However, when our patient was scored, one item, rapidity of developing weakness of legs, was met and the 6-month survival rate was predicted to be 20%. Thus, although the pathogenetic mechanism is different, the survival predicting score developed for gastric cancer patients by Rades et al. may also be applicable for this disease.

We were not able to make a definite diagnosis before surgery, just as it was not previously possible in cases of solitary metastatic epidural tumor from gastric cancer. Surgery

Table 1: Prior case report of solitary spinal epidural metastasis from gastric cancer in Japan.

Author	Year	Age	Gender	Levels	Postoperative survival period
Yoshikawa [5]	1960	73	Female	T4-5	1 M
Yamaguchi and Usumoto [6]	1965	36	Male	L5	2 M
Sato et al. [7]	1990	58	Male	L3	5 M
Our case	2015	79	Male	T2–4	<1 M

was performed to improve the progression of paralysis, but if it could have been diagnosed definitively, avoidance of surgery would have been an option because of the prediction of a poor outcome. In the light of our experience with this patient, when a similar case is encountered, the applicability of surgery should be investigated after obtaining sufficient informed consent.

4. Conclusion

We encountered a patient with a solitary metastatic epidural tumor from gastric cancer. Although it is difficult to make a definite diagnosis, this tumor should be kept in mind to be included in the differential diagnosis when surgery is selected.

Consent

Written informed consent was obtained from the guardian for publication of this case report and accompanying images.

Competing Interests

The authors declare there is no conflict of interests.

References

[1] L.-M. Wu, H.-Y. Gu, J. Zheng et al., "Diagnostic value of whole-body magnetic resonance imaging for bone metastases: a systematic review and meta-analysis," *Journal of Magnetic Resonance Imaging*, vol. 34, no. 1, pp. 128–135, 2011.

[2] H.-L. Yang, T. Liu, X.-M. Wang, Y. Xu, and S.-M. Deng, "Diagnosis of bone metastases: a meta-analysis comparing ^{18}FDG PET, CT, MRI and bone scintigraphy," *European Radiology*, vol. 21, no. 12, pp. 2604–2617, 2011.

[3] O. V. Batson, "The function of the vertebral veins and their role in the spread of metastases," *Annals of Surgery*, vol. 112, pp. 138–149, 1940.

[4] G. Toshkezi, M. A. Galgano, S. Libohova, and S. Marawar, "Isolated spinal metastasis with spinal cord compression leads to a diagnosis of a follicular thyroid carcinoma," *Cureus*, vol. 7, no. 10, article e346, 2015.

[5] K. Yoshikawa, "A case of metastatic spinal epidural cancer," *Seikeigeka*, vol. 11, pp. 972–974, 1960 (Japanese).

[6] H. Yamaguchi and J. Usumoto, "A case of metastatic spinal epidural cancer," *Seikeigeka*, vol. 16, pp. 1170–11174, 1965 (Japanese).

[7] T. Sato, S. Shichino, Y. Akita et al., "A case of metastatic spinal epidural tumor from gastric cancer," *The Japanese Journal of Gastroenterological Surgery*, vol. 23, no. 5, pp. 1144–1148, 1990.

[8] W. G. Spiller, "Rapidly progressive paralysis associated with carcinoma," *Archives of Neurology & Psychiatry*, vol. 13, p. 471, 1925.

[9] J. S. Cole and R. A. Patchell, "Metastatic epidural spinal cord compression," *The Lancet Neurology*, vol. 7, no. 5, pp. 459–466, 2008.

[10] P. R. Algra, J. J. Heimans, J. Valk, J. J. Nauta, M. Lachniet, and B. V. Kooten, "Do metastases in vertebrae begin in the body or the pedicles? Imaging study in 45 patients," *American Journal of Roentgenology*, vol. 158, no. 6, pp. 1275–1279, 1992.

[11] R. W. Gilbert, J. H. Kim, and J. B. Posner, "Epidural spinal cord compression from metastatic tumor: diagnosis and treatment," *Annals of Neurology*, vol. 3, no. 1, pp. 40–51, 1978.

[12] D. Prasad and D. Schiff, "Malignant spinal-cord compression," *The Lancet Oncology*, vol. 6, no. 1, pp. 15–24, 2005.

[13] D. A. Loblaw, N. J. Laperriere, and W. J. Mackillop, "A population-based study of malignant spinal cord compression in Ontario," *Clinical Oncology*, vol. 15, no. 4, pp. 211–217, 2003.

[14] F. Bach, B. H. Larsen, K. Rohde et al., "Metastatic spinal cord compression. Occurrence, symptoms, clinical presentations and prognosis in 398 patients with spinal cord compression," *Acta Neurochirurgica*, vol. 107, no. 1-2, pp. 37–43, 1990.

[15] K. S. Mak, L. K. Lee, R. H. Mak et al., "Incidence and treatment patterns in hospitalizations for malignant spinal cord compression in the United States, 1998–2006," *International Journal of Radiation Oncology, Biology, Physics*, vol. 80, no. 3, pp. 824–831, 2011.

[16] D. Rades and J. L. Abrahm, "The role of radiotherapy for metastatic epidural spinal cord compression," *Nature Reviews Clinical Oncology*, vol. 7, no. 10, pp. 590–598, 2010.

[17] D. Rades, S. Huttenlocher, T. Bartscht, and S. E. Schild, "Predicting the survival probability of gastric cancer patients developing metastatic epidural spinal cord compression (MESCC)," *Gastric Cancer*, vol. 18, no. 4, pp. 881–884, 2015.

17

Bilateral Simultaneous Quadriceps Tendon Rupture in a 24-Year-Old Obese Patient: A Case Report and Review of the Literature

Fahad H. Abduljabbar,[1,2] Abdulaziz Aljurayyan,[1,3] Bayan Ghalimah,[1,2] and Lawrence Lincoln[1]

[1] *Division of Orthopedic Surgery, St. Mary's Hospital Center, McGill University, 3830 Lacombe Avenue, Montreal, QC, Canada H3T 1M5*
[2] *Department of Orthopedic Surgery, King Abdulaziz University, Abdullah Sulayman St., Al Jamiah District, Jeddah 80200, Saudi Arabia*
[3] *Department of Orthopedic Surgery, King Saud University, Riyadh 12372, Saudi Arabia*

Correspondence should be addressed to Fahad H. Abduljabbar; fahad.abduljabbar@mail.mcgill.ca

Academic Editor: Dimitrios S. Karataglis

Introduction. Simultaneous bilateral quadriceps tendon ruptures (SBQTR) are uncommon knee injuries and most frequently occur in male patients, over 50 years of age. It can be associated with one or more predisposing risk factors like obesity, steroids use, and hyperparathyroidism. The main focus of this paper is to review SBQTR in obese patients. *Case Report.* We are reporting the youngest patient in the literature to date, a 24-year-old obese male patient, who presented to the emergency department complaining of bilateral knee pain and inability to walk after a fall during a basketball game. His clinical examination revealed the presence of a palpable suprapatellar gap and loss of knee extension bilaterally. Magnetic resonance imaging (MRI) confirmed that both of his quadriceps tendons were ruptured. A day after his diagnosis, the patient underwent successful operative repair followed by rehabilitation. At the two-year follow-up, the patient had full strength of both quadriceps muscles with no extension lag. *Conclusion.* The diagnosis of SBQTR can be challenging. Early diagnosis and treatment are associated with better functional outcome compared to delayed treatment. Physicians should have a high index of clinical suspicion in order not to miss such an injury and achieve favourable outcomes.

1. Introduction

Quadriceps tendon ruptures are not uncommon and occur typically in men older than 50 years old [1–4]. On the other hand, bilateral quadriceps tendons ruptures are rare [5]. Steiner and Palmer first described this entity in a 67-year-old man in 1949 [6]. However, some cases are reported in young patients with associated chronic illnesses [3, 7, 8]. Predisposing factors for quadriceps tendon rupture are numerous; these include diabetes mellitus, advanced age, obesity, chronic renal failure, hyperparathyroidism, systemic lupus erythematous, steroid use, gout, and pseudogout [9–13]. This report describes a 24-year-old male patient with simultaneous bilateral quadriceps tendons rupture (SBQTR) while playing basketball. To the best of our knowledge, this reports the youngest patient among other reports in the current literature.

2. Case Report

A 24-year-old male patient with a BMI of 35 kg/m^2 (height 185 cm; weight 120 kg) who presented to the emergency department with severe bilateral knee pain and inability to walk. The mechanism of injury was sport-related. While playing basketball, the patient jumped and eccentrically loaded his left knee followed by a popping sound. While trying to maintain his balance by putting his weight on the contralateral leg, he heard a second popping sound, then experienced severe bilateral knee pain, and was not able to stand. His past medical history was unremarkable, and he had no history of steroid or fluoroquinolone intake. He is an active person and plays basketball on weekly basis. He had no history of prodromal knee pain prior to his injury. Clinical examination revealed a palpable gap in the suprapatellar region and loss of knee extension bilaterally. Magnetic resonance imaging (MRI) confirmed the diagnosis, which was bilateral quadriceps tendons rupture (Figure 1).

A day after his diagnosis with SBQTR, he was taken to the operating room for surgical repair. We approached both knees through standard anterior midline incisions. Intra-operatively, we identified both tears at the osteotendinous junction. We debrided all the frayed tissue and then repaired both tendons surgically using number 5 FiberWire® sutures (Arthrex, Naples, Florida) in a Whipstitch fashion. The free ends of the sutures were passed through three drilled holes in each patella using a 2.5 mm drill in a vertical orientation. These 3 holes were drilled using an anterior cruciate ligament (ACL) tibial tunnel guide which is used during this aspect of the procedure to manoeuvre the drill more accurately to the desired endpoint [21]. Using the tunnel guide decreases the risk of violating the articular surface, reduces the number of passes required to obtain an optimal position, minimizes injury to the patellar tendon, and eliminates the additional step of retrieving sutures through drill holes [21]. The drill is then replaced with a Beath pin. The inner limb of each suture is passed through the central tunnel, and then the outer limb is passed through the outer tunnels. All free limbs of the suture on both ends of the tendon were tied with the knee in full extension. We also found a complete retinacular tear in the left knee and only a small longitudinal split in the right knee and both were repaired using a number 1 absorbable suture.

Postoperatively, both knees were protected in a knee immobilizer. The patient was allowed to bear weight as tolerated in full extension with the aid of crutches on both lower extremities. He started physiotherapy at 4 weeks to regain his knee range of motion (ROM) and quadriceps muscle strength. At the two-year follow-up, he had full quadriceps muscle strength with no extension lag (Figure 2), and his ROM was from 0 to 120 degrees bilaterally (Figure 3). At this point, the patient already resumed all his sport activities including playing basketball without limitations.

3. Discussion

Quadriceps tendon rupture (QTR) is not an uncommon occurrence and usually happens in male patients over 50 years old [2, 5, 8, 22]. The overall incidence of quadriceps tendon injuries is 1.37/100.000 [23]. They represent a big percentage of extensor mechanism injuries especially in patients older than 50 years old. Garner et al. reviewed extensor knee injuries over a 25-year period and found that 28.9% of them are quadriceps tendon ruptures [24]. Fortunately, simultaneous bilateral quadriceps tendons rupture (SBQTR) is rare and only 30% to 35% of them are spontaneous [19, 25]. Sometimes SBQTR can be associated with predisposing medical conditions including chronic renal disease, hyperparathyroidism, gout, systemic lupus erythematosus, diabetes mellitus, steroid use, obesity, and advanced age [8, 22, 26, 27]. In addition to that, there are other less common factors such as fluoroquinolones use, severe osteomalacia, and amyloidosis [22, 28]. Despite being associated with known predisposing risk factors, SBQTR can still occur in healthy individuals [8, 27].

In this paper, we are reporting the youngest patient in the literature with SBQRT secondary to a sport-related injury and obesity. The focus of this review will be on all reported cases of SBQRT in obese patients in the current literature. Obesity is one of the common risk factors for SBQRT. In a meta-analysis by Neubauer, obesity represented 10% of all reported risk factors for SBQRT [19]. With the modern sedentary life style and change in diet habits, obesity prevalence is on the rise. According to the National Health and Nutrition Examination Survey (NHANES), the obesity prevalence was relatively low and stable between 1960 and 1980 but more than doubled from 15% in 1980 to 34% in 2006 [29]. The WHO estimates that in 2005 approximately 1.6 billion people worldwide were overweight and that at least 400 million adults were obese. They further project that, by 2015, approximately 2.3 billion adults will be overweight and that at least 700 million will be obese [29]. These numbers are alarming as it could reflect the increased chance of having bilateral quadriceps tendon rupture in those obese patients. Yet there are no epidemiological studies to prove that.

Review of the English literature revealed slightly more than 100 cases of BQRT [9, 30]. Out of all reported patients, we identified 13 obese patients including the patient in this report with a mean age of 53 years (range, 24–75 years) (Table 1) [2, 3, 6, 14–20]. In the remaining 12 patients, the mechanism of injury was a mechanical fall in eleven patients and a spontaneous rupture while climbing stairs in one patient. Shah et al. showed in his review that these injuries happened spontaneously in patients with predisposing medical conditions while the remainder happened secondary to a significant eccentric loading of the tendons with the knee in a flexed position due to falling or participating in sports, more commonly basketball [8, 22, 25, 27, 31]. Six out of the 13 patients had other medical comorbidities in association with obesity. Apart from diagnostic difficulties, obesity itself may have a direct effect on the integrity of the tendon by causing fatty degeneration [7, 8, 28]. More importantly, the increased weight adds significant loading on the tendon, especially if eccentrically loaded (with a semiflexed knee) [18, 32].

Given the rare occurrence of these injuries, early diagnosis can present a challenge to the treating physician. Perfitt et al. reported that 67% of patients were misdiagnosed at their initial presentation [33]. The enlarged soft tissue envelope in obese patients can obscure the suprapatellar gap and make the diagnosis of QTR more challenging. Neubauer et al. reported 23 cases with delayed diagnosis of bilateral simultaneous rupture of the quadriceps tendon and they found that obesity was found most frequently among risk factors (21.4%) [19]. It is also common to misdiagnose ruptures in the elderly population. Strokes, occult fracture, rheumatoid arthritis, bilateral effusion, and other medical causes that may contribute to their inability to move their legs and therefore make

Table 1: Reported obese patients with SBQTR.

References	Age/sex	Mechanism of injury	Location of tear	Time before diagnosis	Risk factor(s)	BMI	Outcome
Steiner and Palmer, 1949 [6]	67/M	Slip and fall	NM	2 days	Obesity	NM	Ambulatory with AD after 5 weeks
Dalal and Whittam, 1966 [14]	63/M	Fall	OT	The same day	Obesity	NM	Extensor lag at 10 weeks
Firooznia et al., 1973 [15]	62/M	Fall	MT	NM	Obesity/DM	NM	NM
Julius, 1984 [3]	58/M	Fall	MT	The same day	Obesity	NM	Full ROM at 4 months
Dhar, 1988 [2]	75/M	Fall	MT	7 days	Obesity/HTN	NM	Extensor lag & ambulatory with AD at 4 months
	61/M	Fall	NM	2 days	Obesity	NM	Full ROM at 5 months
Nabors and Kremchek, 1995 [16]	43/M	Fall	OT & MT	2 weeks	Obesity	NM	Ambulatory with AD at 6 months
El-Zahaar, 1995 [17]	61/F	Fall	NM	The same day	Obesity/osteoporosis	NM	After 7 months, LT knee: 15 degrees of extension lag, RT knee: 20 degrees of extension lag, walks with a cane
Kelly et al., 2001 [18]	52/M	Fall	OT	The same day	Obesity	50.21	After 6 month, LT knee: 10 degrees of extension lag, RT knee: 25 degrees of extension lag
Neubauer et al., 2007 [19]	52/M	Fall	OT	4 weeks	Obesity/HTN	NM	Decreased ROM with good strength at 14 months
	30/M	Fall	OT	3 days	Obesity	NM	Full ROM & strength at 21 months
LaRocco et al., 2008 [20]	52/M	Walking up a flight of stairs	NM	2 days	Obesity/DM/HTN	NM	NM
Abduljabbar et al.	24/M	Sport injury	OT	The same day	Obesity	35	Full ROM & strength with no extension lag at 4 months. Back to sports at 1 year post-op

MT: musculotendinous junction, OT: osteotendinous junction, NM: not mentioned, AD: assistive device, ROM: range of motion, DM: diabetes mellitus, HTN: hypertension, LT: left, and RT: right.

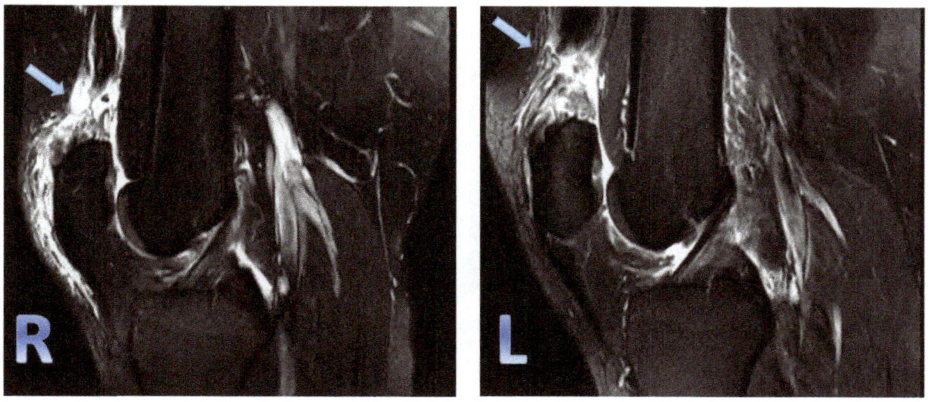

FIGURE 1: MRI of right and left knees showing T2-weighted sagittal image and demonstrating a full-thickness tear of the quadriceps tendon at the osteotendinous junction and fluid within the tendon gap with some retraction of the tendon which is more pronounced on the left side.

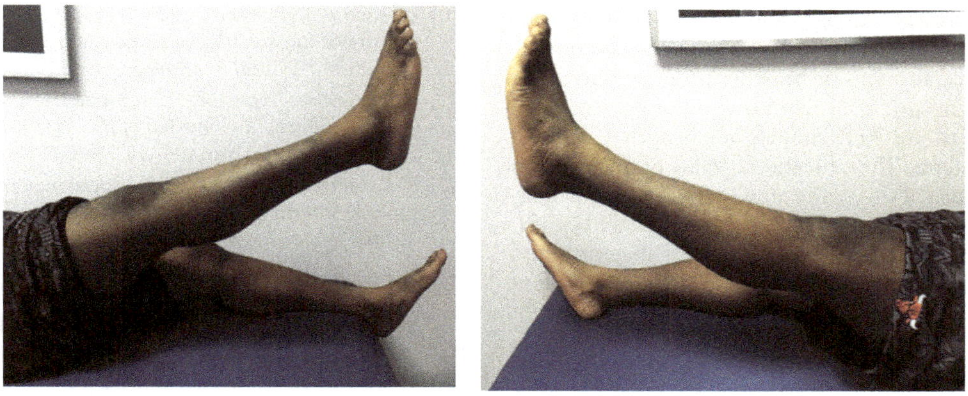

FIGURE 2: Clinical photos showing full active extension 2 years postoperatively without extension lag.

it difficult to perform an appropriate extensor mechanism examination [18]. Failure to diagnose the injury from the initial presentation can delay the appropriate treatment and lead to a suboptimal clinical outcome [5, 27, 34]. To diagnose a quadriceps tendon rupture (QTR), the treating physician must obtain a thorough history and physical examination and supplement it with the appropriate imaging if required. Mechanism of the injury, predisposing medical conditions, and steroid use are key elements of the history. In the physical examination, the presence of knee pain, effusion, palpable suprapatellar gap, and extensor mechanism insufficiency can lead to the diagnosis [22, 26, 27]. Intact extensor mechanism can be misleading at times; this can happen in cases of QTR with intact medial and lateral retinacula; in these cases, further workup is required [35].

The knee extensor mechanism is evaluated while the patient is supine or sitting on the edge of the bed. The patient is asked to actively extend the knee. In some circumstances where the patient can not actively extend the knee, the physician can passively extend the knee lifting the heel off the bed and ask the patient to keep the knee extended. Failure to actively extend the knee or maintain a straight leg can indicate a dysfunction in the extensor mechanism. In the prone position, the knee can be flexed from a 90° position because of an intact hamstring mechanism, but extension will be impaired if the knee is flexed beyond 90° [36]. Further knee examination may show effusion and tenderness to palpation. The patella may be displaced and very mobile. A suprapatellar gap or depression may be palpated. The depression may be increased with active quadriceps muscle contraction. This is useful because an associated hemarthrosis can sometimes mask the suprapatellar gap [37].

Imaging can confirm the diagnosis if, in doubt, plain films, ultrasound (US), and MRI are valid and available options. Plain films are readily available in the emergency room and usually obtained routinely to rule out common differential diagnoses like fractures around the knee and particularly patellar fractures. Paying attention to subtle findings on the plain films like soft tissue defects and avulsed bone fragments at the very end of the quadriceps muscle, patella baja and knee effusion can facilitate the diagnosis of QTR [27, 38, 39]. Ultrasound has the advantages of being cheaper and easier to get compared to MRI; however, it is operator dependent and the diagnosis can be missed if performed by an inexperienced sonographer [20, 39]. MRI remains the modality of choice, as Perfitt et al. showed in his study that it has a 100% sensitivity and specificity with a positive predictive value of 100 in detecting a quadriceps tendon rupture compared to US

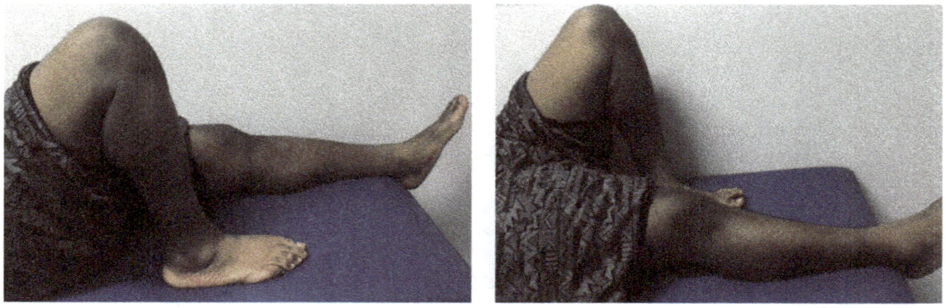

FIGURE 3: Clinical photos 2 years postoperatively showing full range of motion (0–120 degrees).

[33, 35, 39], but increased cost and limited availability of MRI in the emergency setting are major limitations [20, 39].

The goal of the treating physician should be early diagnosis and surgical repair. Several studies suggested that early surgical repair and physiotherapy will result in superior outcomes compared to delayed repair [26, 27]. Emergency physicians, family physicians, and orthopedic surgeons should be familiar with diagnosing QTR from the initial presentation. Although very rare, SBQTR should be suspected even in young healthy patients. The educational value of this paper is to increase awareness of this entity among treating physicians, especially in obese patients in whom diagnosis might be difficult due to increased soft tissue envelope. Early diagnosis and early surgical management are crucial to achieve excellent outcome comparable to unilateral injuries.

Competing Interests

The authors declare that there is no conflict of interests regarding the publication of this paper.

References

[1] M. Chiu and E. S. Forman, "Bilateral quadriceps tendon rupture: a rare finding in a healthy man after minimal trauma," *Orthopedics*, vol. 33, no. 3, 2010.

[2] S. Dhar, "Bilateral, simultaneous, spontaneous rupture of the quadriceps tendon. A report of 3 cases and a review of the literature," *Injury*, vol. 19, no. 1, pp. 7–8, 1988.

[3] A. J. Julius, "Rupture of the quadriceps tendon," *The Netherlands Journal of Surgery*, vol. 36, no. 5, pp. 134–136, 1984.

[4] B. T. Rougraff, C. C. Reeck, and J. Essenmacher, "Complete quadriceps tendon ruptures," *Orthopedics*, vol. 19, no. 6, pp. 509–514, 1996.

[5] P. Ellanti, N. Davarinos, S. Morris, and J. Rice, "Bilateral synchronous rupture of the quadriceps tendon," *Irish Journal of Medical Science*, vol. 181, no. 3, pp. 423–425, 2012.

[6] C. A. Steiner and L. H. Palmer, "Simultaneous bilateral rupture of the quadriceps tendon," *The American Journal of Surgery*, vol. 78, no. 5, pp. 752–755, 1949.

[7] W. J. Ribbans and P. D. Angus, "Simultaneous bilateral rupture of the quadriceps tendon," *The British Journal of Clinical Practice*, vol. 43, no. 3, pp. 122–125, 1989.

[8] M. Shah and N. Jooma, "Simultaneous bilateral quadriceps tendon rupture while playing basketball," *British Journal of Sports Medicine*, vol. 36, no. 2, pp. 152–153, 2002.

[9] M. Lotem, M. D. Robson, and J. B. Rosenfeld, "Spontaneous rupture of the quadriceps tendon in patients on chronic haemodialysis," *Annals of the Rheumatic Diseases*, vol. 33, no. 5, pp. 428–429, 1974.

[10] D. Novoa, R. Romero, and J. Forteza, "Spontaneous bilateral rupture of the quadriceps tendon in uremia and kidney transplantation," *Clinical Nephrology*, vol. 27, no. 1, p. 48, 1987.

[11] E. T. Preston, "Avulsion of both quadriceps tendons in hyperparathyroidism," *The Journal of the American Medical Association*, vol. 221, no. 4, pp. 406–407, 1972.

[12] R. E. Stern and S. F. Harwin, "Spontaneous and simultaneous rupture of both quadriceps tendons," *Clinical Orthopaedics and Related Research*, no. 147, pp. 188–189, 1980.

[13] R. J. Tedd, M. R. Norton, and W. G. Thomas, "Bilateral simultaneous atraumatic quadriceps tendon ruptures associated with 'pseudogout'," *Injury*, vol. 31, no. 6, pp. 467–469, 2000.

[14] V. D. Dalal and D. E. Whittam, "Bilateral simultaneous rupture of the quadriceps tendons," *British Medical Journal*, vol. 2, no. 526, article 1370, 1966.

[15] H. Firooznia, G. Seliger, R. Abrams, and M. Sanz, "Bilateral spontaneous and simultaneous rupture of the quadriceps tendon," *Bulletin of the Hospital for Joint Diseases Orthopaedic Institute*, vol. 34, no. 1, pp. 65–69, 1973.

[16] E. D. Nabors and T. E. Kremchek, "Bilateral rupture of the extensor mechanism of the knee in healthy adults," *Orthopedics*, vol. 18, no. 5, pp. 477–479, 1995.

[17] M. S. El-Zahaar, "Spontaneous rupture of the quadriceps tendon: ten case reports and a review of the literature with a hypothesis of a new classification of causes," *Journal of Neurological and Orthopaedic Medicine and Surgery*, vol. 16, no. 3, pp. 132–136, 1995.

[18] B. M. Kelly, N. Rao, S. S. Louis, B. T. Kostes, and R. M. Smith, "Bilateral, simultaneous, spontaneous rupture of quadriceps tendons without trauma in an obese patient: a case report," *Archives of Physical Medicine and Rehabilitation*, vol. 82, no. 3, pp. 415–418, 2001.

[19] T. Neubauer, M. Wagner, T. Potschka, and M. Riedl, "Bilateral, simultaneous rupture of the quadriceps tendon: a diagnostic pitfall? Report of three cases and meta-analysis of the literature," *Knee Surgery, Sports Traumatology, Arthroscopy*, vol. 15, no. 1, pp. 43–53, 2007.

[20] B. G. LaRocco, G. Zlupko, and P. Sierzenski, "Ultrasound diagnosis of quadriceps tendon rupture," *The Journal of Emergency Medicine*, vol. 35, no. 3, pp. 293–295, 2008.

[21] B. C. Ong and O. Sherman, "Acute patellar tendon rupture: a new surgical technique," *Arthroscopy*, vol. 16, no. 8, pp. 869–870, 2000.

[22] T. Katz, D. Alkalay, E. Rath, D. Atar, and S. Sukenik, "Bilateral simultaneous rupture of the quadriceps tendon in an adult amateur tennis player," *Journal of Clinical Rheumatology*, vol. 12, no. 1, pp. 32–33, 2006.

[23] R. A. E. Clayton and C. M. Court-Brown, "The epidemiology of musculoskeletal tendinous and ligamentous injuries," *Injury*, vol. 39, no. 12, pp. 1338–1344, 2008.

[24] M. R. Garner, E. Gausden, M. B. Berkes, J. T. Nguyen, and D. G. Lorich, "Extensor mechanism injuries of the knee: demographic characteristics and comorbidities from a review of 726 patient records," *The Journal of Bone & Joint Surgery—American Volume*, vol. 97, no. 19, pp. 1592–1596, 2015.

[25] M. K. Shah, "Simultaneous bilateral rupture of quadriceps tendons: analysis of risk factors and associations," *Southern Medical Journal*, vol. 95, no. 8, pp. 860–866, 2002.

[26] M.-F. Gao, H.-L. Yang, and W.-D. Shi, "Simultaneous bilateral quadriceps tendon rupture in a patient with hyperparathyroidism undergoing long-term haemodialysis: a case report and literature review," *The Journal of International Medical Research*, vol. 41, no. 4, pp. 1378–1383, 2013.

[27] A. Assiotis, I. Pengas, and K. Vemulapalli, "Bilateral quadriceps tendon rupture in a seasoned marathon runner with patellar spurs," *Grand Rounds*, vol. 11, no. 1, pp. 77–80, 2011.

[28] S. Kapoor, M. Agrawal, V. Jain, and B. Jain, "Spontaneous, simultaneous, bilateral quadriceps tendon rupture in a 16-year-old girl with severe osteomalacia," *Injury Extra*, vol. 37, no. 7, pp. 267–271, 2006.

[29] D. M. Nguyen and H. B. El-Serag, "The epidemiology of obesity," *Gastroenterology Clinics of North America*, vol. 39, no. 1, pp. 1–7, 2010.

[30] M. Omar, P. Haas, M. Ettinger, C. Krettek, and M. Petri, "Simultaneous bilateral quadriceps tendon rupture following long-term low-dose nasal corticosteroid application," *Case Reports in Orthopedics*, vol. 2013, 5 pages, 2013.

[31] D. I. Ilan, N. Tejwani, M. Keschner, and M. Leibman, "Quadriceps tendon rupture," *Journal of the American Academy of Orthopaedic Surgeons*, vol. 11, no. 3, pp. 192–200, 2003.

[32] M. Boublik, T. F. Schlegel, R. C. Koonce, J. W. Genuario, and J. D. Kinkartz, "Quadriceps tendon injuries in national football league players," *American Journal of Sports Medicine*, vol. 41, no. 8, pp. 1841–1846, 2013.

[33] J. S. Perfitt, M. J. Petrie, C. M. Blundell, and M. B. Davies, "Acute quadriceps tendon rupture: a pragmatic approach to diagnostic imaging," *European Journal of Orthopaedic Surgery and Traumatology*, vol. 24, no. 7, pp. 1237–1241, 2014.

[34] P. Keogh, S. J. Shanker, T. Burke, and R. J. O'Connell, "Bilateral simultaneous rupture of the quadriceps tendons. A report of four cases and review of the literature," *Clinical Orthopaedics and Related Research*, no. 234, pp. 139–141, 1988.

[35] E. Barasch, L. J. Lombardi, L. Arena, and E. Epstein, "MRI visualization of bilateral quadriceps tendon rupture in a patient with secondary hyperparathyroidism: implications for diagnosis and therapy," *Computerized Medical Imaging and Graphics*, vol. 13, no. 5, pp. 407–410, 1989.

[36] K. W. Siwek and J. P. Rao, "Bilateral simultaneous rupture of the quadriceps tendons," *Clinical Orthopaedics and Related Research*, vol. 131, pp. 252–254, 1978.

[37] B. O. Stephens and G. V. Anderson Jr., "Simultaneous bilateral quadriceps tendon rupture: a case report and subject review," *Journal of Emergency Medicine*, vol. 5, no. 6, pp. 481–485, 1987.

[38] A. E. Johnson and S. D. Rose, "Bilateral quadriceps tendon ruptures in a healthy, active duty soldier: case report and review of the literature," *Military Medicine*, vol. 171, no. 12, pp. 1251–1254, 2006.

[39] M. K. Shah, "Simultaneous bilateral quadriceps tendon rupture in renal patients," *Clinical Nephrology*, vol. 58, no. 2, pp. 118–121, 2002.

18

Ultrasound Guidance in Performing a Tendoscopic Surgery to Treat Posterior Tibial Tendinitis: A Useful Tool?

Akinobu Nishimura,[1] Shigeto Nakazora,[2] Aki Fukuda,[2] Ko Kato,[2] and Akihiro Sudo[3]

[1] *Department of Orthopaedic and Sports Medicine, Graduate School of Medicine, Mie University, 2-174 Edobashi, Tsu, Mie 514-8507, Japan*

[2] *Department of Orthopaedic Surgery, Suzuka Kaisei Hospital, 112 Kou, Suzuka, Mie 513-8505, Japan*

[3] *Department of Orthopaedic Surgery, Graduate School of Medicine, Mie University, 2-174 Edobashi, Tsu, Mie 514-8507, Japan*

Correspondence should be addressed to Akinobu Nishimura; meiten@clin.medic.mie-u.ac.jp

Academic Editor: Dimitrios S. Karataglis

A 25-year-old man with a pronation-external rotation type of fracture was surgically treated using a fibular plate. Five years later, he underwent resection of bone hyperplasia because of the ankle pain and limitation of range of motion. Thereafter, the left ankle became intermittently painful, which persisted for about one year. He presented at the age of 43 with persistent ankle pain. Physical and image analysis findings indicated a diagnosis of posttraumatic posterior tibial tendinitis, which we surgically treated using tendoscopy. Endoscopic findings showed tenosynovitis and fibrillation on the tendon surface. We cleaned and removed the synovium surrounding the tendon and deepened the posterior tibial tendon groove to allow sufficient space for the posterior tibial tendon. Full weight-bearing ambulation was permitted one day after surgery and he returned to his occupation in the construction industry six weeks after surgery. The medial aspect of the ankle was free of pain and symptoms at a review two years after surgery. Although tendoscopic surgery for stage 1 posterior tibial tendon dysfunction has been reported, tendoscopic surgery to treat posttraumatic posterior tibial tendinitis has not. Our experience with this patient showed that tendoscopic surgery is useful not only for stage 1 posterior tibial dysfunction, but also for posttraumatic posterior tibial tendinitis.

1. Introduction

Tendoscopy of the tendons around the posterior ankle joint can be technically demanding but can offer a unique perspective of pathological processes. Some tendoscopic procedures have recently been applied to the foot and ankle [1]. An endoscopic tendon procedure was first described by Wertheimer et al. [2] in 1995. van Dijk et al. described the application of tendoscopic surgery for the posterior tibial [3] and peroneal tendons [4]. Tendoscopic synovectomy can provide good control of stage 1 posterior tibial tendon dysfunction (PTTD) [5, 6]. On the other hand, damage to the posterior tibial tendon and/or its retinacula can be associated with ankle fractures [7, 8]. Stenosing tenosynovitis may follow ankle fractures. Here, we applied tendoscopic surgery to treat posttraumatic posterior tibial tendinitis.

2. Case Report

A 43-year-old male construction worker presented with left medial ankle pain. He fell and twisted the left ankle at the age of 25 years. Fibular fracture was diagnosed using simple X-rays and then he was admitted to the emergency department for open reduction and internal fixation using a fibular plate at a hospital near the accident location. Five years later, left ankle pain developed and the range of ankle motion became limited, so he underwent resection of bone hyperplasia. Thereafter, the left ankle became intermittently painful, which persisted for about one year.

The initial examination at our hospital (18 years after the ankle fracture and 43 years old at this time) revealed tenderness along the posterior tibial tendon and a left ankle range of motion from 10° of dorsiflexion to 60° of plantarflexion.

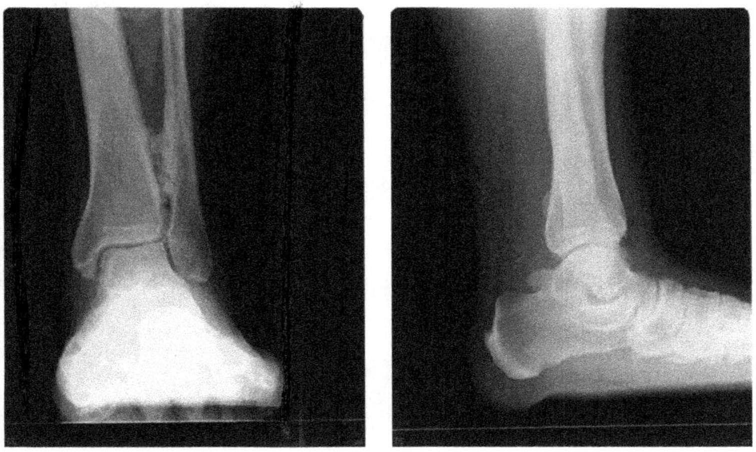

(a) (b)

FIGURE 1: Preoperative radiographic findings. Anteroposterior (a) and lateral (b) views while standing upright.

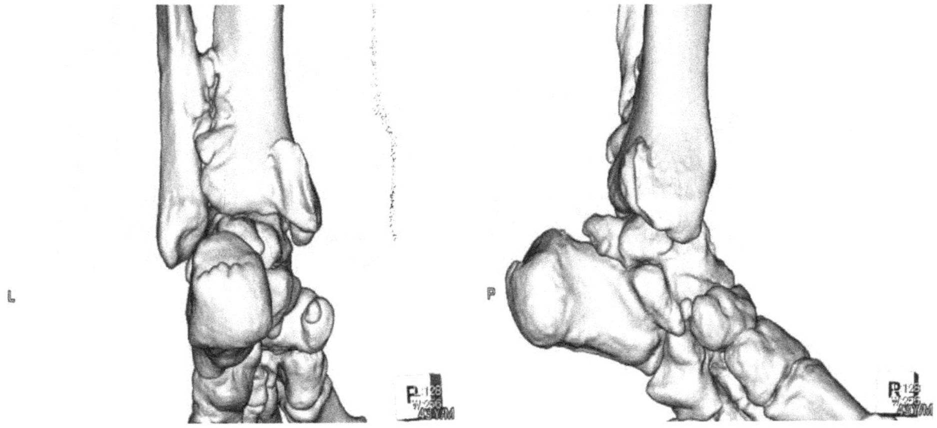

(a) (b)

FIGURE 2: Three-dimensional computed tomography findings. Posteroanterior (a) and medial-lateral (b) views while standing upright.

He was overweight at that time (his body mass index was 35.6 kg/m^2). The left foot was relatively flat, but too much toe sign was not visible and he could perform left single-leg heel raises. X-rays revealed bone hyperplasia between the distal tibia and fibula (Figure 1). Three-dimensional computed tomography (3D-CT) revealed tibial bone hyperplasia along the posterior tibial tendon (Figure 2). The posterior tibial tendon had spotted isointensity in regions of low intensity on T1-weighted magnetic resonance (MR) images and spotted high intensity in low-intensity T2-weighted images (Figure 3). Injecting lidocaine into the posterior tibial tendon sheath relieved the pain. Thus, we diagnosed posttraumatic posterior tibial tendinitis.

We planned a tendoscopic procedure instead of an open procedure because an open procedure needs opening the tendon sheath and postoperative immobilization such as a cast or brace. The patient underwent left posterior tibial tendoscopy using a 2.5 mm 30° arthroscope under spinal anesthesia. We used the two main portals described by van Dijk in 1997 [3]. The distal portal was 2 cm below and anterior to the medial malleolus, whereas the proximal portal was 2 cm posterior and superior to the medial malleolus. An ultrasound machine (Noblus; Hitachi Aloka, Tokyo, Japan) and a high-frequency linear probe (L64 linear probe 18–5 MHz; Hitachi Aloka) are prepared with a sterile ultrasound probe cover and sterile gel. We used an ultrasonography in order to introduce a scope easily, reliably, and safely. Irrigation solution was injected into the posterior tendon sheath under long-axis view along the posterior tibial tendon of sonography just before incising the skin (Figure 4). We opened the tendon sheath via the skin incision by blunt dissection using a hemostat under sonography. Tendoscopic findings revealed tenosynovitis and fibrillation on the surface of the tendon. We cleaned and removed the synovium surrounding the tendon using an arthroscopic shaver system and a radiofrequency wand for small joints (Figure 5). Moreover, we deepened the groove for the posterior tibial tendon using a bone cutter/shaver so as the posterior tibial tendon can move smoothly. After groove

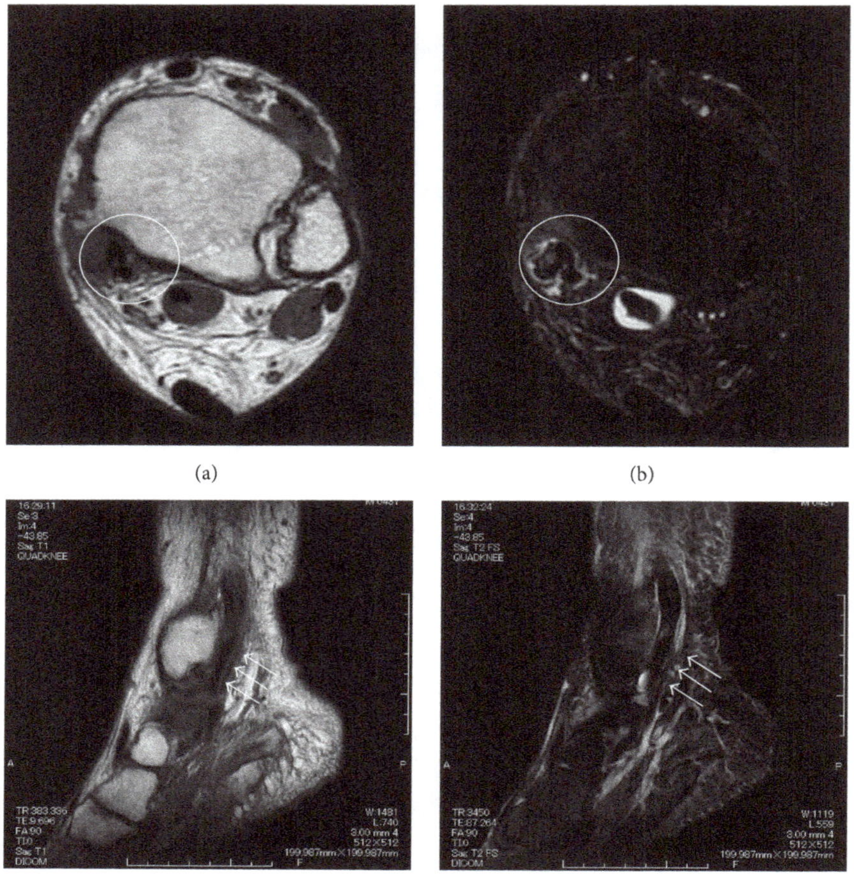

(a) (b) (c) (d)

Figure 3: Magnetic resonance imaging (MRI). (a) T1- and (b) T2-weighted represent axial images. (c) T1- and (d) T2-weighted represent sagittal images. Circle and arrow show the posterior tibial tendon.

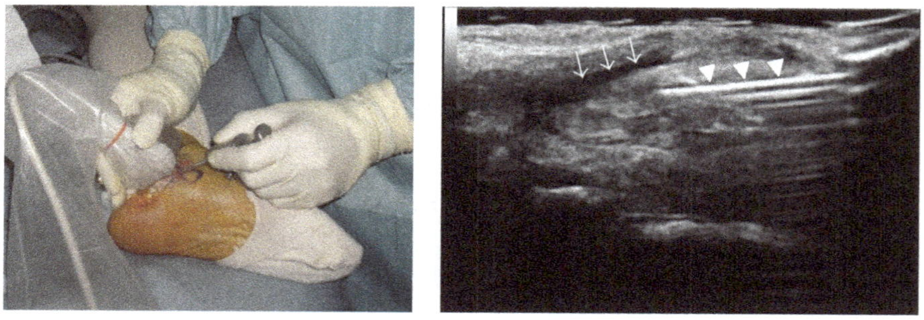

(a) (b)

Figure 4: Sonographic findings. Macroscopic (a) and sonographic (b) findings. Arrows show the irrigation fluid and arrowheads show the needle.

deepening, there was one- or two-millimeter space around the tendon. Weight-bearing ambulation was permitted one day after surgery and the patient returned to full-time work in the construction industry six weeks after surgery. At the most recent review two years after surgery, he had no medial symptoms and he was capable of all types of heavy work despite occasional slight pain related to sinus tarsi syndrome. His preoperative and postoperative scores on the American Orthopaedic Foot and Ankle Society (AOFAS) ankle-hindfoot scale were 71 and 90 points, respectively.

Each author certifies that his or her institution approved the human protocol for this investigation and that all investigations were conducted in conformity with ethical principles of research. The patient and his family were informed that

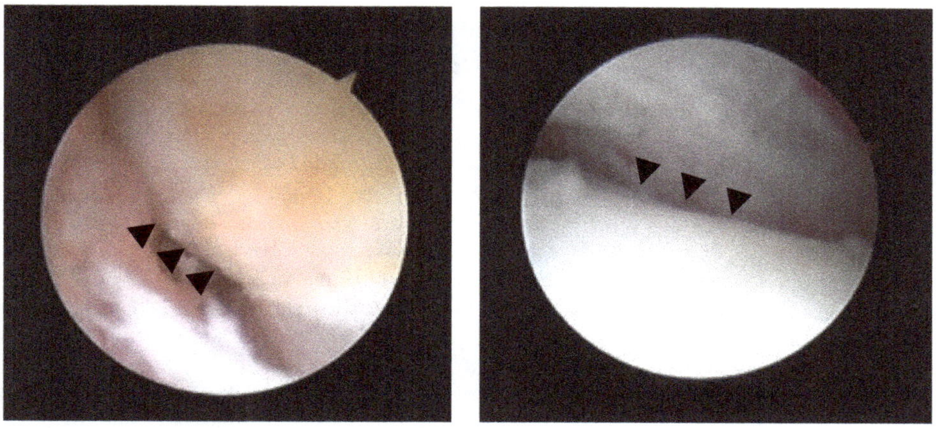

(a) (b)

FIGURE 5: Tendoscopic findings. Before (a) and after (b) synovectomy and groove deepening. Arrowheads show the posterior tibial tendon.

data from the case would be submitted for publication and gave their consent.

3. Discussion

Advances in small joint arthroscopy have led to the development of many effective arthroscopic and endoscopic procedures for foot and ankle conditions [1]. van Dijk et al. [3] first described tendoscopy of the posterior tendon to manage tendon pathology. Chow et al. [5] reported that the results of a case series of tendoscopic synovectomy for six patients with stage 1 PTTD were as good as those reported for open synovectomy [9, 10]. Lui [11] described tendoscopy-assisted posterior tibial tendon reconstruction for stage 2 PTTD, and G. Khazen and C. Khazen [6] reported a case series in which 8 (89%) of 9 patients with stage 1 PTTD reported absent or minor pain after undergoing tendoscopic synovectomy. Bulstra et al. [12] performed 16 procedures in 11 patients that included chronic synovitis ($n = 2$), screw removal from the medial malleolus ($n = 1$), and posterior ankle anatomy ($n = 2$). An irregular sliding channel was smoothed out in two patients and two asymptomatic patients underwent tenosynovectomy and tendon release. The outcome of posterior tibial tendoscopic synovectomy to treat posttraumatic tenosynovitis in our patient was successful.

The posterior tibial tendon that plays an important role in normal hindfoot function lies close to the medial malleolus and beneath the flexor retinaculum, which binds the tendon to the bone. Thus, this tendon can become injured when the ankle is fractured. Crim et al. [13] described a partly torn posterior tibial tendon in 4.2% of hindfoot fractures and that the tendon had become trapped between fracture fragments in 16.1% of them. The initial X-ray image of the ankle of our patient was unavailable, but the later X-ray suggested a relatively proximal fibula fracture and hyperossification between the distal tibia and fibula. These findings indicated a pronation-external rotation (PER) injury, which might have led to a deltoid ligament tear or medial malleolus fracture that may have bled into the posterior tendon sheath, ultimately leading to ossification of the posterior tendon sheath.

Posttraumatic and postsurgical complaints of pain at the posterior margin of the medial malleolus often pose a diagnostic and therapeutic challenge. In the absence of intra-articular pathology, adhesions and irregularities in the tendon sliding channel can be responsible for symptoms in this region. Open tendon release requires postoperative plaster immobilization with the subsequent potential for new adhesion formation [14]. Tendoscopic surgery offers the advantages of decreased morbidity, early range of motion, reduced postoperative pain, and rapid recovery [15].

Our patient had a tendoscopic surgery and it did not require opening the tendon sheath, so postoperative immobilization such as a cast or brace was unnecessary. However, because osteophytes could not be resected along with the posterior tibial tendon by tendoscopic surgery, we enlarged the tendon cavity by deepening the posterior tibial tendon groove. Since postoperative immobilization was not needed, tendon adhesion was not a concern. Tendoscopic surgery enabled range-of-motion exercises to be started immediately, which prevented scar tissue formation and adhesions. Therefore, tendoscopic surgery for this patient was effective and practical.

Tendoscopy is technically demanding. To introduce a scope into the posterior tendon sheath requires experience and finesse, and it is even more difficult in the presence of a subcutaneous irrigation fluid leak. Therefore, we used ultrasonographic guidance. We recommend using ultrasound guidance for especially unexperienced surgeons because it is an easy tool which enable a reliable insertion of an endoscope into the tendon sheath. Yamamoto et al. [16] reported using ultrasonographic assistance to approach a wrist ganglion. Although ultrasonographic resolution is limited, recent improvements in both hardware and software have made it an excellent, noninvasive, and dynamic technique for assessing the musculoskeletal system [17, 18] as it can visualize not only the posterior tibial tendon, but also vessels, nerves, and other tissues such as the long flexor muscles of the toes. These features considerably reduce the risk of serious postprocedural complications. We consider that sonography combined with endo/arthroscopy represents a useful and practical approach to soft tissue surgery.

In conclusion, ultrasonography-assisted tendoscopic synovectomy is useful for posterior tendon synovitis. Tendoscopic synovectomy requires specific skills, but it is more favorable than open synovectomy in terms of postoperative rehabilitation and cosmetic aspects. Ultrasonographic assistance also facilitates the introduction of a scope into the tendon sheath.

Competing Interests

The authors did not receive any outside funding or grants and have no commercial associations that might pose a conflict of interests in connection with the submitted paper.

References

[1] T. H. Lui, "Arthroscopy and endoscopy of the foot and ankle: indications for new techniques," *Arthroscopy*, vol. 23, no. 8, pp. 889–902, 2007.

[2] S. J. Wertheimer, C. A. Weber, B. G. Loder, D. R. Calderone, and S. T. Frascone, "The role of endoscopy in treatment of stenosing posterior tibial tenosynovitis," *Journal of Foot and Ankle Surgery*, vol. 34, no. 1, pp. 15–22, 1995.

[3] C. N. van Dijk, N. Kort, and P. E. Scholten, "Tendoscopy of the posterior tibial tendon," *Arthroscopy*, vol. 13, no. 6, pp. 692–698, 1997.

[4] C. N. van Dijk and N. Kort, "Tendoscopy of the peroneal tendons," *Arthroscopy*, vol. 14, no. 5, pp. 471–478, 1998.

[5] H. T. Chow, K. B. Chan, and T. H. Lui, "Tendoscopic debridement for stage I posterior tibial tendon dysfunction," *Knee Surgery, Sports Traumatology, Arthroscopy*, vol. 13, no. 8, pp. 695–698, 2005.

[6] G. Khazen and C. Khazen, "Tendoscopy in stage I posterior tibial tendon dysfunction," *Foot and Ankle Clinics*, vol. 17, no. 3, pp. 399–406, 2012.

[7] J. G. Anderson and S. T. Hansen, "Fracture-dislocation of the ankle with posterior tibial tendon entrapment within the tibiofibular interosseous space: a case report of a late diagnosis," *Foot & Ankle International*, vol. 17, no. 2, pp. 114–118, 1996.

[8] M. A. West, C. Sangani, and E. Toh, "Tibialis posterior tendon rupture associated with a closed medial malleolar fracture: a case report and review of the literature," *Journal of Foot and Ankle Surgery*, vol. 49, no. 6, pp. 565.e9–565.e12, 2010.

[9] T. C. Beals, G. C. Pomeroy, and A. Manoli II, "Posterior tendon insufficiency: diagnosis and treatment.," *The Journal of the American Academy of Orthopaedic Surgeons*, vol. 7, no. 2, pp. 112–118, 1999.

[10] R. D. Teasdall and K. A. Johnson, "Surgical treatment of stage I posterior tibial tendon dysfunction," *Foot & Ankle International*, vol. 15, no. 12, pp. 646–648, 1994.

[11] T. H. Lui, "Endoscopic assisted posterior tibial tendon reconstruction for stage 2 posterior tibial tendon insufficiency," *Knee Surgery, Sports Traumatology, Arthroscopy*, vol. 15, no. 10, pp. 1228–1234, 2007.

[12] G. H. Bulstra, P. G. M. Olsthoorn, and C. N. van Dijk, "Tendoscopy of the posterior tibial tendon," *Foot and Ankle Clinics*, vol. 11, no. 2, pp. 421–427, 2006.

[13] J. Crim, M. Enslow, and J. Smith, "CT assessment of the prevalence of retinacular injuries associated with hindfoot fractures," *Skeletal Radiology*, vol. 42, no. 4, pp. 487–492, 2013.

[14] P. W. Lapidus and H. Seidenstein, "Chronic non-specific tenosynovitis with effusion about the ankle; report of three cases," *The Journal of Bone & Joint Surgery—American Volume*, vol. 32, no. 1, pp. 175–179, 1950.

[15] J. C. Christensen and T. D. Lanier, "Tendoscopy of the ankle," *Clinics in Podiatric Medicine and Surgery*, vol. 28, no. 3, pp. 561–570, 2011.

[16] M. Yamamoto, S. Kurimoto, N. Okui, M. Tatebe, T. Shinohara, and H. Hirata, "Sonography-guided arthroscopy for wrist ganglion," *The Journal of Hand Surgery*, vol. 37, no. 7, pp. 1411–1415, 2012.

[17] S. Bianchi, D. Della Santa, T. Glauser, J.-Y. Beaulieu, and J. van Aaken, "Sonography of masses of the wrist and hand," *American Journal of Roentgenology*, vol. 191, no. 6, pp. 1767–1775, 2008.

[18] H. T. Harcke, L. E. Grissom, and M. S. Finkelstein, "Evaluation of the musculoskeletal system with sonography," *American Journal of Roentgenology*, vol. 150, no. 6, pp. 1253–1261, 1988.

19

A Rare Case of Progressive Palsy of the Lower Leg Caused by a Huge Lumbar Posterior Endplate Lesion after Recurrent Disc Herniation

Masatoshi Morimoto, Kosaku Higashino, Shinsuke Katoh, Tezuka Fumitake, Kazuta Yamashita, Fumio Hayashi, Yoichiro Takata, Toshinori Sakai, Akihiro Nagamachi, and Koichi Sairyo

Department of Orthopedics, Institute of Health Biosciences, University of Tokushima Graduate School, Tokushima, Japan

Correspondence should be addressed to Masatoshi Morimoto; masa_m_089034@yahoo.co.jp

Academic Editor: Yuichi Kasai

A lesion of the lumbar posterior endplate is sometimes identified in the spinal canal of children and adolescents; it causes symptoms similar to those of a herniated disc. However, the pathology of the endplate lesion and the pathology of the herniated disc are different. We present a rare case of a 23-year-old woman who developed progressive palsy of the lower leg caused by huge lumbar posterior endplate lesion after recurrent disc herniation.

1. Introduction

A lesion of the lumbar posterior endplate is sometimes identified in the spinal canal of children and adolescents; it causes symptoms similar to those of a herniated disc [1–4]. However, the pathology of the endplate lesion and the pathology of the herniated disc are different [5]. The lesion of the posterior endplate lesion is usually not absorbed [6]; on the other hand lumbar disc herniation is usually absorbed. Our previous study described that the long-term outcome is good, in patients treated either conservatively or surgically for an endplate lesion [6]. We present a rare case of progressive palsy of the lower leg caused by huge lumbar posterior endplate lesion after recurrent disc herniation.

2. Case Report

This 14-year-old junior high school female had low back pain during ordinary daily activities. She was otherwise healthy without any other medical complications. She did not have hyperostosis disease, such as ossification of posterior longitudinal ligament or diffuse idiopathic skeletal hyperostosis. Neurological examination did not show obvious deficit at the first examination. Radiographic findings revealed lumbar disc degeneration with posterior end plate lesions at L4/5 and L5/S1 (Figure 1). She was treated with conservative therapy. The low back pain subsided after conservative therapy and she was able to return to ordinary daily life.

At age 18 she had low back pain again. Radiographic findings showed a lumbar posterior lesion at L4/5 (Figure 2). We diagnosed lumbar disc herniation at L4/5. MRI showed posterior lumbar disc herniation connecting the nucleus pulposus tissue at L4/5. The lumbar disc herniation at L5/S1 was absorbed, although the posterior endplate lesion still remained at L5/S1. The endplate lesion at L5/S1 involved the cartilage or bony tissue of the growth plate and the tissue of the annulus and nucleus [5, 6]. She was treated with conservative therapy again. The low back pain disappeared completely. She worked at a metal plant factory after graduating from high school.

At age 23 she visited her general physician due to muscle weakness of the right lower leg without low back pain. Manual muscle testing (MMT) of the right tibialis anterior muscle (TA) and that of the right extensor hallucis longus muscle (EHL) were both 4/5 at this first examination. On the seventh day her neurological deficit deteriorated. She

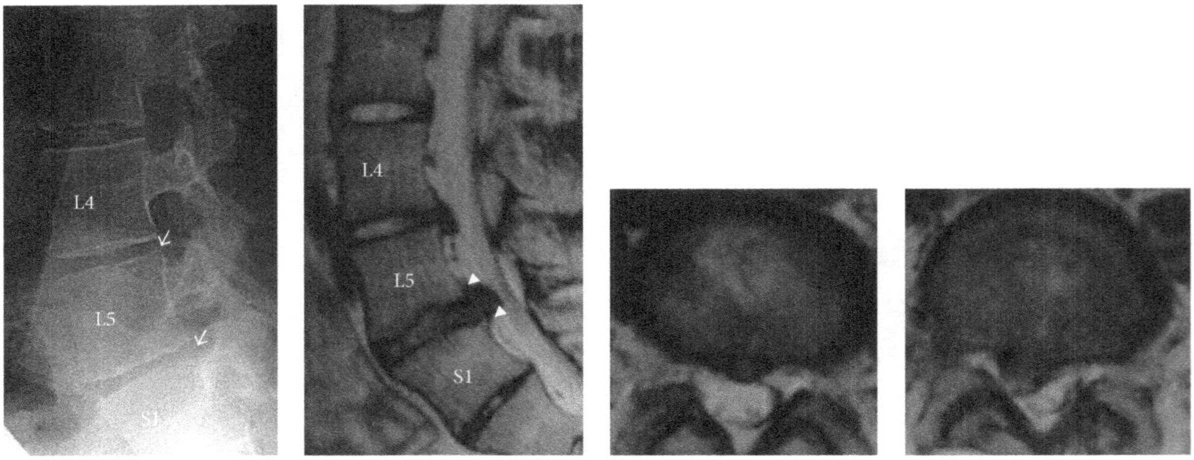

(a) (b) (c) (d)

Figure 1: Radiographs showed lumbar posterior endplate lesions at L4/5 and L5/S1 at 14 years of age ((a), white arrows). Sagittal (b) and axial ((c) and (d)) T2-weighted MR images revealed L4/5 and L5/S1 lumbar disc herniation with endplate lesion. White arrow head showed irregular shape of the posterior end plate at the corner of S1 and L5 vertebrae.

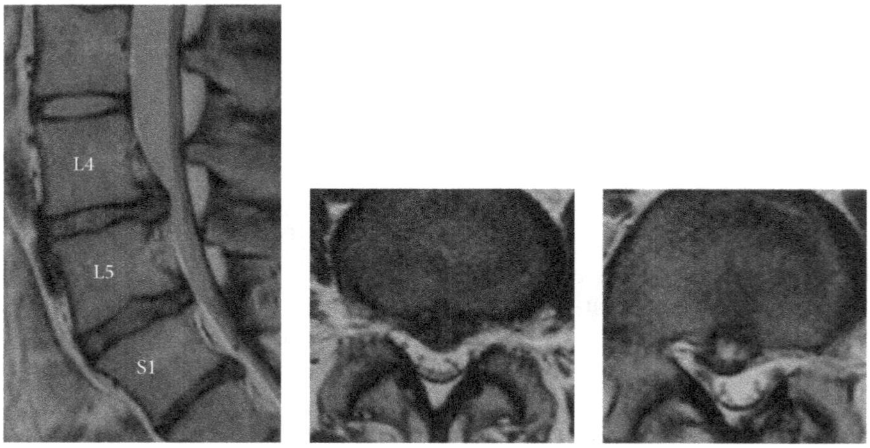

(a) (b) (c)

Figure 2: MRI showed posterior lumbar disc herniation connecting the nucleus pulposus tissue at L4/5 at the age of 18 years ((a) and (b)). The lumbar disc herniation at L5/S1 was absorbed, although the posterior endplate lesion still remained at L5/S1 ((a) and (c)).

had difficulty in walking with the right foot drop. On the thirteenth day she was referred to our hospital. At that time physical examination showed that MMT of both the right TA and the right EHL was 0/5. The straight leg raising test was restricted within 30 degrees. Sensory impairment at the right area of L4, L5, and S1 was presented. Computer tomography (CT) showed a huge ossification on the dorsal of annulus fibrosus of intervertebral disc at L4/5. CT did not show an abnormal ossification of annulus fibrosus or posterior longitudinal ligament at the other levels (Figure 3). MRI, compared to those taken when she was 18 years old, revealed severe stenosis at L4/5 and the lesion of the posterior endplate lesion still remained at L5/S1. She had progressive urinary retention.

She underwent surgery of L4 total laminectomy and L5 partial laminectomy with posterolateral fusion at L4/5. The huge ossification compressed the dura matter and adhered to L5 nerve root completely, so that the ossification was not able to be removed.

The postoperative course was satisfactory, her neurological deficit improved, and she had no difficulty in daily activities. Physical examination carried out 2 years later showed MMT of the TA to be 4/5 and EHL to be 2/5; sensory impairment had disappeared.

3. Discussion

The lumbar vertebral ring apophysis starts to ossify at about 6 years of age before ossification of ring apophysis. The vertebral ring apophysis appears as a secondary ossification center at approximately 10 years of age. Fusion to the vertebral body usually occurs between 17 and 20 years of age [5, 7–9].

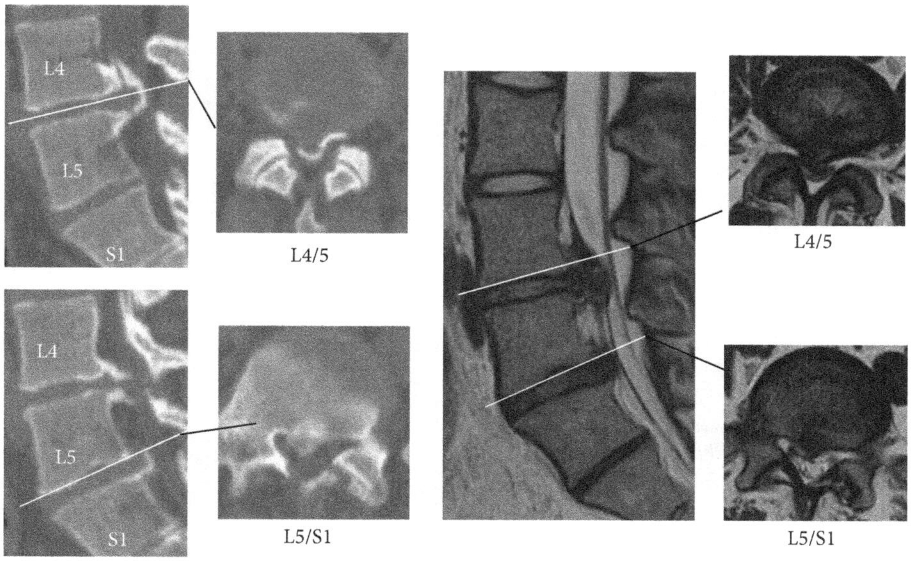

FIGURE 3: Computed tomography (CT) showed a huge ossification on the dorsal of annulus fibrosus of intervertebral disc at L4/5 at the age of 23 years. Ossification at L4/5 was larger than that at L5/S1. The ossification was consecutive with the posterior end plate at L4/5 and L5/S1. CT did not show an abnormal ossification of annulus fibrosus or posterior longitudinal ligament at the other levels. MRI revealed severe stenosis at L4/5 and the lesion of the posterior endplate lesion still remained at L5/S1.

A relative weak point exists between ring apophysis and the vertebral body until the fusion completes [10, 11]. Faizan et al. reported that the apophyseal ring experienced twice as much stress in the ossified stage as compared to the cartilaginous stage. This may be the cause of frequent fractures at the interface of bone and cartilage [12].

Terai et al. reported that the posterior region of the lumbar vertebrae in the pediatric model had higher stresses, as compared to the adult model. The most marked differences between the pediatric and adult models were found in the apophyseal ring [13].

In our previous study twenty-four consecutive patients with endplate lesions for 13.8 years in average were studied [5]. We concluded the long-term outcome for patients with a posterior endplate lesion is favorable. However radiographs showed degenerative changes at the lumbar disc and endplate lesion. Histological examination of the endplate lesion removed surgically showed an abnormal endplate with degeneration and some chondrocytes without a nucleus [6]. The endplate lesion seemed not able to remodel or not able to become resorbed.

The abnormal mechanical stress at the posterior lumbar lesion occurred twice at the age of 14 and 17 in this case. We think the huge ossification was a part of end plate lesion, because CT images of Figure 3 showed ossification was consecutive with the posterior end plate. Although we are not able to prove the pathological mechanism to induce the huge ossification of the end plate lesion, we speculated that multiple injuries might induce hyperossification of endplate lesion.

In summary, we report on a rare case of progressive palsy of the lower leg caused by huge lumbar posterior endplate lesion after recurrent disc herniation.

Competing Interests

The authors declare that there is no conflict of interests regarding the publication of this paper.

References

[1] A. Hellstadius, "A contribution to the question of the origin of anterior paradiscal defects and so-called persisting apophyses in the vertebral bodies," *Acta Orthopaedica*, vol. 18, no. 1–4, pp. 377–386, 1949.

[2] J.-D. Laredo, M. Bard, J. Chretien, and M.-F. Kahn, "Lumbar posterior marginal intra-osseous cartilaginous node," *Skeletal Radiology*, vol. 15, no. 3, pp. 201–208, 1986.

[3] K. Lindblom, "Discography of dissecting transosseous ruptures of intervertebral discs in the lumbar region," *Acta Radiologica*, vol. 36, no. 1, pp. 12–16, 1951.

[4] K. Takata, S.-I. Inoue, K. Takahashi, and Y. Ohtsuka, "Fracture of the posterior margin of a lumbar vertebral body," *The Journal of Bone & Joint Surgery—American Volume*, vol. 70, no. 4, pp. 589–594, 1988.

[5] T. Ikata, T. Morita, S. Katoh, K. Tachibana, and H. Maoka, "Lesions of the lumbar posterior end plate in children and adolescents. An MRI study," *The Journal of Bone & Joint Surgery—British Volume*, vol. 77, no. 6, pp. 951–955, 1995.

[6] K. Higashino, K. Sairyo, S. Katoh, S. Takao, H. Kosaka, and N. Yasui, "Long-term outcomes of lumbar posterior apophyseal end-plate lesions in children and adolescents," *The Journal of Bone & Joint Surgery—American Volume*, vol. 94, no. 11, article e74, 2012.

[7] J. G. Edelson and H. Nathan, "Stages in the natural history of the vertebral end-plates," *Spine*, vol. 13, no. 1, pp. 21–26, 1988.

[8] K. Sairyo, S. Katoh, T. Ikata, K. Fujii, K. Kajiura, and V. K. Goel, "Development of spondylolytic olisthesis in adolescents," *The Spine Journal*, vol. 1, no. 3, pp. 171–175, 2001.

[9] C. H. Yen, S. K. Chan, Y. F. Ho, and K. H. Mak, "Posterior lumbar apophyseal ring fractures in adolescents: a report of four cases," *Journal of Orthopaedic Surgery*, vol. 17, no. 1, pp. 85–89, 2009.

[10] A. Baranto, L. Ekström, M. Hellström, O. Lundin, S. Holm, and L. Swärd, "Fracture patterns of the adolescent porcine spine: an experimental loading study in bending-compression," *Spine*, vol. 30, no. 1, pp. 75–82, 2005.

[11] R. Savini, M. Di Silvestre, G. Gargiulo et al., "Posterior lumbar apophyseal fractures," *Spine*, vol. 16, pp. 1118–1123, 1991.

[12] A. Faizan, K. Sairyo, V. K. Goel, A. Biyani, and N. Ebraheim, "Biomechanical rationale of ossification of the secondary ossification center on apophyseal bony ring fracture: a biomechanical study," *Clinical Biomechanics*, vol. 22, no. 10, pp. 1063–1067, 2007.

[13] T. Terai, K. Sairyo, V. K. Goel et al., "Biomechanical rationale of sacral rounding deformity in pediatric spondylolisthesis: a clinical and biomechanical study," *Archives of Orthopaedic and Trauma Surgery*, vol. 131, no. 9, pp. 1187–1194, 2011.

20

Difficulty in Fixation of the Volar Lunate Facet Fragment in Distal Radius Fracture

Hiroyuki Obata,[1] Tomonori Baba,[2] Kentaro Futamura,[1] Osamu Obayashi,[1] Atsuhiko Mogami,[1] Hideki Tsuji,[3] Yoshiaki Kurata,[3] and Kazuo Kaneko[2]

[1]*Department of Orthopaedic Surgery, Juntendo University Shizuoka Hospital, Shizuoka, Japan*
[2]*Department of Orthopaedic Surgery, Juntendo University School of Medicine, Tokyo, Japan*
[3]*Orthopaedic Trauma Center, Sapporo Tokushukai Hospital, Sapporo, Japan*

Correspondence should be addressed to Tomonori Baba; tobaba@juntendo.ac.jp

Academic Editor: Andreas Panagopoulos

Recent reports suggest the presence of a rare fracture type for which reduction and fixation cannot be achieved with volar locking plate (VLP). In particular, it is difficult to achieve reduction and fixation with volar lunate facet (VLF) fragments present on the volar ulnar aspect of the lunate facet, because of the anatomical structure and biomechanics in this region. Herein, we report two challenging cases of difficulty in fixation of the VLF fragment in distal radius fracture. For this fracture type, it is most important to identify the volar ulnar bone fragment before surgery; it may also be necessary to optimize distal placement of the VLP via a dual-window approach and to apply additional fixations, such as a small plate, anchor, and/or external fixation.

1. Introduction

Volar locking plate (VLP) fixation has become the gold standard for surgical treatment of distal radius fracture over the last 10 years because of its favorable postoperative outcomes. However, the presence of a rare fracture type has recently been suggested, in which a fragment is present on the volar ulnar aspect and reduction and fixation are difficult with VLPs. In 2004, Harness et al. reported that fixation of the volar lunate facet (VLF) fragment with a VLP is difficult because of the shape of the bone, which is flat on the sagittal view and slopes towards the ulnar side on the axial view [1]. Furthermore, in 2014 Beck et al. reported the risk factors for displacement of a VLF fragment based on various plain radiography parameters [2]. Reduction and fixation of a VLF fragment in distal radius fracture with VLPs are difficult anatomically (bone shape, approach) and biomechanically (distraction by ligaments) [1]. Reports focusing on VLF fragments have occasionally been published [2–4]. However, because this fracture type is very rare, no consensus has been reached on the definition of the fracture type, risk factors for displacement, or appropriate reduction and fixation methods. We encountered two patients with distal radius fracture with a VLF fragment and report these cases with a review of the literature.

2. Case Presentation

Patient 1. A 54-year-old woman presented with right distal radius fracture (AO classification 23C3.1). A 10 × 8 mm VLF fragment was observed on plain radiography, with volar displacement (Figure 1). In the first surgery, reduction and fixation were achieved with a MODE VLP for proximal placement (Medical Dynamic Marketing Inc., Tokyo, Japan), used as a buttress plate (Figure 2(a)). However, redisplacement was noted 2 weeks after surgery (Figure 2(b)). At reoperation via a dual-window approach, reduction and fixation were achieved again with an Acu-Loc 2 VLP for distal placement (Acumed Co., Oregon, USA) (Figure 2(c)). However, redisplacement was again noted 5 days after surgery (Figure 2(d)). At second reoperation via a dual-window approach, the displaced VLF fragment was reduced from the ulnar side and fixed with a VariAx handplate (Stryker Co., Michigan, USA) used as a buttress plate; concomitant external fixation was applied for

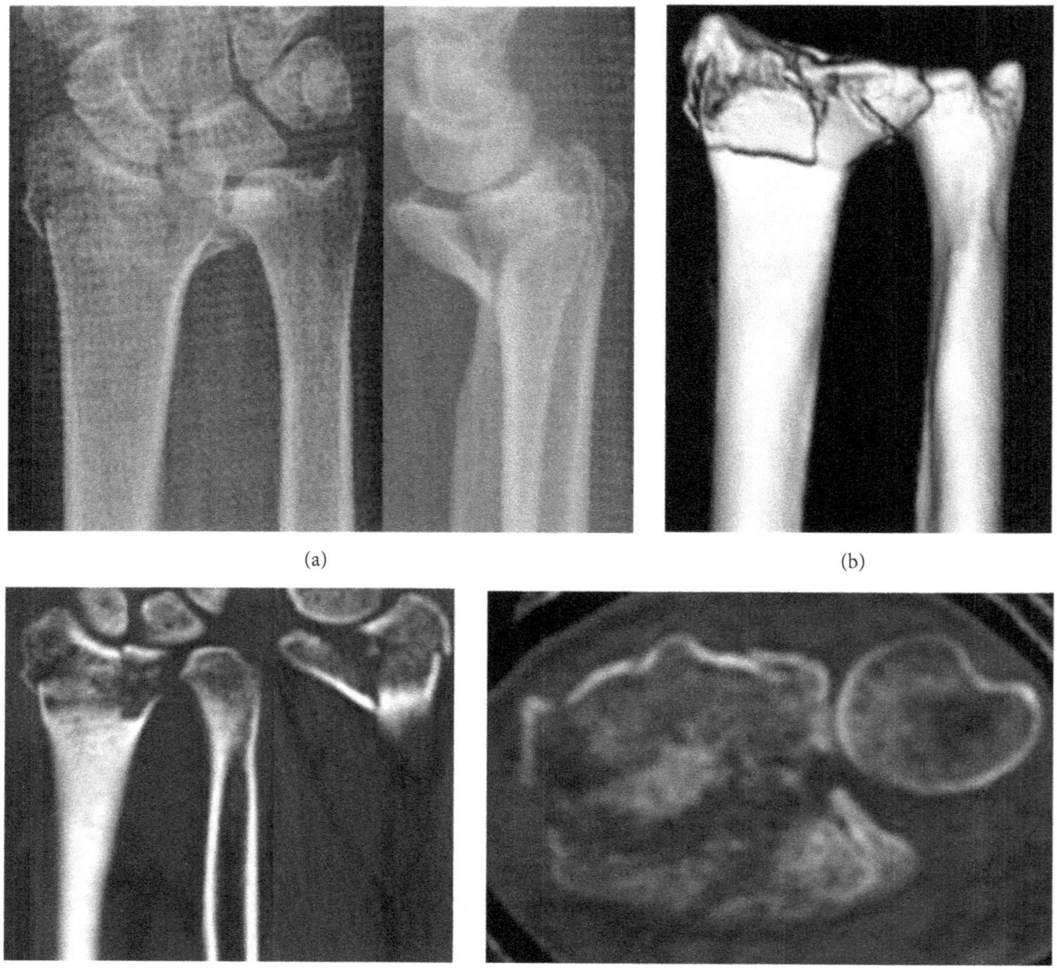

(a) (b) (c) (d)

FIGURE 1: Patient 1. Plain radiographs (a) and CT (b, c, d) at the time of injury. A 10 × 8 mm VLF fragment is observed, with volar displacement.

4 weeks (Figure 2(e)). At 1 year after surgery, bone union was achieved without redisplacement (Figure 2(f)).

Patient 2. A 58-year-old woman presented with right distal radius fracture (AO classification 23C3.1). A 12 × 12 mm VLF fragment was observed on plain radiography, with volar displacement (Figure 3). In the first surgery, reduction and fixation were achieved with a VA-TCP VLP for proximal placement (Depuy Synthes Co., Zuchwil, Switzerland), used as a buttress plate (for the distal screw, monoaxial screws were inserted over the guide block); however, redisplacement was noted after surgery (Figures 4(a) and 4(b)). Because 10 weeks had passed at the time of reoperation and malunion of the displaced VLF fragment was observed, corrective osteotomy was performed, followed by reduction and fixation which were achieved with an Acu-Loc 2 VLP for distal placement (Acumed Co., Oregon, USA) (Figure 4(c)). Concomitant external fixation was applied for 5 weeks. At 9 months after surgery, bone union was achieved without redisplacement (Figure 4(d)).

3. Discussion

The VLF fragment was first described by Harness et al. in 2004 [1]. That study reported difficulty in reduction and fixation of the VLF fragment with a VLP because of the anatomical structure and biomechanics in this region. In 2014 Beck et al. reported the risk factors for displacement of VLF fragments based on various plain radiography parameters [2]. However, plate coverage of the VLF fragment and the number of inserted screws were not associated with risk of displacement, suggesting the presence of a rare fracture type for which reduction and fixation cannot be achieved with VLPs. There have been several reports of reduction and fixation of VLF fragments [2–5], redisplacement resulting from inappropriate early treatment because of a lack of preoperative understanding of the VLF fragment. Because it is very rare for redisplacement with appropriate plate selection and positioning, it is difficult to objectively evaluate risk factors (e.g., size, shape, and position of the fragment) for VLF fragment displacement and to determine appropriate

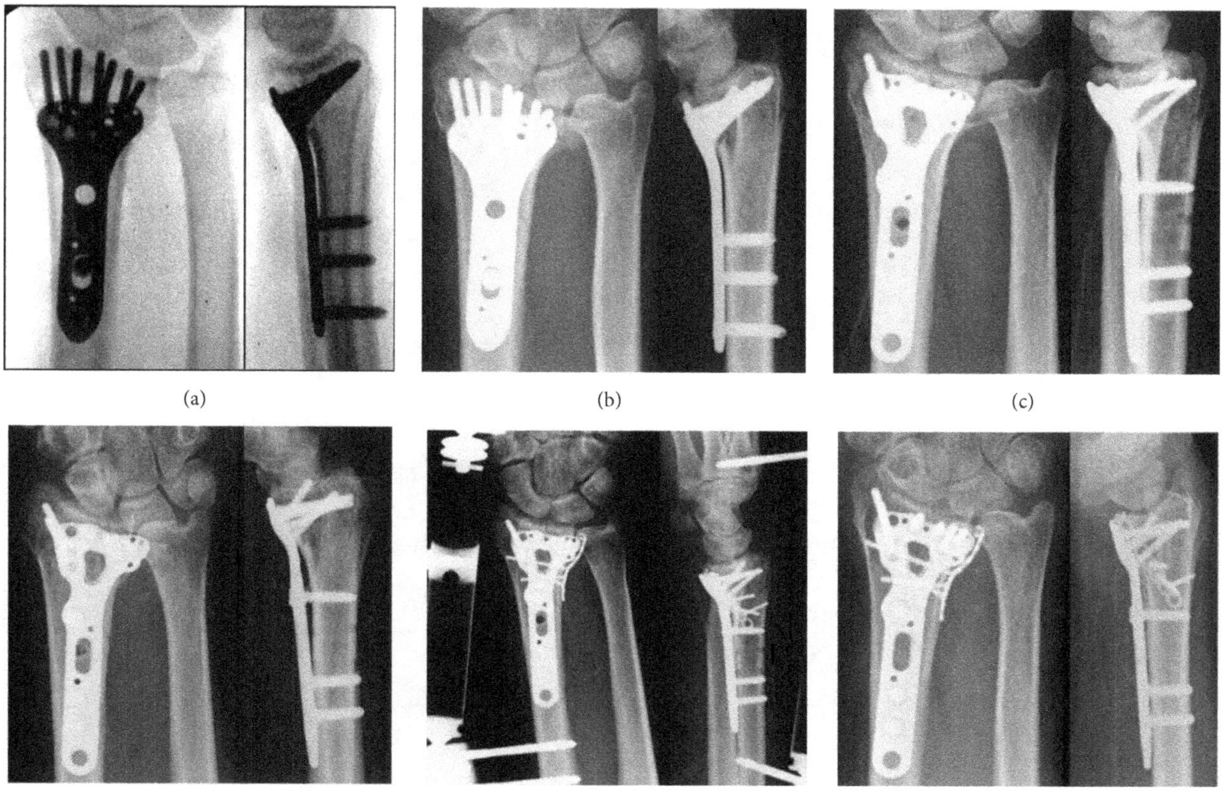

FIGURE 2: Plain radiographs of Patient 1. (a) Immediately after the first surgery. (b) Two weeks after the first surgery; redisplacement is seen. (c) Immediately after reoperation. (d) Five days after reoperation; redisplacement is seen. (e) Immediately after the third surgery. (f) One year after the third surgery; bone union was achieved without redisplacement.

reduction and fixation methods. Many VLPs have been designed to provide double-tiered subchondral support: their structures support the dorsal subchondral bone at the center of the joint surface, because supporting the volar subchondral bone with screws is difficult [6]. Our first choice of VLP is the monoaxial mode, since we think that the stability of the monoaxial mode is higher than the polyaxial one. Both cases were stabilized by the monoaxial mode and it was possible for them to cover the lunate facet fragment by preoperative template. But support with a plate may also not be possible when the VLF fragment is small. On 3DCT, when a VLF fragment is present in the region contained within a straight line connecting the volar radial margin of the lunate facet and the proximal end of the distal radioulnar joint and the center of the distal radioulnar joint, instability occurs towards the volar ulnar side because the VLF fragment provides the attachment sites for the short radiolunate ligament and the distal radioulnar ligament. Of 177 cases of distal radius fracture treated surgically at our hospital, VLF fragment was present in five patients; the AO classification was C3 in each case. Two had volar displacement and three had dorsal displacement. Two had redisplacement after surgery. Both of these cases had volar displacement, and the fracture type was relatively simple, with mild crushing of the joint surface. Loads on the VLF fragment may be dispersed in fractures with marked joint surface crushing, whereas loads may be concentrated in relatively simple fractures with less joint surface crushing. In addition, loads may be more markedly concentrated in cases of volar displacement. The following characteristics may be risk factors for displacement: (1) a VLF fragment is present, (2) the joint surface is less crushed, and (3) the displacement is volar.

Regarding the reduction and fixation method, additional fixation with a miniscrew, K wire, soft wire, and hook plate has been reported [3]. However, these methods are likely to provide insufficient fixation force and to result in refracture. Therefore, when instability is marked and concomitant external fixation is applied it may be appropriate to apply a suture to the articular capsule with a small buttress plate and anchor as a basic procedure. The conventional trans-FCR approach can visualize VLF fragment adequately. However, when we have to place the buttress plate on the juxta-DRUJ, dual-window approach allows for the procedure of the buttress plating. This procedure cannot be achieved by trans-FCR approach. Stryker hand plating system was placed in bone slope towards DRUJ, so the edge of this small plate would not extend to the joint surface of DRUJ actually. Moreover, intraoperatively we confirmed pronation and

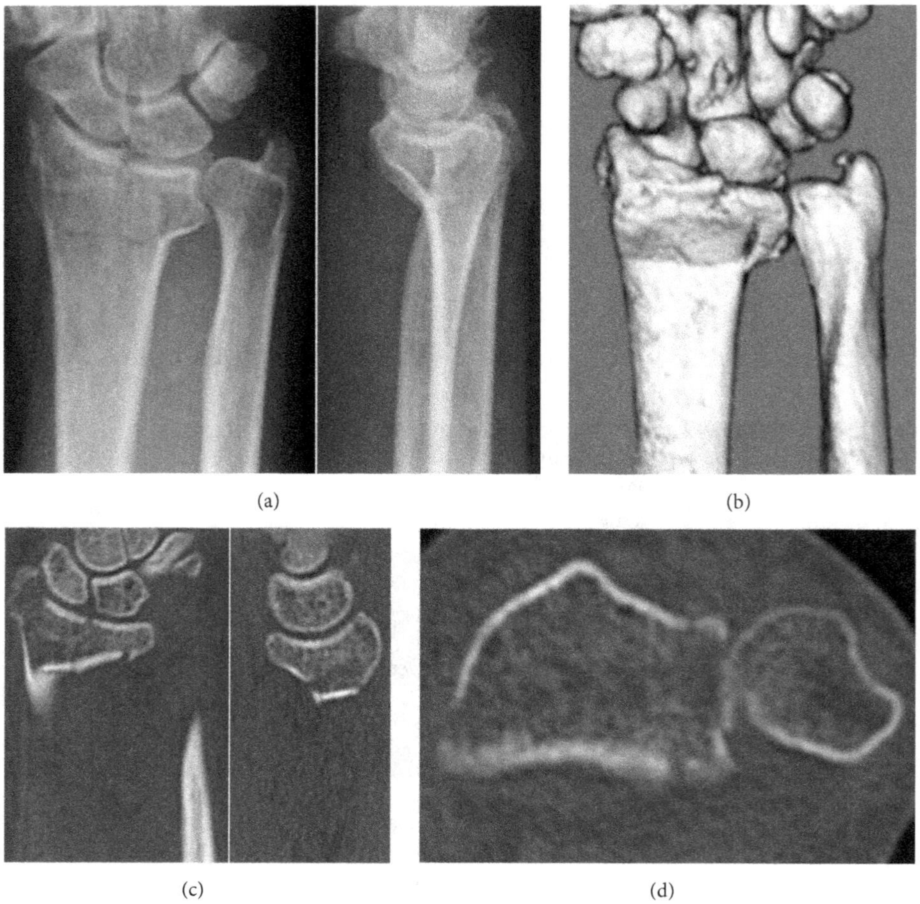

FIGURE 3: Patient 2. Plain radiographs (a) and CT (b, c, d) at the time of injury. A 12 × 12 mm VLF fragment is observed, with volar displacement.

supination of the forearm smoothly without the impingement of the implant. However postoperatively the limitation of supination occurred, so the placement of this small plate would cause some kind of factor (e.g., the adhesion of the soft tissue, the bulkiness of the plate). In fact, the limitation of the supination improved by the implant removal. Thus, if the limitation of supination and pronation occurred, we would have to remove the implant.

Redisplacement occurred in the current patients because a lack of preoperative understanding of the volar ulnar bone fragment resulted in inappropriate plate selection. Both cases were operated on in the different institutions. So the criteria for use of VLP differed in each institution. Redisplacement occurred despite optimal distal VLP placement, suggesting that reduction and fixation with available VLPs alone are difficult and that additional fixations are necessary, such as a small plate and external fixation. For fractures with a volar lunate facet fragment, it is necessary to identify the volar ulnar bone fragment. In the case of small volar lunate facet fragment, we suture the ligament on to the plate hole by using the anchor. In case of relative large volar lunate facet fragment, we think the small plate as a buttress plate from volar ulnar side is useful. As to the indication for the external fixator, if the stabilization of the internal fixation may be not enough, we use it in order to avoid the redisplacement. Both cases were operated on multiple times for the displacement of the volar lunate facet fragment. We had to immobilize the wrist joint by using the external fixation system in order to avoid the redisplacement.

For fractures with a VLF fragment, it is necessary to (1) identify the VLF fragment, (2) optimally place a VLP for distal placement via a dual-window approach, and (3) apply additional fixation (small plate, anchor, and/or external fixation).

Ethical Approval

The study was carried out in accordance with the Declaration of Helsinki and the appropriate ethical framework.

Consent

Written informed consent was obtained from the patient for publication of this case report and any accompanying images.

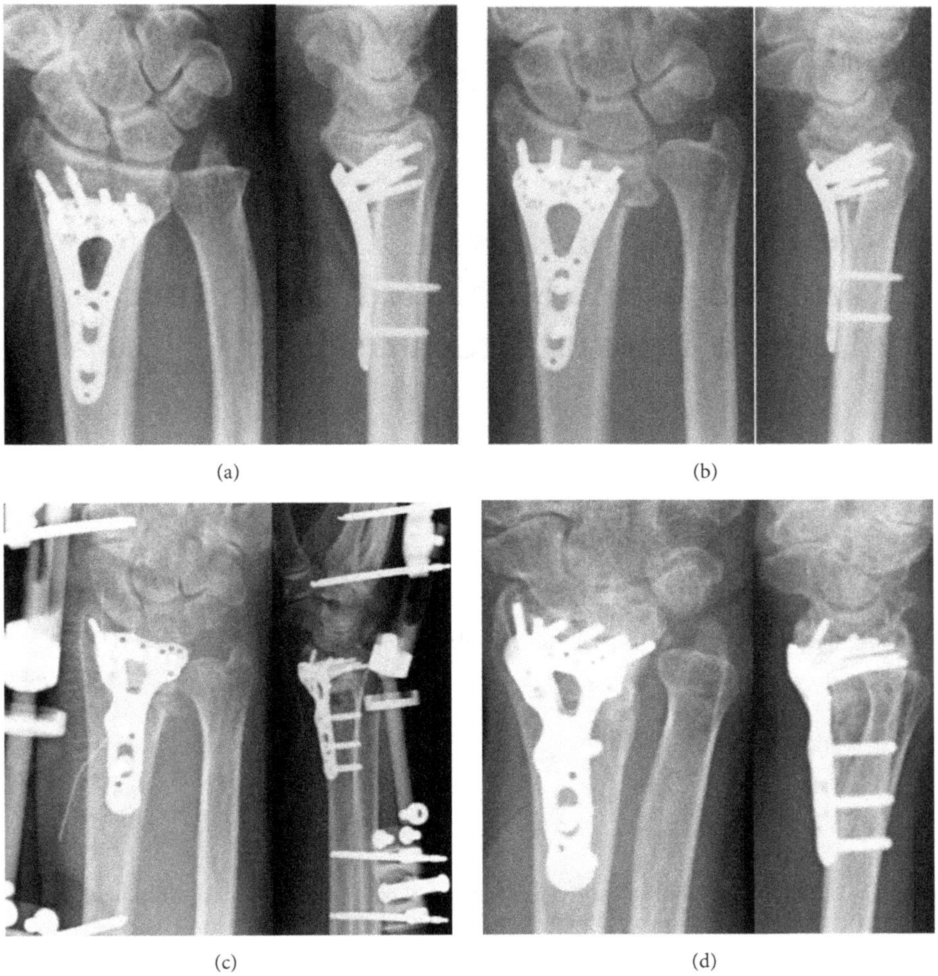

FIGURE 4: Plain radiographs of Patient 2. (a) Immediately after the first surgery. (b) Six weeks after the first surgery; redisplacement is seen. (c) Immediately after reoperation. (d) Nine months after reoperation; bone union was achieved without redisplacement.

Competing Interests

The authors declare that they have no competing interests.

References

[1] N. G. Harness, J. B. Jupiter, J. L. Orbay, K. B. Raskin, and D. L. Fernandez, "Loss of fixation of the volar lunate facet fragment in fractures of the distal part of the radius," *The Journal of Bone & Joint Surgery—American Volume*, vol. 86, no. 9, pp. 1900–1908, 2004.

[2] J. D. Beck, N. G. Harness, and H. T. Spencer, "Volar plate fixation failure for volar shearing distal radius fractures with small lunate facet fragments," *Journal of Hand Surgery*, vol. 39, no. 4, pp. 670–678, 2014.

[3] A. Marcano, D. P. Taormina, R. Karia, N. Paksima, M. Posner, and K. A. Egol, "Displaced intra-articular fractures involving the volar rim of the distal radius," *Journal of Hand Surgery*, vol. 40, no. 1, pp. 42–48, 2015.

[4] A. J. Bakker and A. Y. Shin, "Fragment-specific volar hook plate for volar marginal rim fractures," *Techniques in Hand and Upper Extremity Surgery*, vol. 18, no. 1, pp. 56–60, 2014.

[5] K. R. Chin and J. B. Jupiter, "Wire-loop fixation of volar displaced osteochondral fractures of the distal radius," *Journal of Hand Surgery*, vol. 24, no. 3, pp. 525–533, 1999.

[6] K. Kawasaki, T. Nemoto, K. Inagaki, K. Tomita, and Y. Ueno, "Variable-angle locking plate with or without double-tiered subchondral support procedure in the treatment of intra-articular distal radius fracture," *Journal of Orthopaedics and Traumatology*, vol. 15, no. 4, pp. 271–274, 2014.

21

Gait Analysis of Conventional Total Knee Arthroplasty and Bicruciate Stabilized Total Knee Arthroplasty Using a Triaxial Accelerometer

Takenori Tomite,[1] Hidetomo Saito,[2] Toshiaki Aizawa,[1] Hiroaki Kijima,[2] Naohisa Miyakoshi,[2] and Yoichi Shimada[2]

[1]*Kitaakita Municipal Hospital, 16-29 Shimosugiaza Kamishimizusawa, Kitaakita City, Akita 018-4221, Japan*
[2]*Department of Orthopedic Surgery, Akita University Graduate School of Medicine, Hondou 1-1-1, Akita City, Akita 010-8543, Japan*

Correspondence should be addressed to Takenori Tomite; takenoritomite@yahoo.co.jp

Academic Editor: Bayram Unver

One component of conventional total knee arthroplasty is removal of the anterior cruciate ligament, and the knee after total knee arthroplasty has been said to be a knee with anterior cruciate ligament dysfunction. Bicruciate stabilized total knee arthroplasty is believed to reproduce anterior cruciate ligament function in the implant and provide anterior stability. Conventional total knee arthroplasty was performed on the right knee and bicruciate stabilized total knee arthroplasty was performed on the left knee in the same patient, and a triaxial accelerometer was fitted to both knees after surgery. Gait analysis was then performed and is reported here. The subject was a 78-year-old woman who underwent conventional total knee arthroplasty on her right knee and bicruciate stabilized total knee arthroplasty on her left knee. On the femoral side with bicruciate stabilized total knee arthroplasty, compared to conventional total knee arthroplasty, there was little acceleration in the x-axis direction (anteroposterior direction) in the early swing phase. Bicruciate stabilized total knee arthroplasty may be able to replace anterior cruciate ligament function due to the structure of the implant and proper anteroposterior positioning.

1. Introduction

Conventional total knee arthroplasty (TKA) can include preservation of the posterior cruciate ligament (PCL) (cruciate-retaining, CR), removal of the PCL (posterior stabilized, PS), and substitution of the PCL (cruciate-substituting or cruciate-sacrificing, CS), but the anterior cruciate ligament (ACL) is still removed, and the knee after TKA has ACL dysfunction. Therefore, there are cases that experience paradoxical motion, in which the femur exhibits anterior slipping in early flexion; this is considered one of the causes of poor results after TKA [1].

Victor and Bellemans developed bicruciate stabilized (BCS) TKA to solve this problem [2]. BCS TKA is believed to reproduce ACL function in the implant and provide anterior stability. Changing the shape of the articulating surfaces and the thickness of the polyethylene reportedly causes medial pivot motion and roll back close to that of a normal knee joint [3].

Conventional TKA on the right knee and BCS TKA on the left knee were performed in the same patient. A triaxial accelerometer was then fitted to both knees after surgery, and gait analysis was performed.

2. Case Presentation

A 78-year-old woman had experienced pain in both knees since around 2005. Conservative medical treatment at a nearby clinic failed to mitigate her symptoms, and she was referred to our hospital in 2012. Preoperative range of motion was −10° and 130° in right knee extension and flexion, respectively, and −5° and 130° in left knee extension and flexion, respectively. The preoperative X-ray showed equivalent deformation on the left and right (Figure 1).

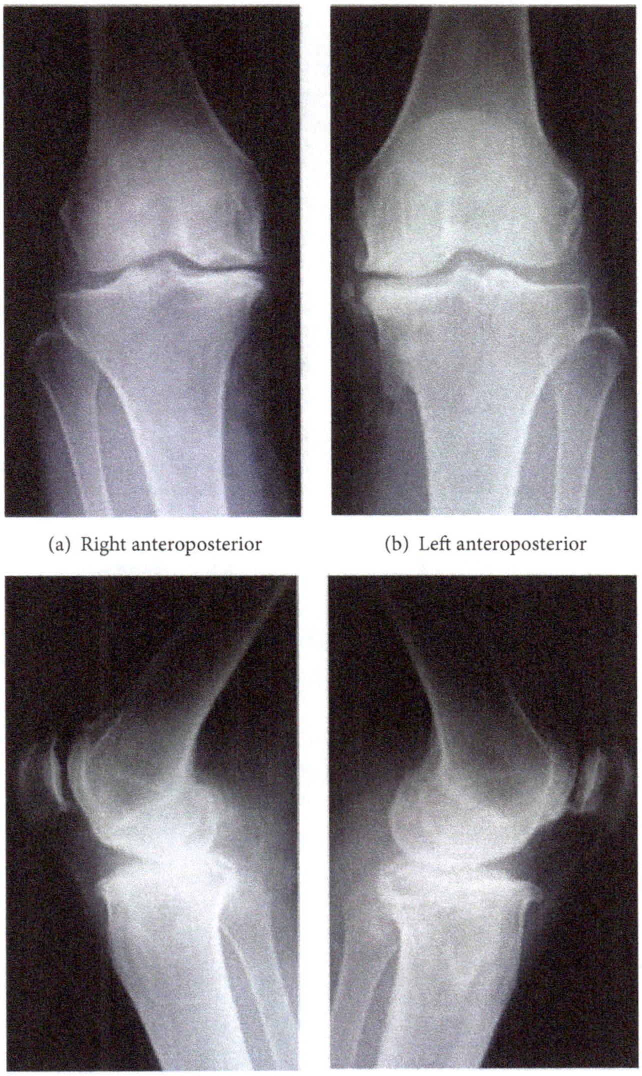

(a) Right anteroposterior (b) Left anteroposterior

(c) Right lateral (d) Left lateral

FIGURE 1: Preoperative X-ray.

In 2012, she underwent right TKA, for which the implant was the Scorpio NRG (Stryker, Mahwah, NJ, USA). It was performed with a medial parapatellar incision, followed by PS and cement fixation, without patellar resurfacing. In 2015, she underwent left TKA, for which the implant was the Journey II (Smith and Nephew, Memphis, TN, USA). That procedure was also performed with a medial parapatellar incision, followed by BCS, cement fixation, and patellar resurfacing.

Postoperative lateral X-ray images of the extended position showed that the posterior offset ratio (POR) was 12.1% with conventional TKA and 0% with BCS TKA. This POR is the POR ($a/b \times 100\%$) calculated with the knee joint in the extended position, reported by Onodera et al. (Figure 2) [4]. The POR of a normal knee is reportedly 5.63% ± 5.34%, and BCS TKA is believed to yield anteroposterior positioning that is close to that of a normal knee.

TABLE 1: New knee society score.

	Right conventional	Left bicruciate stabilized
Indicators	63	66
Symptoms	25	25
Satisfaction	36	36
Expectations	8	10
Activities	50	48

The range of motion of the knee joint was 5° to 130° for the right knee and 0° to 145° for the left knee at three months after the BCS TKA. The new Knee Society Score (2011 KSS) was used for postoperative assessment, yielding equivalent results for the left and right knees (Table 1). Objective knee indicators show higher points in left knee, because the range of motion

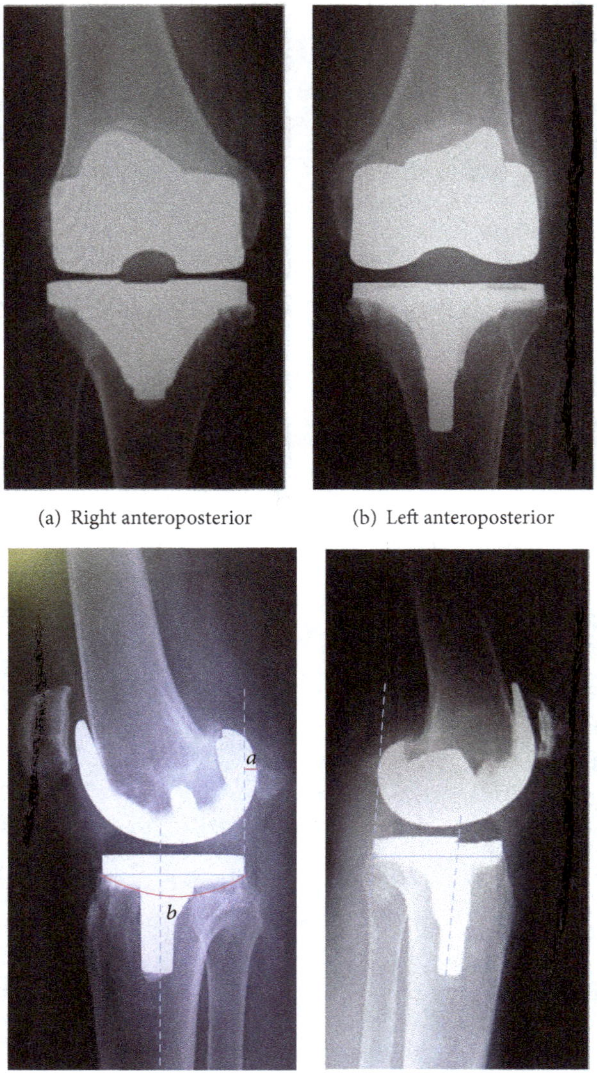

(a) Right anteroposterior (b) Left anteroposterior

(c) Right lateral (d) Left lateral

FIGURE 2: Postoperative X-ray.

is better in left knee than right knee. And expectation also shows higher points in left knee, because left knee has better pain relief than right knee. In terms of activity, points of walking on an uneven surface and climbing up or down a flight or stairs are fewer in left knee than right knee.

After surgery, the patient was asked to walk with a triaxial accelerometer (Hitachi H48C 3-Axis Accelerometer Module, Hitachi Metals Co., Ltd., Tokyo, Japan) (Figure 3(a)) placed on the upper end of the patella on the femoral side and on the tibial tubercle on the tibial side and a heel sensor (Click BP, Tokyo Sensor Co., Ltd., Tokyo, Japan) (Figure 3(b)) placed on the heel in order to determine the stance phase and the swing phase. For gait conditions, the patient was instructed to walk at normal speed and to walk a flat straight path without using a walking aid.

The resulting data were collected into a data logger (Memory HiLogger LR8431, Hioki E. E. Co., Nagano, Japan). A graph of the actual walking data is presented (Figure 4(a)). The horizontal axis is time, and the vertical axis is voltage (volts (V)). The straight line shown in the graph is the signal of the heel sensor, making it possible to determine the stance phase and swing phase. The accelerometer has an output power of 1.5 V when stopped; in a resting state, 1.5 V is 0 g (gravity) and 1.833 V is 1 g (gravity) ($1\,g = 9.81\,m/s^2$). Acceleration can be interpreted as being positive or negative with reference to 1.5 V. The definition of each acceleration axis is that the x-axis is the anteroposterior direction, the y-axis in the superoinferior direction, and the z-axis is the horizontal direction (Figure 4(b)).

Results from walking while wearing the accelerometers on the femur and tibia of the conventional TKA and BCS TKA legs showed a difference in the x-axis of the anteroposterior direction, which is presented in more detailed graphs (Figures 5 and 6). The femur of conventional TKA was found to have

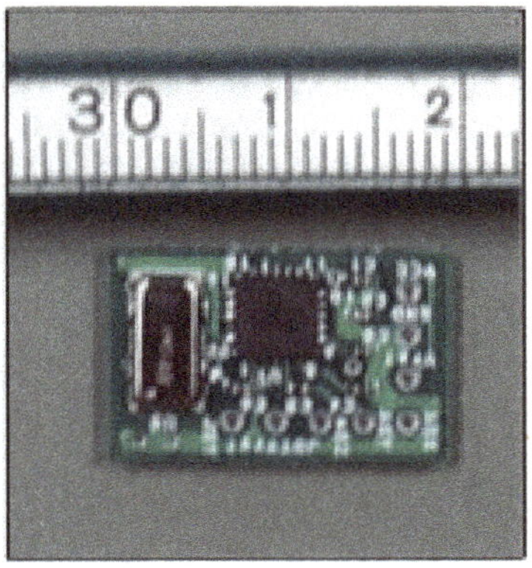

(a) Accelerometer

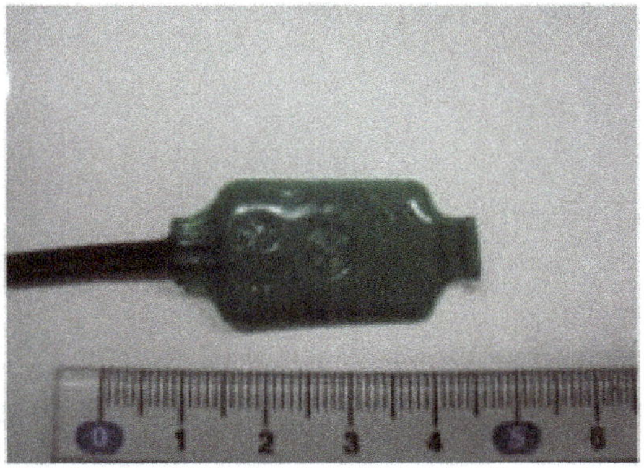

(b) Heel sensor

FIGURE 3: Sensors.

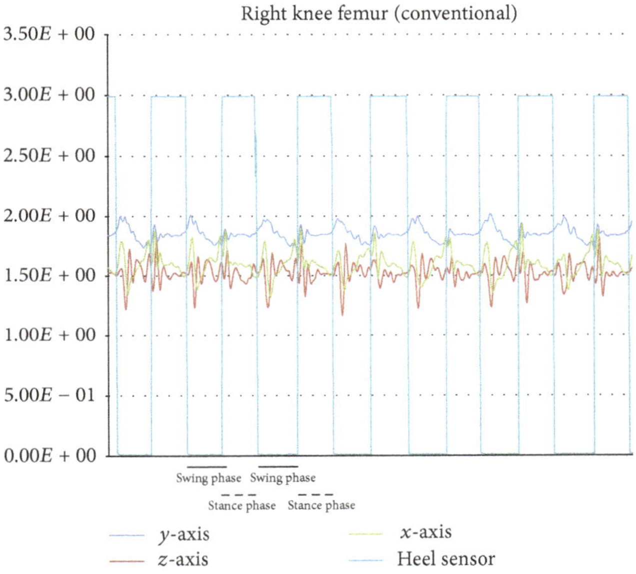

(a) Data of accelerometer and heel sensor

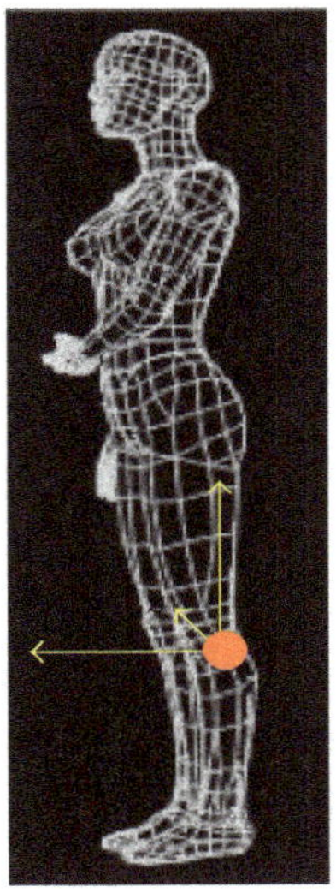

(b) A definition of the axis of acceleration

FIGURE 4: Data of sensors and a definition of the axis.

a greater amplitude of voltage than the femur of BCS TKA. A similar trend was observed on the tibial side, though not as great as the femoral side. When the maximum amplitude is measured with 1.5 V, which is the output power when stopped, as the baseline, then the femoral side and tibial side for conventional TKA were 1.902 V and 1.741 V, respectively, while the femoral side and tibial side for BCS TKA were 1.685 V and 1.612 V, respectively. A left/right comparison showed that, on the femoral side with BCS TKA, compared to conventional TKA, there was little acceleration in the x-axis direction (anteroposterior direction) in the early swing phase ($P < 0.05$ paired t-test). A similar trend was also observed on the tibial side (Figure 7). All analyses were performed using SPSS ver. 23.0 (IBM Corp., Armonk, NY, USA).

3. Discussion

BCS TKA has been said to provide anterior stability, but few reports have quantitatively assessed stability. In this report, accelerometers were used to quantitatively assess anterior stability with left/right comparisons made between conventional TKA and BCS TKA in the same patient.

There have been some reports on motion analysis of the knee using accelerometers, and they are reportedly effective tools for motion analysis [5–7].

Staab et al. used accelerometers and gyroscopes to conduct gait analysis in OA patients and reported that these sensors were approximately the same as the Vicon [5]. Khan et al. conducted gait analysis with accelerometers in a TKA group and a control group, and they reported that the TKA

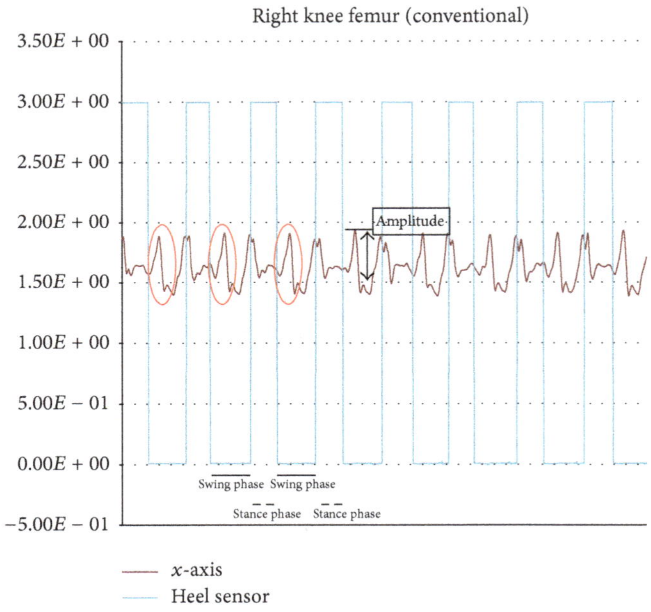

(a) Conventional femur

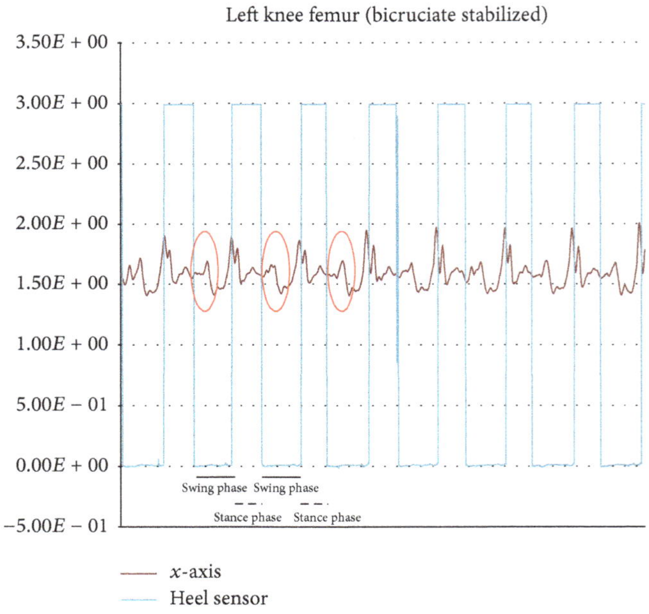

(b) Bicruciate stabilized femur

FIGURE 5: Acceleration of the femur.

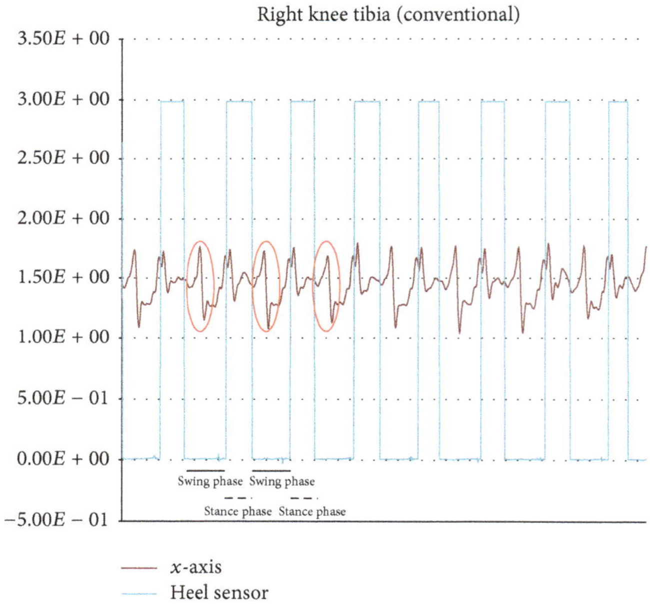

(a) Conventional tibia

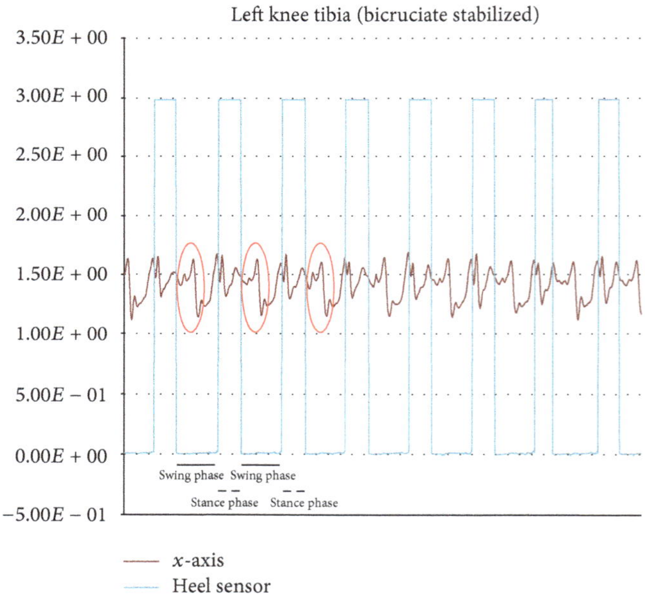

(b) Bicruciate stabilized tibia

FIGURE 6: Acceleration of the tibia.

group showed greater acceleration changes than the control group in step-down and turning motions [6]. Liikavainio et al. reported that skin-mounted accelerometers above and below knee had good repeatability in healthy young men [7].

The ACL is said to act as a stabilizer in the early flexion phase [8]. In this study, the analysis confirmed that, in the early swing phase (early flexed phase), there was less acceleration in the anteroposterior direction on the femoral side with BCS TKA than with conventional TKA. This suggests that, with BCS TKA, the knee joint was stabilized in the anteroposterior direction in the early flexion phase, reducing the so-called paradoxical motion said to occur in the early flexion phase with conventional TKA, where the femur exhibits anterior slipping.

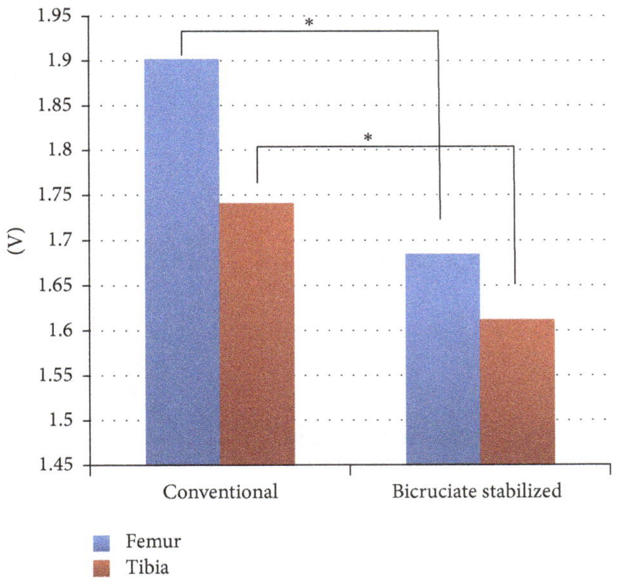

FIGURE 7: Acceleration of the conventional and bicruciate stabilized total knee arthroplasty. $^{*}P < 0.05$ paired t-test.

4. Conclusion

BCS TKA may be able to replace ACL function due to the structure of the implant and proper anteroposterior positioning.

Consent

The authors state that the patient has given their informed consent for the case report to be published.

Competing Interests

The authors declare that they have no competing interests.

References

[1] D. A. Dennis, R. D. Komistek, M. R. Mahfouz, B. D. Haas, and J. B. Stiehl, "Multicenter determination of in vivo kinematics after total knee arthroplasty," *Clinical Orthopaedics and Related Research*, vol. 416, pp. 37–57, 2003.

[2] J. Victor and J. Bellemans, "Physiologic kinematics as a concept for better flexion in TKA," *Clinical Orthopaedics and Related Research*, no. 452, pp. 53–58, 2006.

[3] F. Catani, A. Ensini, C. Belvedere et al., "In vivo kinematics and kinetics of a bi-cruciate substituting total knee arthroplasty: a combined fluoroscopic and gait analysis study," *Journal of Orthopaedic Research*, vol. 27, no. 12, pp. 1569–1575, 2009.

[4] T. Onodera, T. Majima, O. Nishiike, Y. Kasahara, and D. Takahashi, "Posterior femoral condylar offset after total knee replacement in the risk of knee flexion contracture," *The Journal of Arthroplasty*, vol. 28, no. 7, pp. 1112–1116, 2013.

[5] W. Staab, R. Hottowitz, C. Sohns et al., "Accelerometer and gyroscope based gait analysis using spectral analysis of patients with osteoarthritis of the knee," *Journal of Physical Therapy Science*, vol. 26, no. 7, pp. 997–1002, 2014.

[6] H. Khan, P. S. Walker, J. D. Zuckerman et al., "The potential of accelerometers in the evaluation of stability of total knee arthroplasty," *The Journal of Arthroplasty*, vol. 28, no. 3, pp. 459–462, 2013.

[7] T. Liikavainio, T. Bragge, M. Hakkarainen, J. S. Jurvelin, P. A. Karjalainen, and J. P. Arokoski, "Reproducibility of loading measurements with skin-mounted accelerometers during walking," *Archives of Physical Medicine and Rehabilitation*, vol. 88, no. 7, pp. 907–915, 2007.

[8] A. E. Ellison and E. E. Berg, "Embryology, anatomy, and function of the anterior cruciate ligament," *Orthopedic Clinics of North America*, vol. 16, no. 1, pp. 3–14, 1985.

22

Double-Layered Lateral Meniscus in an 8-Year-Old Child: Report of a Rare Case

Susumu Araki,[1,2] Mitsuhiko Kubo,[1] Kosuke Kumagai,[1] and Shinji Imai[1]

[1]*Department of Orthopaedic Surgery, Shiga University of Medical Science, Otsu, Shiga 520-2192, Japan*
[2]*Public Interest Incorporated Foundation, Toyosato Hospital, No. 12, 8 Moku, Toyosato-cho, Inukami, Shiga 529-1158, Japan*

Correspondence should be addressed to Susumu Araki; arakisu@belle.shiga-med.ac.jp

Academic Editor: Dimitrios S. Karataglis

Reports of congenital abnormalities of the lateral meniscus include discoid meniscus, accessory meniscus, double-layered meniscus, and ring-shaped meniscus. Particularly, only a few cases of double-layered meniscus have been reported. We report a case of double-layered lateral meniscus, in which an additional semicircular meniscus was observed under the normal lateral meniscus. The accessory hemimeniscus was resected by means of arthroscopic surgery. This case demonstrates an interesting and extremely rare anatomical abnormality of the lateral meniscus.

1. Introduction

The overall incidence of meniscal anomalies is rather small. These anomalies are more frequent in East Asian populations and tend to be more prevalent in the lateral meniscus. Discoid meniscus is the most common aberration, but other meniscus malformations are rare [1]. Among them, cases of accessory lateral meniscus in the form of a double-layered meniscus are extremely uncommon. To our knowledge, only a few such cases have been described to date [2–10]. Furthermore, our report involves the second youngest case patient thus far [10]. We report on a rare case that we diagnosed as double-layered lateral meniscus and operated on the patient by performing partial resection with arthroscopy. A physical examination of the left knee revealed pain and catching at the lateral aspect on deep flexion.

2. Case Report

2.1. History of Present Illness. An 8-year-old boy presented with pain in the left knee during baseball practice. He had no history of knee injury. At presentation at our institution (1 week after the onset of pain), his left knee pain and hydrarthrosis had become too severe to continue playing baseball well. On physical examination, full range of motion, tenderness at the lateral joint line, pain and catching on deep flexion, and a positive McMurray test on the lateral side were observed. His gait was normal and there was no sign of giving way of the affected knee. The valgus and varus stress tests, anterior drawer test, pivot-shift test, and posterior drawer test had negative results, indicating an absence of ligamentous abnormalities. The neurovascular examination showed normal findings. The radiographs and magnetic resonance images (MRIs) were normal (Figure 1).

2.2. Past Medical History. There was no history of injury and any other illness.

2.3. Family History. There was no relevant family history.

2.4. Athletic Experience. The patient had been playing baseball (position: catcher) for 3 years.

2.5. Surgical Operation and Postoperative Course. We performed follow-up examination on the patient for 2 weeks; however, his symptoms did not improve (especially the knee pain and catching on deep flexion). Therefore, he underwent arthroscopy of the left knee. On examination of the lateral compartment, a second semicircular meniscus was seen

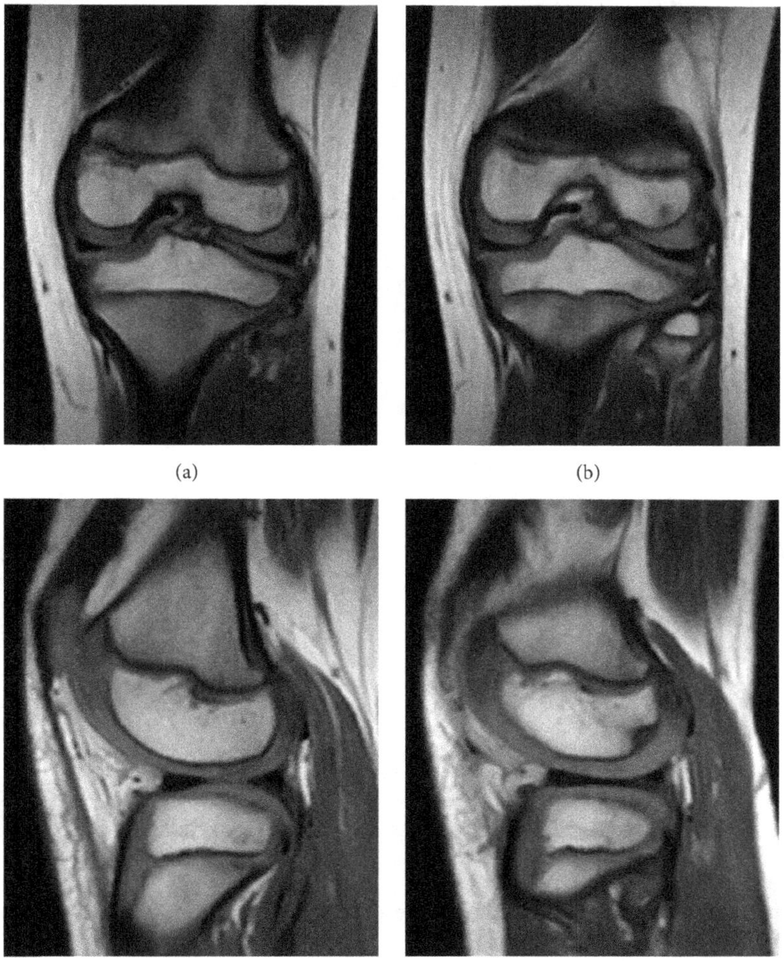

FIGURE 1: T1-weighted magnetic resonance images. Coronal (a, b) and sagittal (c, d) sections showing normal findings of the lateral meniscus.

under the original lateral meniscus, and it could be pulled forward easily on probing (Figure 2). There were no other joint abnormalities. The second semicircular meniscus of the left knee was resected arthroscopically, resulting in the complete relief of symptoms. The patient has now been able to return to baseball practice without restrictions.

The patient and his family members were informed that data from the case would be submitted for publication and provided their consent.

2.6. Histological Findings. In the lower layer of the meniscus, no disorder was seen in the arrangement of collagen fibers, which were dense and parallel (Figure 3).

3. Discussion

After the operation, we rechecked the previous MRIs; however, we could not find any lesion from those images. However, before the operation, the patient had been experiencing sharp pain and catching of the posterolateral side of his left knee on deep flexion. This finding made us suspect the presence of a meniscus lesion (e.g., lateral meniscus injury or a hypermobile meniscus), a synovium mass lesion, or a cartilage lesion. Furthermore, the possibility of an inflammatory lesion from his knee hydrarthrosis was considered. However, in this case, we judged it to be absent because the sharp pain and catching of the left knee occur only during motion. The patient frequently played baseball as a catcher. This position often requires a full range of motion of the knee. Therefore, we considered that this fact was closely related to the symptoms.

In this case, as mentioned above, a second semicircular meniscus was seen under the original lateral meniscus. Furthermore, the middle part of the abnormal meniscus was attached to the normal meniscus and the posterior horn was attached to the tibial articular cartilage surface. Concerning the movement of a normal lateral meniscus, it is believed that the lateral femoral condyle rolls back in the knee flexure, and at the same time the lateral meniscus recedes following the femoral condyle. However, in this case, the patient felt clicking and pain in the left knee because his abnormal

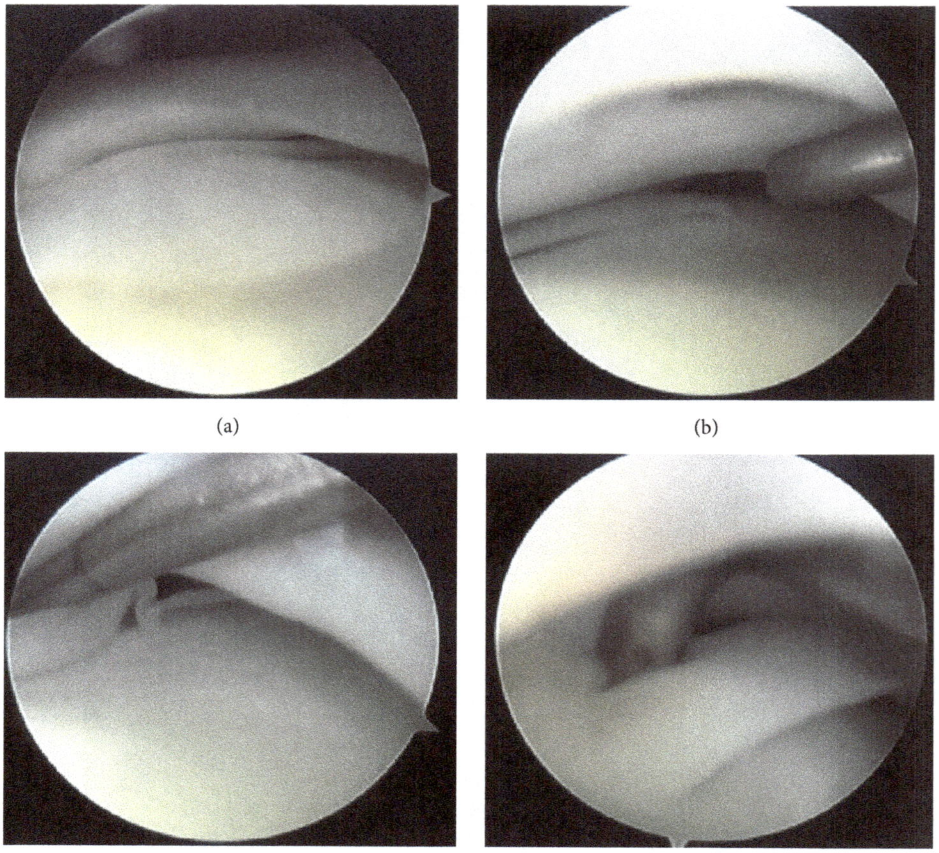

(a) (b) (c) (d)

FIGURE 2: Arthroscopic findings. (a) Lateral meniscus of the left knee. (b) A second semicircular meniscus is seen under the original lateral meniscus. It could be pulled forward easily on probing (c, d).

(a) (b)

FIGURE 3: Histological findings of the second semicircular meniscus. No disorder was seen in the arrangement of collagen fibers, which were dense and parallel. Hematoxylin and eosin staining, ×40 (a) and ×100 (b).

meniscus was attached to the tibial plateau and it was left against the lateral femoral condyle.

A discoid lateral meniscus is the most common abnormality of the lateral meniscus. However, cases of accessory lateral meniscus in the form of a double-layered meniscus are extremely uncommon (reported with a prevalence of 0.06% to 0.09% [2, 3]) and, when present, are believed to potentially contribute to the symptoms of patients [2]. To our knowledge, only nine such cases have been described to date [2–10]. All patients were young and had malformation of the lateral meniscus. Furthermore, in all nine cases, an accessory meniscus was overlying the normal lateral meniscus. This case demonstrates an interesting and extremely rare anatomical abnormality of the lateral meniscus. This is the first reported case of an accessory meniscus under a layered original meniscus.

As with other meniscus malformations, a double-layered meniscus is believed to develop in the early fetal periods [11]. At the age of 8 years, the present patient is the second youngest case patient in the literature [10]. The age at presentation of the patient coincides with the start of competition activities in school club teams in Japan and thus correlates with an increase in physical activity compared with children in lower grades. Furthermore, it was considered that the nature of the movements of the patient as a baseball catcher induced his symptoms. The presence of an abnormally shaped meniscus may lead to significantly altered biomechanics of the lateral compartment. The clinical significance of such altered biomechanics is not always clear; however, they have often been associated with pain and clicking. In addition, it is clinically important to differentiate such symptoms from any other pain and/or clicking in the knee in children.

4. Conclusions

We reported a case of double-layered lateral meniscus in the second youngest patient thus far. Furthermore, this is the first reported case of an accessory meniscus located under the normal lateral meniscus. Arthroscopic partial meniscectomy resulted in patient satisfaction and a return to normal daily activities, which included baseball practice. In the case of suspicion of a meniscal lesion or its symptoms on physical examination, meniscal malformation/injury should be considered even if the MRI does not show any injury/morphological aberration.

Competing Interests

All authors have no conflict of interests.

References

[1] K. Ryu, T. Iriuchishima, M. Oshida et al., "Evaluation of the morphological variations of the meniscus: a cadaver study," *Knee Surgery, Sports Traumatology, Arthroscopy*, vol. 23, no. 1, pp. 15–19, 2015.

[2] S. Suzuki, F. Mita, and H. Ogishima, "Double-layered lateral meniscus: a newly found anomaly," *Arthroscopy*, vol. 7, no. 3, pp. 267–271, 1991.

[3] K. Okahashi, K. Sugimoto, M. Iwai, M. Oshima, Y. Fujisawa, and Y. Takakura, "Double-layered lateral meniscus," *Journal of Orthopaedic Science*, vol. 10, no. 6, pp. 661–664, 2005.

[4] D. Karataglis, A. Dramis, and D. J. A. Learmonth, "Double-layered lateral meniscus. A rare anatomical aberration," *Knee*, vol. 13, no. 5, pp. 415–416, 2006.

[5] K. Takayama, R. Kuroda, T. Matsumoto et al., "Bilateral double-layered lateral meniscus: a report of two cases," *Knee Surgery, Sports Traumatology, Arthroscopy*, vol. 17, no. 11, pp. 1336–1339, 2009.

[6] N. Komatsu, K. Yamamoto, and E. Chosa, "Bilateral congenital separation of the lateral meniscus. A case report," *Knee*, vol. 15, no. 4, pp. 330–332, 2008.

[7] Q. Wang, X.-M. Liu, S.-B. Liu, and Y. Bai, "Double-layered lateral meniscus," *Knee Surgery, Sports Traumatology, Arthroscopy*, vol. 19, no. 12, pp. 2050–2051, 2011.

[8] K. W. Lee, D. S. Yang, and W. S. Choy, "Dislocated double-layered lateral meniscus mimicking the bucket-handle tear," *Orthopedics*, vol. 36, no. 10, pp. e1333–e1335, 2013.

[9] A. Fukuda, A. Nishimura, S. Nakazora, K. Kato, and A. Sudo, "Double-layered lateral meniscus accompanied by meniscocapsular separation," *Case Reports in Orthopedics*, vol. 2015, Article ID 357463, 5 pages, 2015.

[10] W. H. Bailey and G. E. Blundell, "An unusual abnormality affecting both knee joints in a child: case report," *The Journal of Bone & Joint Surgery—American Volume*, vol. 56, no. 4, pp. 814–816, 1974.

[11] C. R. Clark and J. A. Ogden, "Development of the menisci of the human knee joint. Morphological changes and their potential role in childhood meniscal injury," *Journal of Bone and Joint Surgery—Series A*, vol. 65, no. 4, pp. 538–547, 1983.

A Case of Legg-Calvé-Perthes Disease due to Transient Synovitis of the Hip

Tadahiko Ohtsuru, Yasuaki Murata, Yuji Morita, Yutaro Munakata, and Yoshiharu Kato

Department of Orthopedic Surgery, Tokyo Women's Medical University, 8-1 Kawada-cho, Shinjuku Ward, Tokyo 162-8666, Japan

Correspondence should be addressed to Tadahiko Ohtsuru; tada0403@gmail.com

Academic Editor: Johannes Mayr

Transient synovitis (TS) of the hip develops spontaneously in childhood; it usually has a good prognosis and is a self-limiting disease. However, its pathology is not well known. We describe a case of Legg-Calvé-Perthes disease (LCPD) that seemingly developed due to TS. Even if TS is diagnosed on the basis of the patient's medical history and imaging findings, physicians should consider the possibility of LCPD and perform a careful observation if joint effusion continues and/or a symptom does not improve within 4 weeks.

1. Introduction

Transient synovitis (TS) of the hip has a good prognosis, and it is a self-limiting disease. However, if the diagnosis of TS is delayed, it may progress to Legg-Calvé-Perthes disease (LCPD), which has a poor prognosis. The causal association between TS and LCPD is not well understood. We describe a case of LCPD that was seemingly due to TS and present a literature review.

2. Case Presentation

A 7-year-old girl complained of pain in her left thigh, and she was limping. She had no history of trauma, disease, or surgery. She had left thigh pain for 3 weeks before visiting the outpatient clinic. The ranges of left hip motion were as follows: flexion, 130°; abduction, 30°; extension, 10°; internal rotation, 45°; and external rotation, 10°. The circumferences of the right and left thighs were 29.5 cm and 28.5 cm, respectively. Plain radiographs obtained at the initial visit showed no abnormalities (Figure 1). T2-weighted magnetic resonance imaging (MRI) scan of the hip joints showed no abnormal findings, except left hip joint effusion (Figure 2). TS was diagnosed on the basis of the patient's medical history and imaging findings, and we continued follow-up. She was on bedrest for 4 weeks, and we instructed her to avoid weight bearing during this time. However, her left thigh pain and limping did not improve. The ultrasonic joint spaces (distance from the anterior cortex of the femoral neck to the front of the capsule [the width of the joint space]) measured 6.0 mm on the right side and 8.7 mm on the left side at 4 weeks after the initial visit. Joint effusion was diagnosed on the basis of anechoic findings of the left hip joint space. T1-weighted and T2-weighted MRI scans of the hip joints showed a linear low-signal-intensity region at the left femoral capital epiphysis 2 months after the initial visit (Figure 3). Although no abnormalities were found, follow-up continued. The ultrasonic joint space measured 11.6 mm on the left side 2 months after the initial visit (Figure 4). Synovitis was diagnosed on the basis of echoic findings of the left hip joint space. A culture of the joint aspirate showed negative results. The laboratory data showed no abnormalities. The ultrasonic joint space measured 12.3 mm on the left side 3 months after the initial visit. Hence, we determined that synovitis progressed. Plain radiograph showed bone resorption at the left femoral capital epiphysis 3 months after the initial visit (Figure 5). Bone scintigraphy findings showed a cold-in-hot pattern at the left femoral capital epiphysis (Figure 6). We diagnosed the patient as having LCPD on the basis of these imaging findings. We instructed her to wear a hip abduction and non-weight-bearing brace. We categorized the disease as Catterall group II and Herring group B according to the

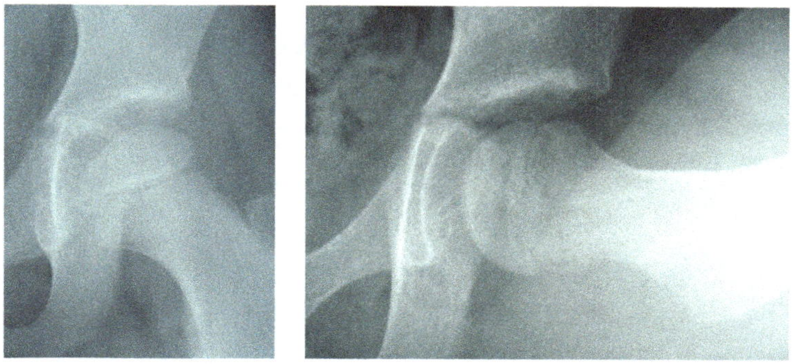

(a) (b)

Figure 1: Plain radiographs of the hip joints at the initial visit. (a) Anteroposterior image. (b) Lateral image. No abnormalities were observed.

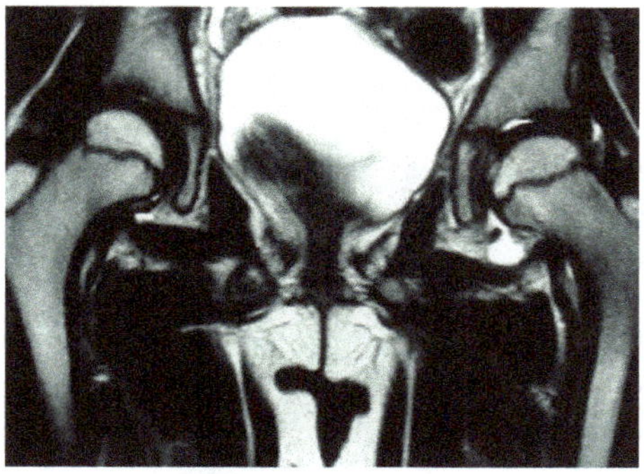

Figure 2: Coronal, T2-weighted magnetic resonance imaging scan at the initial visit. No abnormal findings, except left hip joint effusion, were observed.

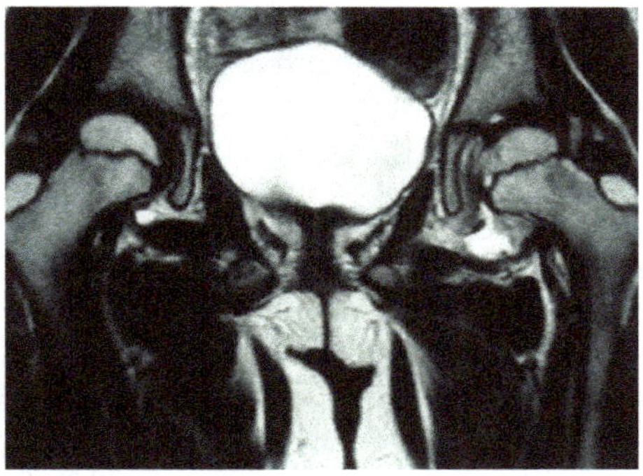

Figure 3: Coronal, T2-weighted magnetic resonance imaging scan of the hip joints 2 months after the initial visit. A linear low-signal-intensity region was found at the left femoral capital epiphysis.

findings from plain radiographs 8 months after the initial visit (Figure 7). Plain radiographs showed a continuous subchondral bone 15 months after the initial visit. We removed her brace and continued follow-up. Plain radiographs showed good remodeling of the necrotic area at the left femoral capital epiphysis 7 years after the initial visit. She did not have a lower limb discrepancy, left thigh pain, or limping (Figure 8).

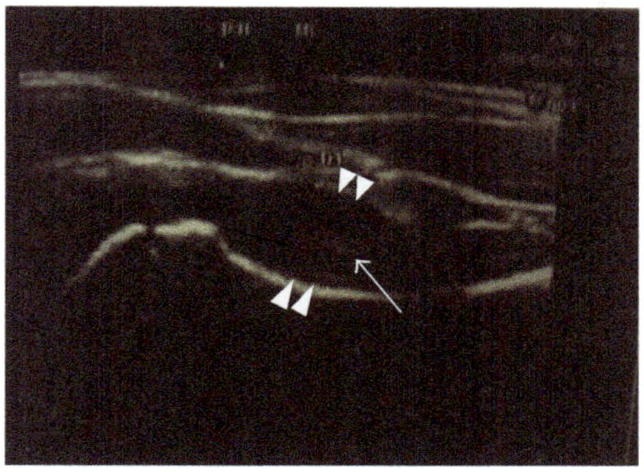

Figure 4: Ultrasonic joint space (distance from the anterior cortex of the femoral neck to the front of the capsule [the width of the joint space]) 2 months after the initial visit. It was 11.6 mm for the left hip (arrowheads). The intracapsular space showed echoic findings (arrow).

3. Discussion

Hip diseases in school-age children are categorized as a good-prognosis or poor-prognosis disease. TS is a self-limiting, good-prognosis disease, whereas LCPD, slipped capital femoral epiphysis, and septic arthritis of the hip are poor-prognosis diseases if the diagnosis is delayed. Although most hip diseases in school-age children can be easily diagnosed, some cases are difficult to diagnose. In addition, the association between TS and LCPD is still unclear.

Plain radiographs of the present patient showed no abnormalities at the time of pain onset. T2-weighted MRI scans and ultrasonogram of the hip joints showed no abnormal findings, except left hip joint effusion. Thus, we diagnosed the present patient as having TS. However, her left thigh pain and limping did not improve. Although T1-weighted and T2-weighted MRI scans of the hip joints showed a linear low-signal-intensity region at the left femoral capital epiphysis 2 months after the initial visit, we determined that these findings did not indicate anything significant. Finally, LCPD was diagnosed on the basis of the findings from plain radiographs and bone scintigraphy 3 months after the initial visit.

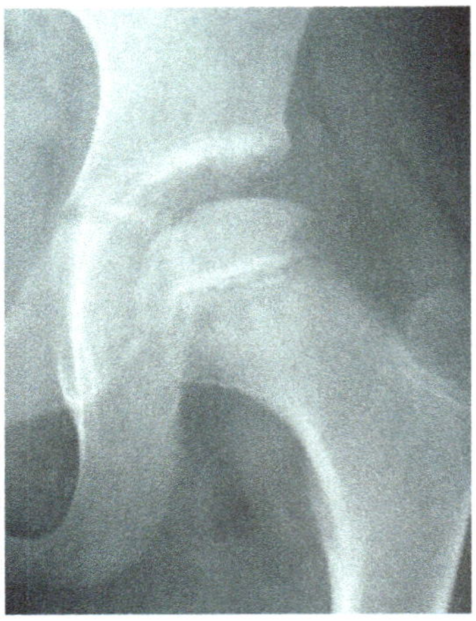

FIGURE 5: Plain radiograph of the hip joint 3 months after the initial visit. Bone resorption was observed at the left femoral capital epiphysis.

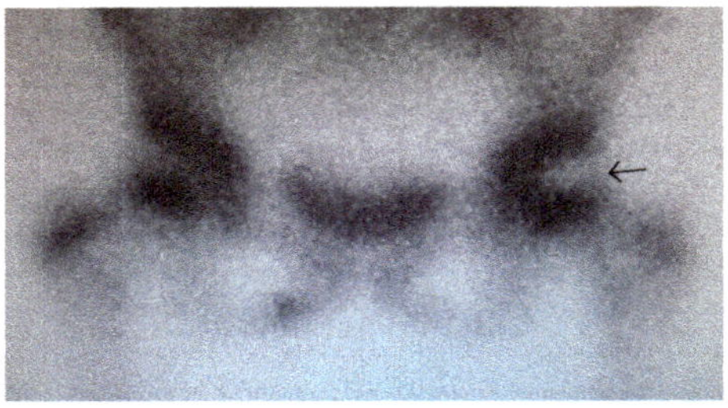

FIGURE 6: Bone scintigraphy findings. A cold-in-hot pattern is shown at the left femoral capital epiphysis (arrow).

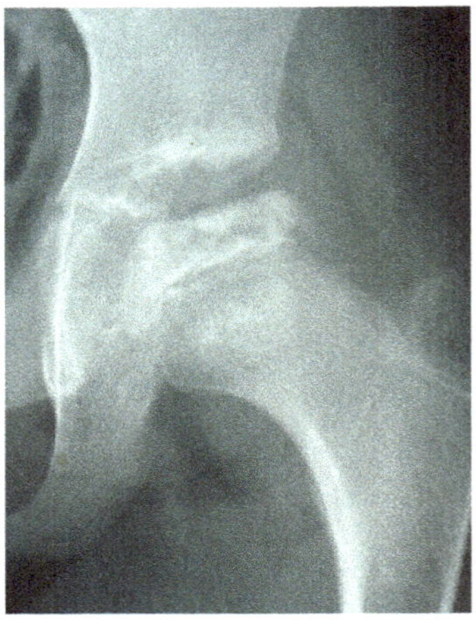

FIGURE 7: Plain radiograph of the left hip joint 8 months after the initial visit. We categorized the disease as Catterall group II and Herring group B.

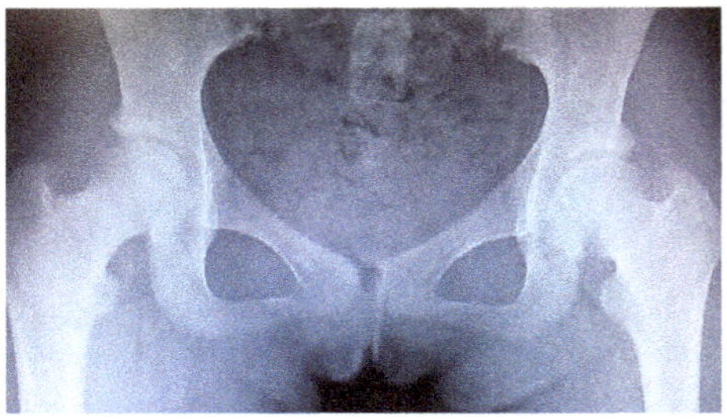

FIGURE 8: Plain radiograph of the hip joints 7 years after the initial visit. Good remodeling of the necrotic area at the left femoral capital epiphysis was observed.

In 1984, Wilson et al. first reported the usefulness of ultrasonography for diagnosing coxarthrosis in childhood [1]. Zieger et al. reported that if the intracapsular intensity on an ultrasonogram was anechoic, it indicated effusion or fresh blood, and if the intracapsular intensity on an ultrasonogram was echoic, it indicated septic arthritis, old blood, synovitis, or a tumor [2]. The period between the onset and disappearance of symptoms was about 2 weeks in cases of TS [1, 3, 4]. Hattori et al. reported on discriminating between early LCPD and TS by measuring the ultrasonic joint space [5]. They concluded that although the ultrasonic joint space normalized within 2 weeks in cases of TS, it did not improve for more than 4 weeks in cases of LCPD. The normal values of the ultrasonic joint space in children reportedly range from 5 to 6 mm [5, 6]. Thus, the ultrasonic joint spaces on both sides of the hip must be compared, because the spaces may be large in a healthy patient [7].

Considering these previous reports, a patient with symptoms that do not improve within more than 4 weeks should be considered as having LCPD. As the present patient had a typical clinical course and imaging findings of TS for the initial 4 weeks and those of LCPD for more than 4 weeks later (Figure 9), we suspected that there was an association between these two diseases.

The causal association between TS and LCPD is not well understood. Bickerstaff et al. [4], Terjesen and Østhus [8], and Landin et al. [9] reported cases that have likely developed LCPD due to TS [4, 8, 9]. In contrast, Kallio et al. did not support the association between TS and LCPD [3]. Futami et al. described the case of a 10-year-old boy who developed right LCPD during follow-up for left LCPD [10]; MRI was performed incidentally 5 weeks before right LCPD developed. T1-weighted MRI scan showed a low-intensity band region at the femoral capital epiphysis, and T2-weighted MRI scan showed a high-intensity band region at the femoral capital epiphysis. They reported that these findings indicated bone marrow edema. Similarly, MRI was performed before necrosis developed in the present case, and T1-weighted and T2-weighted MRI scans showed a linear low-signal-intensity region at the femoral capital epiphysis (Figure 3). As the findings of this region coincided with the medial margin of necrosis, which developed later, we considered that this finding indicated a small portion of the necrotic region just after it began to develop.

Trueta reported that LCPD was caused by vascular insufficiency of the lateral epiphyseal artery (the branch of the medial circumflex femoral artery) [11]. We considered that avascular necrosis of the femoral capital epiphysis was caused

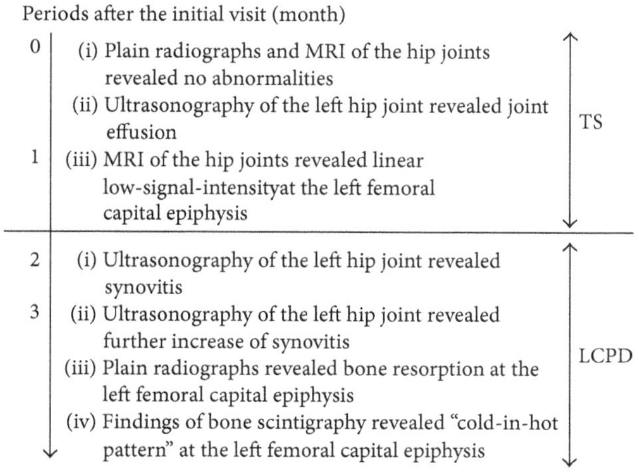
Periods after the initial visit (month)
0
(i) Plain radiographs and MRI of the hip joints revealed no abnormalities
(ii) Ultrasonography of the left hip joint revealed joint effusion
1
(iii) MRI of the hip joints revealed linear low-signal-intensityat the left femoral capital epiphysis
TS
2
(i) Ultrasonography of the left hip joint revealed synovitis
3
(ii) Ultrasonography of the left hip joint revealed further increase of synovitis
(iii) Plain radiographs revealed bone resorption at the left femoral capital epiphysis
(iv) Findings of bone scintigraphy revealed "cold-in-hot pattern" at the left femoral capital epiphysis
LCPD

FIGURE 9: Flowchart of the imaging findings in the present case. MRI: magnetic resonance imaging, TS: transient synovitis, and LCPD: Legg-Calvé-Perthes disease.

by the increase in intracapsular pressure due to prolonged effusion and synovitis, as reported by Wlngstrand et al. [12].

In conclusion, we described a case of LCPD seemingly due to TS. Even if TS is diagnosed on the basis of a patient's medical history and imaging findings, physicians should consider LCPD and perform careful observation if joint effusion continues and/or a symptom does not improve within 4 weeks.

Consent

The authors obtained written informed consent from the patient's next of kin for the publication of this case report.

Competing Interests

The authors declare no competing interests.

References

[1] D. J. Wilson, D. J. Green, and J. C. MacLarnon, "Arthrosonography of the painful hip," *Clinical Radiology*, vol. 35, no. 1, pp. 17–19, 1984.

[2] M. M. Zieger, U. Dörr, and R. D. Schulz, "Ultrasonography of hip joint effusions," *Skeletal Radiology*, vol. 16, no. 8, pp. 607–611, 1987.

[3] P. Kallio, S. Ryoppy, and I. Kunnamo, "Transient synovitis and Perthes' disease. Is there an aetiological connection?" *The Journal of Bone & Joint Surgery—British Volume*, vol. 68, no. 5, pp. 808–811, 1986.

[4] D. R. Bickerstaff, L. M. Neal, A. J. Booth, P. O. Brennan, and M. J. Bell, "Ultrasound examination of the irritable hip," *The Journal of Bone & Joint Surgery—British Volume*, vol. 72, no. 4, pp. 549–553, 1990.

[5] T. Hattori, Y. Yoshihashi, S. Tanaka, F. Ito, T. Miura, and Y. Yamada, "Ultrasonography in hip disease in children," *The Journal of the Japanese Society of Orthopedic Ultrasonics*, vol. 1, no. 1, pp. 26–29, 1989 (Japanese).

[6] V. T. Valley and S. A. Stahmer, "Targeted musculoarticular sonography in the detection of joint effusions," *Academic Emergency Medicine*, vol. 8, no. 4, pp. 361–367, 2001.

[7] J. Y. Jung, G.-U. Kim, H.-J. Lee, E.-C. Jang, I. S. Song, and Y.-C. Ha, "Diagnostic value of ultrasound and computed tomographic arthrography in diagnosing anterosuperior acetabular labral tears," *Arthroscopy*, vol. 29, no. 11, pp. 1769–1776, 2013.

[8] T. Terjesen and P. Østhus, "Ultrasound in the diagnosis and follow-up of transient synovitis of the hip," *Journal of Pediatric Orthopaedics*, vol. 11, no. 5, pp. 608–613, 1991.

[9] L. A. Landin, L. G. Danielsson, and C. Wattsgard, "Transient synovitis of the hip. Its incidence, epidemiology and relation to Perthes' disease," *The Journal of Bone & Joint Surgery—British Volume*, vol. 69, no. 2, pp. 238–242, 1987.

[10] T. Futami, K. Ishida, K. Tamura, and S. Suzuki, "Features of early Perthes' disease," *Orthopedic Surgery*, vol. 32, pp. 358–394, 1997 (Japanese).

[11] J. Trueta, "The normal vascular anatomy of the human femoral head during growth," *The Journal of Bone & Joint Surgery—British Volume*, vol. 39, no. 2, pp. 358–394, 1957.

[12] H. Wlngstrand, N. Egund, N. O. Carlin, L. Forsberg, T. Gustafson, and G. Sundén, "Intracapsular pressure in transient synovitis of the hip," *Acta Orthopaedica Scandinavica*, vol. 56, no. 3, pp. 204–210, 1985.

24

Unusual Closed Traumatic Avulsion of Both Flexor Tendons in Zones 1 and 3 of the Little Finger

Marie-Aimée Päivi Soro, Thierry Christen, and Sébastien Durand

Department of Plastic and Hand Surgery, Lausanne University Hospital, rue du Bugnon 46, 1011 Lausanne, Switzerland

Correspondence should be addressed to Marie-Aimée Päivi Soro; paivi.soro@gmail.com

Academic Editor: Johannes Mayr

Closed tendon avulsion of both flexor tendons in the same finger is an extremely rare condition. We encountered the case of a patient who presented a rupture of the flexor digitorum profundus in zone 1 and flexor digitorum superficialis in zone 3 in the little finger. This occurrence has not been reported previously. We hereby present our case, make a review of the literature of avulsion of both flexor tendons of the same finger, and propose a treatment according to the site of the ruptures.

1. Introduction

Closed tendon avulsion is a well recognized injury in hand surgery. Also called *Jersey finger*, it usually involves the flexor digitorum profundus (FDP) tendon. The typical mechanism is a forced hyperextension on a fully flexed finger. It is often encountered in contact sports like rugby, American football, or judo when a player grabs his opponent's shirt with the tip of his finger while the opponent is running away.

Closed avulsion of the flexor digitorum superficialis (FDS) associated with an avulsion of the FDP is a rare occurrence. Only 8 cases have been reported since 1984 [1–9].

We encountered an unusual case of closed avulsion of both flexor tendons of the little finger with a rupture of the FDP in zone 1 and FDS in zone 3. Combination of simultaneous avulsion in zones 1 and 3 has not been reported previously. We will present our case, review the literature, and propose a treatment according to the site of the ruptures.

2. Case Report

A 30-year-old patient presented to the emergency unit after a rugby game with the impossibility to flex his fifth finger on the left hand. Surgical exploration was performed the same day; it demonstrated a rupture of the FDP a few millimetres from its insertion and a laceration of the FDS in the mid-palm (Figure 1). No previous trauma or other pathology could explain this double rupture.

The FDP was reinserted using a pull-out technique. In order to avoid flexion deformity of the distal interphalangeal (DIP) joint related to excessive tension of the FDP, the procedure was completed with a lengthening Z-plasty of the FDP in the forearm proximal to the carpal tunnel.

As the rupture of the FDS occurred in the mid-palm, a reconstruction would not interfere with the course of the FDP in the digital canal. Therefore the suture of the FDS was reinforced with a palmaris longus tendon graft.

The patient was immobilized in a Duran splint and underwent the usual rehabilitation protocol for flexor tendon lesions with physical therapists.

Follow-up at 6 months showed the patient was able to touch his palm with his little finger (Figures 2 and 3) and return to work. The mobility of the finger in extension/flexion was as follows: metacarpophalangeal (MCP) joint: 0/0/95°, proximal interphalangeal (PIP) joint: 0/10/85°, and distal interphalangeal (DIP) joint: 0/10/25°. Active flexion of the PIP joint was observed when action of the FDP was prevented.

3. Discussion-Review of the Literature

We found 8 case reports (11 fingers) of closed avulsion of both flexor tendons in a single finger [1–9]. The characteristics of the patients, injury type, surgical repair technique, and results are summarized in Table 1.

TABLE 1: Closed avulsion of both flexors in the same finger.

Author	Patient age, sex, HD	Mechanism	Finger(s)	Site of rupture	Days before surgery	Technique	Months of postsurgery follow-up	Success
Our case	30, ♂, R	Jersey finger	D5 L	FDS: zone 3 FDP: zone 1	0	FDP: pull-out, FDS: suture reinforced by a tendon graft	6	E/F MCP: 0/0/95°, PIP: 0/10/85° DIP: 0/10/22°. Back to work.
Cheung and Chow [3]	24, ♂, R	Jersey finger	D4 R	FDS: zone 2 FDP: zone 1	4	Both tendons sutured to a periosteal flap and FDP reinforced by pull-out	3.5	Full range of motion MP + PIP, flexum 4° DIP. Back to work.
Oğün et al. [8]	21, ♂, NM	Jersey finger	D4 R	FDS: zone 2 FDP: zone 1	0	FDP: pull-out, FDS: resected	19	Total active range of motion = 230°, flexum PIP, DIP stiffness.
Naohito et al. [7]	49, ♂, L	Direct shock	D5 R	FDS: zone 2 FDP: zone 2	20	FDP: end-to-end suture, FDS resected	4	E/F: MCP: 30/0/80; PIP: 0/40/85, DIP: 0/5/60. Back to work.
Matthews and Walton [6]	28, ♂, R	Repeated microtrauma	D3 R	FDS: zone 2 mi-P1 FDP: zone 2 mi-P1	14	Two-stage repair: resection, silicone rod, reoperation at 10 weeks, palmaris longus graft.	3.5	Good result: normal flexion PIP, DIP stiffness. Back to work.
Cañadas Moreno et al. [2]	16, ♂, NM	Blast	D2 L: FDP + FDS D3 L: FDP + FDS D4 + D5: FDP	FDS: zone 2 FDP: zone 1	0	4 FDP: pull-out, 2 FDS: anchor suture technique	4 months 3 years	IPD: flexum 30° D2, D3, D5 Completely recovered.
Toussaint et al. [9]	23, ♂, R	Blast	D4 L D5 L	FDS: zone 2 FDP dilacerated in zone 1 + volar plate pull-out	D1	FDP: pull-out, FDS: resected	7	D4: PID: flexum 15°, PIP: flexum 10°. D5: PID flexum 40°, PIP flexum 10°. Back to work.
Backe and Posner [1]	23, ♂, NM	Traction-hyperextension	D4 R	FDS: zone 2 FDP: zone 1	4 weeks	Palmaris longus tendon graft	NM	Complete extension and active flexion to within 1.5 cm of the midpalmar crease. DIP stiffness. Back to work as truck driver.
Lanzetta and Conolly [4, 5]	28, ♂, R	Traction-hyperextension	D4 R	FDS: zone 2 FDP: zone 1	3	Two-stage repair: excision of both tendons, left plantaris tendon graft 9 weeks after the 1st surgery	4	Recovery of full extension and flexion. Back to work as a mechanic 4 months after 2nd surgery.

HD = hand dominance, R = right, L = left, NM = not mentioned, E/F = extension/flexion, MCP = metacarpophalangeal joint, PIP = proximal interphalangeal joint, and DIP = distal interphalangeal joint.

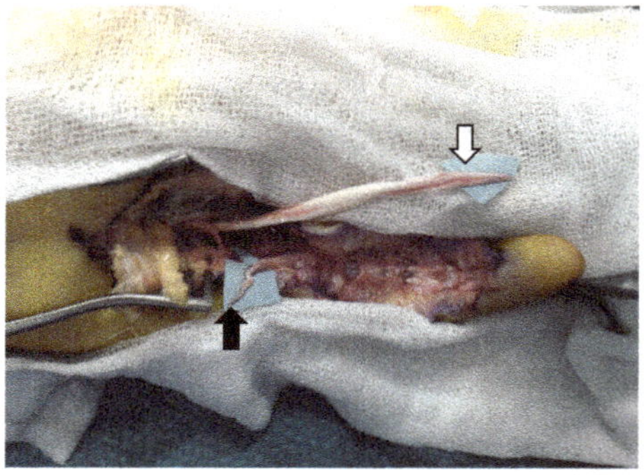

Figure 1: The white arrow indicates the proximal stump of the FDP, and the black arrow the distal dilacerated stump of the FDS.

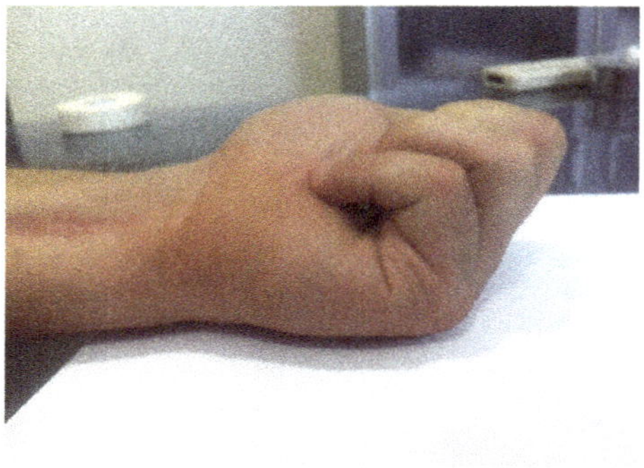

Figure 2: 6 months after surgery.

The mean age of the patients was 26.9 years. They were all men. The dominant hand was affected in 42% of patients (three authors did not mention the hand dominance). The ring finger (5/11 fingers) was the most commonly affected. Six different mechanisms of injury were encountered. Two patients presented with a typical Jersey finger [3, 8]. Two others suffered a blast injury [2, 9] and had several fingers affected. Two patients had a mechanism of traction-hyperextension [1, 4, 5]. The patient from Naohito et al. [7] hurt his fifth finger in a fall without further details. Repeated microtraumas were responsible for the rupture in one case [6]. The mean interval between traumatism and surgical exploration was 7.8 days (median 3 days). Five patients underwent surgery in the first week after trauma and 3 patients after 2 weeks.

One author used ultrasonography as a diagnostic help [9]. Their localisation of the rupture was accurate.

All FDS tendons were ruptured in zone 2 except in our case (zone 3).

All FDP including our case were ruptured in zone 1 except for two in zone 2 [6, 7].

Six authors chose to resect the FDS [1, 4–9]. In the other two cases [2, 3], the rupture was not intratendinous but at the insertion and associated with a bony avulsion. Both authors reinserted it with a transosseous suture.

Four authors reinserted the FDP through a pull-out suture [2, 3, 8, 9]. Naohito et al. [7] performed an end-to-end suture for a zone 2 rupture. Three authors [1, 4–6] performed

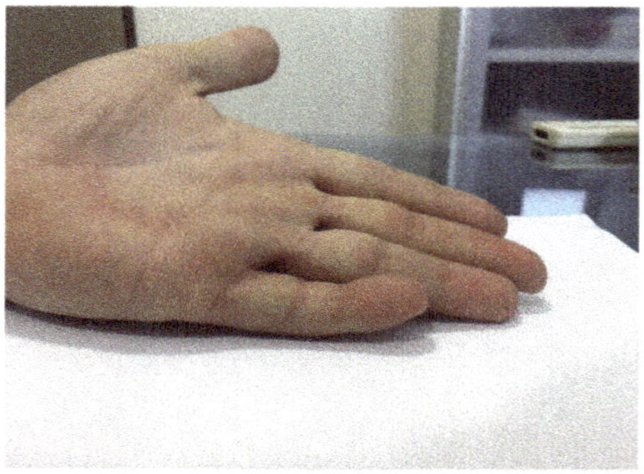

Figure 3: 6 months after surgery.

an FDP resection followed by a tendon graft in a one- or two-stage procedure when rupture was in zone 2 or in cases of delayed presentation.

The outcome was reported as good to excellent in 4 cases out of 8. In the other four cases, the results were poorer due to an FDP lesion in zone 2 or dilacerated in zone 1. Seven out of nine patients went back to work with no or little disability [1, 3–7, 9]. Two authors did not mention whether their patients were able to return to normal activity [2, 8].

Our case is unusual as the FDS was dilacerated in zone 3. The literature shows that few patients (2 out of 8) benefited from an FDS repair [2, 3]. This is probably due to the fact that both flexor tendon sutures in zone 2 are known to result in poorer outcome than more proximal lesions [10]. The rupture in zone 3 allowed for an FDS suture reinforced by a tendon graft. The other distinctive characteristic that our case presents is that the FDP pull-out suture was completed with a lengthening Z-plasty in the forearm which prevented tension deformity from the DIP and PIP joint. We were able to repair both tendons and avoid a suture in zone 2. The result was good at the 6-month follow-up visit and the patient was able to return to work.

Only one author used ultrasonography as a diagnostic tool before surgery [9]. Its utility has been shown as a diagnostic help for flexor tendon injuries [11, 12]. Double flexor tendon injury in the same finger is a rare occurrence and the usefulness of ultrasonography still needs to be explored in this indication. However, it might be an interesting tool to assess the zones in which the tendons have ruptured in order to define preoperatively surgical strategy.

In conclusion:

(1) When FDS is ruptured in zone 3 and FDP in zone 1, an FDS repair is recommended as it will not impair the FDP function in the digital canal and reinforces the action of the FDP. The FDP can benefit from a pull-out suture. If the FDP is dilacerated and the pull-out suture prevents full extension of the DIP or PIP joint we recommend a lengthening Z-plasty in the forearm so as to avoid a resection-graft which has worse outcomes.

(2) When the FDS is ruptured in zone 2 and the FDP in zone 1, we recommend to reinsert the FDP with

a pull-out suture. An FDS reinsertion could be considered in particular conditions [2, 3].

(3) If both tendons are ruptured in zone 2, whenever possible, both tendons should be repaired, as long as the FDP is gliding freely. If the tendons are severely dilacerated or oedematous and the FDS suture impairs the FDP course in the digital canal, the FDS should be resected [10]. The FDP, depending on the dilacerations and extension of the lesions, could be either sutured or grafted [6, 7]. Another surgical option is the transfer of a hemi-FDP-tendon from an adjacent finger [13].

Competing Interests

The authors declare that they have no competing interests.

Acknowledgments

The authors warmly thank Miss Robin Avona Hampton for her careful read-through of our manuscript.

References

[1] H. Backe and M. A. Posner, "Simultaneous rupture of both flexor tendons in a finger," *The Journal of Hand Surgery*, vol. 19, no. 2, pp. 246–248, 1994.

[2] O. Cañadas Moreno, R. Martínez González-Escalada, and F. J. Lara García, "Multiple closed avulsions of flexor tendons of the hand caused by a firecracker blast," *Annals of Plastic Surgery*, vol. 68, no. 2, pp. 158–160, 2012.

[3] K. M. C. Cheung and S. P. Chow, "Closed avulsion of both flexor tendons of the ring finger," *Journal of Hand Surgery*, vol. 20, no. 1, pp. 78–79, 1995.

[4] M. Lanzetta and W. B. Conolly, "Simultaneous rupture of both flexor tendons in a finger," *The Journal of Hand Surgery*, vol. 21, no. 6, pp. 1114–1115, 1996.

[5] M. Lanzetta and W. B. Conolly, "Biomechanical explanation of a simultaneous closed rupture of both flexor tendons in the same digit," *Australian and New Zealand Journal of Surgery*, vol. 66, no. 3, pp. 191–194, 1996.

[6] R. N. Matthews and J. N. Walton, "Spontaneous rupture of both flexor tendons in a single digit," *The Journal of Hand Surgery*, vol. 9, no. 2, pp. 134–136, 1984.

[7] H. Naohito, A. Masato, A. Rui, H. Daisuke, Y. Yusuke, and I. Koichi, "Closed rupture of both flexor digitorum profundus and superficialis tendons of the small finger in zone II: case report," *Journal of Hand Surgery*, vol. 36, no. 1, pp. 121–124, 2011.

[8] T. C. Oğün, H. M. Ozdemir, and H. Senaran, "Closed traumatic avulsion of both flexor tendons in the ring finger," *The Journal of Trauma*, vol. 60, no. 4, pp. 904–905, 2006.

[9] B. Toussaint, E. Lenoble, O. Roche, C. Iskandar, J. Dossa, and Y. Allieu, "Subcutaneous avulsion of the flexor digitorum profundus and flexor digitorum superficialis tendons of the ring and little fingers by blast injury," *Annales de Chirurgie de la Main et du Membre Supérieur*, vol. 9, no. 3, pp. 232–235, 1990.

[10] J. B. Tang, "Flexor tendon repair in zone 2C," *The Journal of Hand Surgery*, vol. 19, no. 1, pp. 72–75, 1994.

[11] T. S. Sügün, N. Karabay, T. Toros, K. Özaksar, M. Kayalar, and E. Bal, "Validity of ultrasonography in surgically treated zone 2 flexor tendon injuries," *Acta Orthopaedica et Traumatologica Turcica*, vol. 44, no. 6, pp. 452–457, 2010.

[12] S. B. Cohen, A. B. Chhabra, M. W. Anderson, and M. E. Pannunzio, "Use of ultrasound in determining treatment for avulsion of the flexor digitorum profundus (rugger jersey finger): a case report," *American Journal of Orthopedics*, vol. 33, no. 11, pp. 546–549, 2004.

[13] S. Durand, C. Oberlin, and A. MacQuillan, "FDP to FDP hemitendon transfer—a new technique for delayed repair of the flexor digitorum profundus in zones I and II of the finger," *The Journal of Hand Surgery*, vol. 35, no. 8, pp. 677–678, 2010.

Combined Isolated Laugier's Fracture and Distal Radial Fracture: Management and Literature Review on the Mechanism of Injury

Walid Osman,[1] Meriem Braiki,[1] Zeineb Alaya,[2] Nader Naouar,[1] and Mohamed Ben Ayeche[1]

[1] *Department of Orthopedic Surgery, Sahloul University Hospital, Sousse, Tunisia*
[2] *Department of Rheumatology, Farhat Hached University Hospital, Sousse, Tunisia*

Correspondence should be addressed to Meriem Braiki; m-braiki@live.fr

Academic Editor: Johannes Mayr

Introduction. Isolated fracture of the trochlea is an uncommon condition requiring a particular mechanism of injury. Its association with a distal radial fracture is rare. We aimed through this case report to identify the injury mechanism and to assess surgical outcomes. *Case Presentation*. We report a 26-year-old female who was admitted to our department for elbow trauma following an accidental fall on her outstretched right hand with her elbow extended and supinated. On examination, the right elbow was swollen with tenderness over the anteromedial aspect of the distal humerus. The elbow range was restricted. Standard radiographs showed an intra-articular half-moon-shaped fragment lying proximal and anterior to the distal humerus. There was a comminuted articular fracture of the distal radius with an anterior displacement. A computed tomography revealed an isolated shear fracture of the trochlea without any associated lesion of the elbow. The patient was surgically managed. Anatomical reduction was achieved and the fracture was fixed with 2 Kirschner wires. The distal radial fracture was treated by open reduction and plate fixation. The postoperative course was uneventful with a good recovery. *Conclusion*. Knowledge of such entity would be useful to indicate the suitable surgical management and eventually to obtain good functional outcomes.

1. Introduction

Coronal shear fractures of distal humerus usually involve the capitellum and a variable part of the trochlea [1]. Fracture of the humeral trochlea is usually associated with elbow dislocation or capitellum fracture [2–4]. The trochlea rarely fractures in isolation because of its location deep within the elbow joint and thus is protected from direct trauma [5]. Also called Laugier's fracture, isolated fractures of the articular surface of the trochlea are very uncommon and are sporadically mentioned in the literature as case reports [5–15].

We aimed to document a rare combination of isolated displaced trochlea fracture associated with a distal radial fracture that was successfully managed with open reduction and internal fixation. The literature was discussed and reviewed.

2. Case Report

A 26-year-old female was admitted to our department for elbow trauma following an accidental fall on her outstretched right hand with her elbow extended and supinated. She presented with pain and swelling in her right elbow. On examination, the right elbow was swollen with tenderness over the anteromedial aspect of the distal humerus. The elbow range was restricted and too painful. Neurovascular examination was unremarkable. Lateral radiograph (Figure 1) showed an intra-articular half-moon-shaped fragment lying proximal and anterior to the distal humerus simulating a capitellar fracture without associated elbow dislocation. But, on anteroposterior view, the fracture appeared to involve the trochlea showing irregularity of the medial joint space. There was a comminuted articular fracture of the distal radius with an anterior displacement (Figure 2).

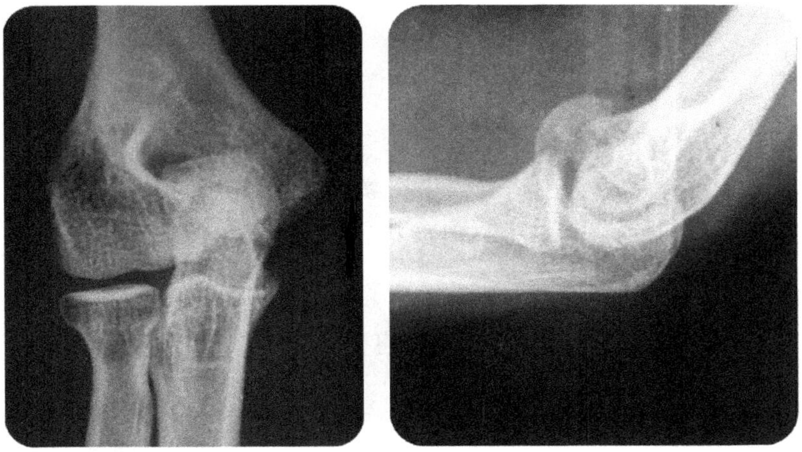

(a) (b)

FIGURE 1: (a) Anteroposterior and (b) lateral radiographs showing an intra-articular half-moon-shaped fragment lying proximal and anterior to the distal humerus simulating a capitellar fracture with irregularities over the trochlear-olecranon articulation surface.

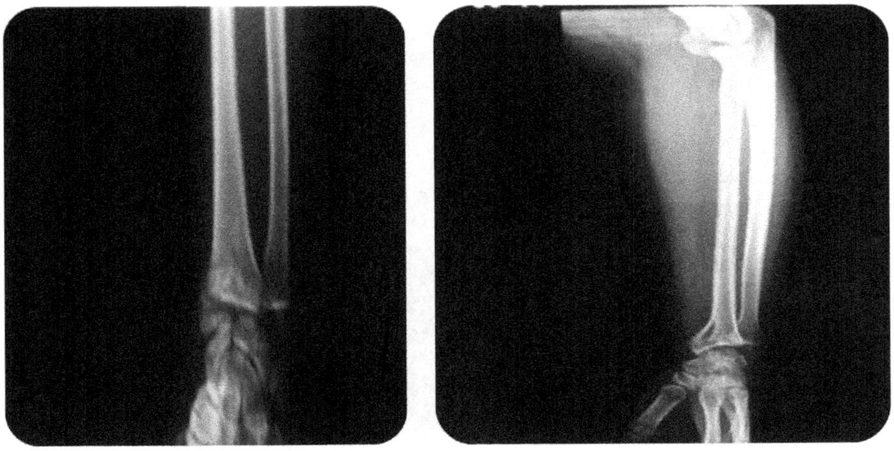

(a) (b)

FIGURE 2: (a) Anteroposterior and (b) lateral radiographs showing comminuted articular fracture of the distal radius with an anterior displacement.

A computed tomography (CT) scan (Figure 3) allowed better analysis of the fracture. It showed an isolated shear fracture of the trochlea without any bony associated lesion of the elbow. The patient was surgically managed. Open reduction and internal fixation were planned for our patient. The fracture site was initially exposed through a medial approach. The ulnar nerve was identified and protected, the common flexors were detached from the medial epicondyle, and the capsule was incised. An osteochondral fragment was displaced proximally. Anatomical reduction was achieved and the fracture was fixed with one Kirschner wire which was directed perpendicular to the fracture line. The reduction of fracture was confirmed preoperatively by direct visualization and fluoroscopic examination (Figure 4). Then, stability and range of movements were checked after the fixation. Common flexors were reattached to the medial epicondyle using nonabsorbable sutures. Subsequently, the distal radial fracture was treated by open reduction and plate fixation through an anterior approach. Postoperatively the limb was immobilized in 90° flexion with an above-elbow back splint for two weeks in order to allow soft tissues healing. Gradual mobilization was started after its removal. The follow-up period was 2 years. At the last control, she was symptoms-free. She turned back to her initial employment. We report excellent functional outcomes according to Dash score which was 83,25/100 (Figure 5). No signs of osteonecrosis or arthritis were found on follow-up radiographs (Figure 6).

3. Discussion

Fracture of the trochlea has been previously described as part of the complex fracture of distal end of humerus and

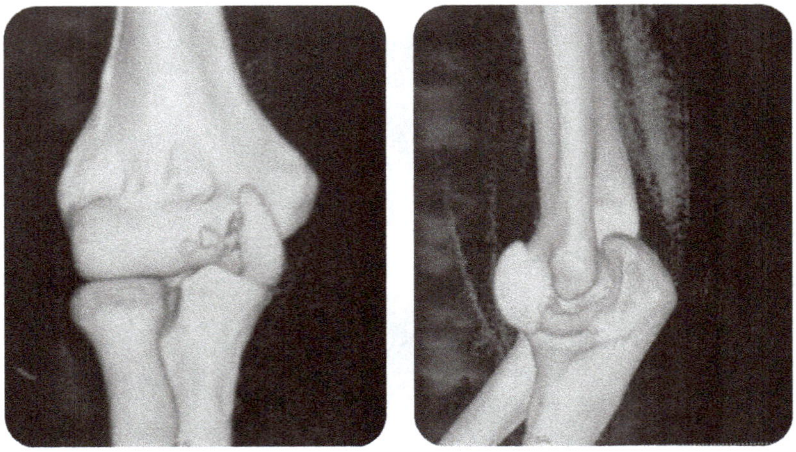

(a) (b)

FIGURE 3: Computed tomography of the elbow with 3D reconstruction showed an isolated shear fracture of the trochlea with no other bony abnormality.

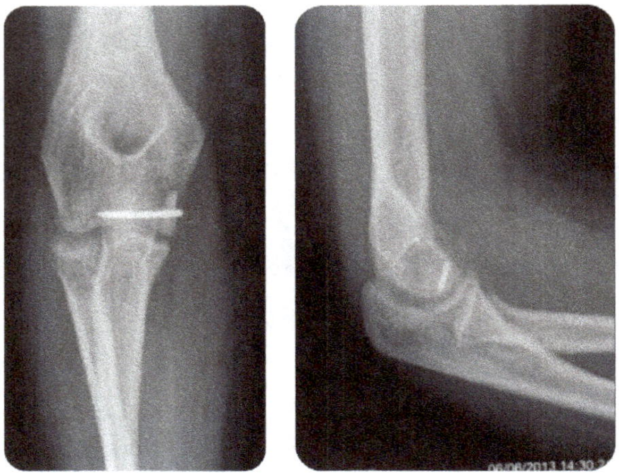

(a) (b)

FIGURE 4: Immediate postoperative radiographs after fixation (a, b) anteroposterior and lateral views of the elbow.

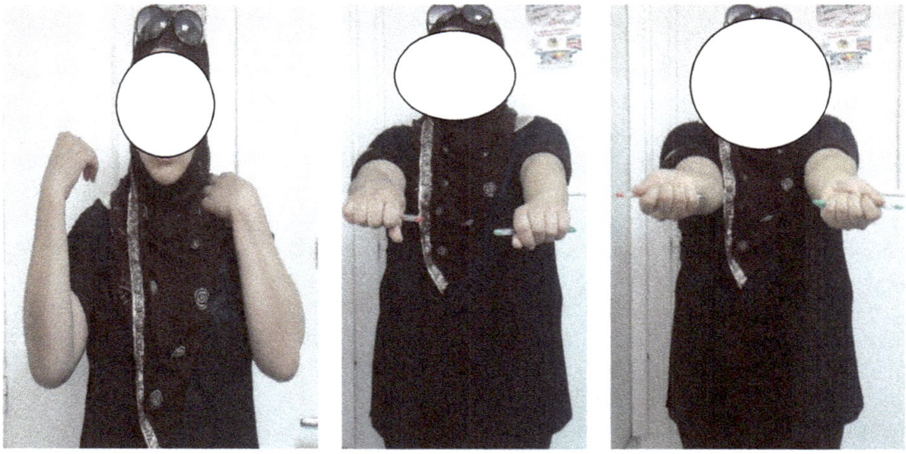

FIGURE 5: Recovery with excellent functional outcomes.

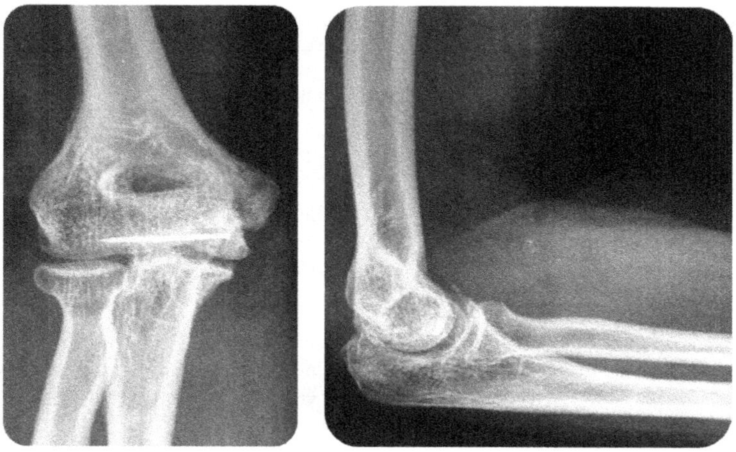

(a) (b)

FIGURE 6: Two years after fixation with Kirschner wires: anteroposterior view (a) and lateral view (b) showing bone union without degenerative changes.

dislocation of elbow [1, 7]. However, the trochlea rarely fractures in isolation. This fracture seems to be occurring for several reasons. The trochlea has no muscular or ligamentous attachments and the ulnohumeral joint is not subject to shear forces that occur at the radiocapitellar [5]. Moreover, the trochlea is located deep in the elbow joint; therefore, it is not directly exposed to trauma and usually remains intact in direct elbow injuries [13]. In addition to that, forces transmitted from the ulna across the trochlea tend to produce more a wedging action than shearing forces [8].

Numerous theories were advanced regarding the injury mechanism. Dhurve et al. [15] reported 2 cases of isolated fracture of the trochlea with review of the literature on the mechanism of injury. Authors found three different mechanisms that could be responsible for the occurrence of this fracture: axial load in flexion, axial load in extension, and direct impact of the elbow in flexion. Nakatani et al. [5] suggested the role of varus stress with axial loading in isolated trochlear fracture. Thus, it was documented that varus stress displaces the compressive forces of the radio-humeral compartment in the ulnohumeral compartment [12]. Back to our case, the fracture occurred following an axial load while the elbow was in an extended position.

The mechanisms described in the literature are for isolated fracture of the trochlea. There is only one case report describing a rare combination of an ipsilateral simultaneous fracture of the trochlea involving the lateral end clavicle and distal end radius [7]. In our current case, we think that the possible mechanism might be the preaxial loading stresses in forearm that went to postaxial border of arm and transmitted through elbow which caused fracture of the trochlea with fracture at end distal radius. The patient fell on his hand with his elbow extended; an axial load from the coronoid process and varus stress could have impacted the trochlea.

Clinically, a fracture of the trochlea is atypical with pain, minimal swelling, and tenderness on the medial side of the elbow.

Diagnosis is based on plain radiographs of the injured elbow. It is difficult to detect isolated trochlear fracture on anteroposterior radiograph. However, careful inspection may show an irregularity at the ulnohumeral joint [5, 10, 11] but the image can be interpreted "normal" [6, 8, 13]. A half-moon-shaped osteochondral fragment can be seen on the lateral view which is difficult to distinguish from capitellar fracture. If there is still a doubt, computed tomography (CT) scan can be helpful to make correct diagnosis. In fact, three-dimensional CT reconstructions are very useful for delineating the size and the extent of the fracture more accurately. Moreover, this exam helps rule out other bony injury guiding surgical treatment procedures but cannot show osteochondral damage which is predictive of outcome [3, 6, 9]. In our case report CT scan was useful for surgical planning.

All the cases reported in literature were surgically managed with good outcomes (Table 1). As the osteochondral fracture of the trochlea has no muscular or ligamentous attachments, osteonecrosis is expected in these cases by conventions. However, there is no evidence of osteonecrosis in the reported cases in literature. Conservative treatment has been recommended for undisplaced humeral fracture [4, 11], whereas unsatisfactory results were noted: arthrosis, contracture, and elbow stiffness. If left untreated, the bony fragment can cause mechanical block to elbow flexion by obstructing the coronoid fossa [7]. Excision of irreparable small fragments has been described as a method of treatment. But this may result in a significant loss of articular surface, possibly causing elbow pain and unstability of the ulno-humeral joint [11]. The mainstay of treatment of displaced trochlear fracture is surgical stabilization. Open reduction and stable internal fixation combined with early motion exercises can achieve optimal results [5, 8, 11, 13]. After open reduction, various materials, including Kirschner wires, AO compression screws, and headless compression screws, have been used in the treatment of trochlear fractures with various

Table 1: Surveys found in the literature reporting details of patients managed for isolated fracture of the trochlea.

Authors	Patients number	Mechanism of injury	Position of elbow during injury	Fixation method	Results
Sen et al. (2013) [6]	5	—	—	Screw fixation and Kirschner wire.	Excellent outcomes in 4 patients and good results in 1 patient.
Gupta et al. (2014) [7]	1	Road traffic accident.	Fall on the outstretched hand. Lying in extending position.	Internal fixation with lag screws.	Good functional outcomes.
Kaushal et al. (2005) [8]	1	Road traffic accident.	Fall on the outstretched hand with the elbow in extension.	Internal fixation with screws.	Excellent functional result according to functional rating scale of Broberg and Morrey.
Somanna et al. (2008) [9]	1	Road traffic accident.	—	Reduction and internal fixation using Kirschner wires.	Excellent functional results.
Foulk et al. (1995) [11]	1	Accidental Fall.	Fall on the outstretched hand with the elbow in extension.	Open reduction with internal fixation.	Good functional results.
Nakatani et al. (2005) [5]	1	Road traffic accident.	Landing on the outstretched hand.	Reduction and internal fixation with Herbert screws.	Good functional results.
Abbassi et al. (2015) [12]	1	Accidental fall.	Landing on the palm of his right hand with his elbow extending and supinated.	Internal fixation.	Good functional results.
Kwan et al. (2007) [13]	2	Road traffic accident.	Landing in a prone position with his elbow in flexed position.	Reduction and internal fixation with Herbert screws.	Good functional results.
Zimmerman et al. (2015) [14]	1	Accidental fall.	Fall on the outstretched hand with the elbow in extension.	Open reduction and internal fixation with two headless Herbert screws.	Good outcomes.

degrees of success [6]. The choice of materials of fixation depends on the size of the fragment and comminution. Screw fixation allows compression at fracture site with good stability and early motion. Wire fixation is advocated in case of small osteochondral fragment not amenable to screw fixation. After review of the literature, we noticed 15 reported cases, all treated by ORIF. The medial approach was most used in cases. The anterior approach was used only twice. Screw fixation was used in 12 cases and K-wires fixation was used only in 3 cases because of the small size of the fragments. For the same reason, we opted for this type of osteosynthesis and achieved good functional outcomes.

4. Conclusion

We treated successfully combined isolated Laugier's fracture and distal radial fracture. A fall on outstretched hand with elbow extended can cause this injury. This case exemplify the excellent functional outcome that is possible with internal fixation and early-range-of-motion exercises.

Additional Points

Clinical Message. Isolated Laugier's fractures are uncommon, and their association with distal radial fracture is exceptional. Knowledge about this injury and its mechanism of occurrence is essential to manage adequately this condition. Open reduction and internal fixation are well indicated.

Competing Interests

The authors report that there is no conflict of interests regarding the publication of this manuscript.

Acknowledgments

The authors acknowledge that no benefits in any form have been or will be received from a commercial party related directly or indirectly to the subject of this article.

References

[1] J. H. Dubberley, K. I. Faber, J. C. MacDermid, S. D. Patterson, and G. J. W. King, "Outcome after open reduction and internal fixation of capitellar and trochlear fractures," *The Journal of Bone & Joint Surgery—American Volume*, vol. 88, no. 1, pp. 46–54, 2006.

[2] I. R. Grant and J. H. Miller, "Osteochondral fracture of the trochlea associated with fracture-dislocation of the elbow," *Injury*, vol. 6, no. 3, pp. 257–260, 1975.

[3] M. D. Mckee, J. B. Jupiter, and H. B. Bamberger, "Coronal shear fractures of the distal end of the humerus," *The Journal of Bone & Joint Surgery—American Volume*, vol. 78, no. 1, pp. 49–54, 1996.

[4] H. Mehdian, H. Mehdian, M. D. McKee, and M. D. McKee, "Fractures of capitellum and trochlea," *Orthopedic Clinics of North America*, vol. 31, no. 1, pp. 115–127, 2000.

[5] T. Nakatani, S. Sawamura, Y. Imaizumi et al., "Isolated fracture of the trochlea: a case report," *Journal of Shoulder and Elbow Surgery*, vol. 14, no. 3, pp. 340–343, 2005.

[6] R. K. Sen, S. K. Tripahty, T. Goyal, and S. Aggarwal, "Coronal shear fracture of the humeral trochlea," *Journal of Orthopaedic Surgery*, vol. 21, no. 1, pp. 82–86, 2013.

[7] R. K. Gupta, R. Singh, V. Verma et al., "Ipsilateral simultaneous fracture of the trochlea involving the lateral end clavicle and distal end radius: a rare combination and a unique mechanism of injury," *Chinese Journal of Traumatology*, vol. 17, no. 4, pp. 246–248, 2014.

[8] R. Kaushal, A. Bhanot, P. N. Gupta, and R. Bahadur, "Isolated shear fracture of humeral trochlea," *Injury Extra*, vol. 36, no. 6, pp. 210–211, 2005.

[9] M. S. Somanna, S. D. Amarnath, S. M. Sudhakar, and M. P. Umanand, "A rare case of isolated fracture of trochlea—a case report," *Journal of Orthopaedics*, vol. 5, no. 3, p. 5, 2008.

[10] P. S. Ajay, K. D. Ish, K. D. Anil, and J. Saurabh, "Neglected isolated fracture of the trochlea humeri," *Chinese Journal of Traumatology*, vol. 13, no. 4, pp. 247–249, 2010.

[11] D. A. Foulk, P. A. Robertson, and L. A. Timmerman, "Fracture of the trochlea," *Journal of Orthopaedic Trauma*, vol. 9, no. 6, pp. 530–532, 1995.

[12] N. Abbassi, N. Abdeljaouad, A. Daoudi, and H. Yacoubi, "Isolated fracture of the humeral trochlea: a case report and review of the literature," *Journal of Medical Case Reports*, vol. 9, no. 1, article 121, 2015.

[13] M. K. Kwan, E. H. Khoo, Y. P. Chua, and A. Mansor, "Isolated displaced fracture of humeral trochlea: a report of two rare cases," *Injury Extra*, vol. 38, no. 12, pp. 461–465, 2007.

[14] L. J. Zimmerman, J. J. Jauregui, and C. E. Aarons, "Isolated shear fracture of the humeral trochlea in an adolescent: a case report and literature review," *Journal of Pediatric Orthopaedics Part B*, vol. 24, no. 5, pp. 412–417, 2015.

[15] K. Dhurve, V. S. Patil, A. S. Chandanwale, and R. G. Puranik, "Isolated fracture of the trochlea: report of two cases with review of the literature on the mechnism of injury," *Journal of Evolution of Medical and Dental Sciences*, vol. 26, no. 2, pp. 4805–4812, 2013.

26

Resection and Resolution of Bone Marrow Lesions Associated with an Improvement of Pain after Total Knee Replacement: A Novel Case Study Using a 3-Tesla Metal Artefact Reduction MRI Sequence

Thomas Kurien,[1,2] Robert Kerslake,[1,3] Brett Haywood,[1,4] Richard G. Pearson,[1,2] and Brigitte E. Scammell[1,2,3]

[1] *Arthritis Research UK Pain Centre, Nottingham University, Nottingham, UK*
[2] *Academic Orthopaedics, Trauma and Sports Medicine, School of Medicine, The University of Nottingham, Queen's Medical Centre, Derby Road, Nottingham NG7 2UH, UK*
[3] *Nottingham University Hospitals NHS Trust, Queen's Medical Centre, Nottingham NG7 2UH, UK*
[4] *Academic Radiology, The University of Nottingham, Queen's Medical Centre, Derby Road, Nottingham NG7 2UH, UK*

Correspondence should be addressed to Thomas Kurien; thomas.kurien@nottingham.ac.uk

Academic Editor: Dimitrios S. Karataglis

We present our case report using a novel metal artefact reduction magnetic resonance imaging (MRI) sequence to observe resolution of subchondral bone marrow lesions (BMLs), which are strongly associated with pain, in a patient after total knee replacement surgery. Large BMLs were seen preoperatively on the 3-Tesla MRI scans in a patient with severe end stage OA awaiting total knee replacement surgery. Twelve months after surgery, using a novel metal artefact reduction MRI sequence, we were able to visualize the bone-prosthesis interface and found complete resection and resolution of these BMLs. This is the first reported study in the UK to use this metal artefact reduction MRI sequence at 3-Tesla showing that resection and resolution of BMLs in this patient were associated with an improvement of pain and function after total knee replacement surgery. In this case it was associated with a clinically significant improvement of pain and function after surgery. Failure to eradicate these lesions may be a cause of persistent postoperative pain that is seen in up to 20% of patients following TKR surgery.

1. Introduction

Painful osteoarthritis (OA) is the 4th largest cause of ill health and disability in the United Kingdom [1]. Subchondral noncystic bone marrow lesions (BMLs) have been identified as key biomarkers in the pathogenesis of osteoarthritis and are characterised as ill-defined areas of low signal intensity compared to normal marrow on T1-weighted images or hyperintense signal change within the subchondral bone on T2-weighted, fat saturated, or short tau inversion recovery MR images [2]. BMLs are not visible on plain radiographs; hence the discovery of these changes on MRI, and their correlation with pain, is of significant clinical interest. Over 75% of patients with painful osteoarthritis of the knee have subchondral BMLs on MRI, and several large studies have reported the correlation of subchondral BMLs with pain [3]. Recent work has also demonstrated that BMLs are a predictor for adjacent cartilage loss in the same knee compartment and that the pain experienced in patients corresponds to the change in size of the BMLs present [4].

Total knee replacement surgery (TKR) is one of the most common orthopaedics procedures performed worldwide and is generally a very successful and cost-effective treatment for improving pain and function in patients with severe painful OA. In the United Kingdom nearly 84,000 primary total knee replacement procedures were performed in 2014.

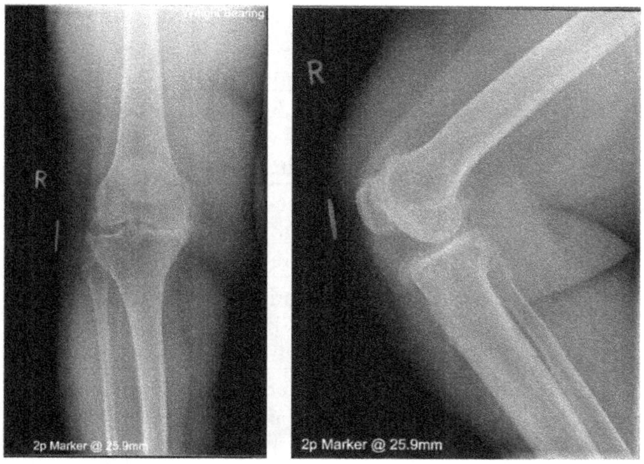

FIGURE 1: Preoperative weight-bearing AP and lateral radiographs clearly showing tricompartmental knee OA (K-L Grade IV).

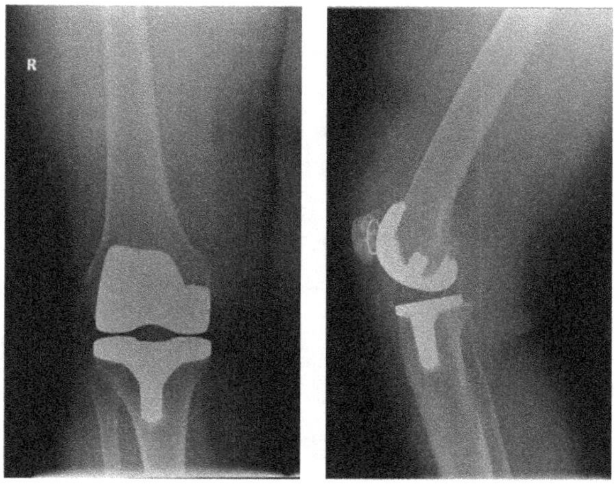

FIGURE 2: Postoperative AP and lateral radiographs of right Columbus TKR.

For many patients, TKR is an effective surgical intervention; however, unfortunately up to 20% of all patients who undergo this surgery report severe dissatisfaction and chronic postoperative pain in spite of objective measures of surgical success [5]. Chronic postoperative pain is defined by the International Association for the Study of Pain (IASP) as pain that is present in a subject six months after surgery. Risk factors associated with the development of chronic postoperative pain after TKR include female gender, lower age, greater preoperative pain, pain at remotes sites, pain catastrophizing, depression, anxiety, and sleep disturbance. The presence of BMLs after TKR has not previously been explored, primarily due to the fact that, even with optimisation of conventional MR sequences, tissues in the immediate vicinity of metallic implants are largely obscured due to image distortion and artefact. However, considerable reduction in artefacts around metallic implants has been achieved using recently introduced MR pulse sequences [6]. We report our early finding using a novel metal artefact reduction MRI sequence showing the complete resection and resolution of BMLs 12 months after TKR surgery with an associated improvement of pain and function of the knee.

2. Case Details

The Nottinghamshire Research Ethics Committee gave ethical approval for this patient to receive a metal artefact reduction MRI scan as part of a wider study (REC ref number 10/H0408/115). The patient (female, aged 72, BMI 33.8) awaiting right total knee replacement surgery was recruited after taking informed consent as part of the pilot study. The patient had severe tricompartmental osteoarthritis of the knee with radiographic (Kellegren-Lawrence grade IV) and symptomatic OA prior to the joint replacement surgery (Figure 1). The patient had suffered from progressively worsening symptoms of pain in the right knee for over 15 years. She described pain on standing and on movement as well as disturbance of her normal sleep pattern. On clinical examination she had a varus knee with a mild fixed flexion deformity. Her range of movement was limited to 90° flexion and she was tender on palpation around the medial joint line.

Preoperative questionnaires were administered within 2 weeks of the total joint replacement and were repeated 12 months after the operation. The questionnaires included assessment of pain severity, pain catastrophizing, knee function, anxiety, depression, and a measure of the neuropathic pain-like symptoms. The questionnaires included are outlined in Table 1. A navigated Columbus total knee replacement (B. Braun) prosthesis was used as the implant in the case (Figure 2).

3. Preoperative Knee MRI Methods

MRI was performed on a 3.0 T system (GE MR 750, GE Healthcare, Waukesha, WI) using an 8-channel phased array transmit-receive knee coil. The knee was scanned in sagittal and axial planes using a proton-density fat-suppressed sequence (2.5 mm thickness, spacing 0.3 mm, repetition time (T_R) 3321 ms, effective echo time (T_E) 41 ms, echo train length (ETL) 7, and pixel bandwidth (BW) 162) and a coronal T1-weighted sequence (2.5 mm thickness, spacing 0.3 mm, T_R 580 ms, T_E 11 ms, ETL 1, and BW 244).

4. Postoperative Knee MRI Methods

Twelve months following knee arthroplasty, the patient was imaged again using the same 3 T MR system and coil. On this occasion, the knee was scanned in sagittal, axial, and coronal planes using an inversion-recovery fat saturated MAVRIC STIR SL sequence (T_R/T_E 5000/7.4 ms, inversion time 175 ms, ETL 20, BW 976, slice thickness 4 mm, and zero spacing).

5. Bone Marrow Lesion Assessment

Subchondral BMLs (defined as areas of altered subchondral marrow signal adjacent to the underlying the medial tibia, medial femoral, lateral tibia, lateral femoral, and patellar aspects of the knee joint) were assessed quantitatively using

Table 1: Pre- and postoperative questionnaires.

Assessment	Questionnaire	Comments
Pain severity	Visual Analogue Scale (VAS)	Used to categorise individuals with high or low pain. Scores range from 0 to 100, with score ≥ 60 representing high pain intensity.
Pain catastrophizing	Pain Catastrophizing Scale (PCS)	This 13-item scale uses questions about coping with pain. Scores range from 0 to 52 with a higher score seen in individuals that are high catastrophizers.
Depression	Beck Depression Inventory (BDI)	21-question assessment rating inventory attitudes and symptoms of depression. The score ranges from 0 to 63 with a score ≥ 19 indicative of clinical depression.
Anxiety	State-Trait Anxiety (STAI)	Assesses how patients feel and reflects situational factors, which influence anxiety levels. Scores range from 20 to 80 with higher scores associated with higher anxiety.
Neuropathic pain-like symptoms	PainDetect	Individuals are categorised as having neuropathic pain based on the results of a joint-specific version of the PainDetect questionnaire. Scores range from 0 to 39 with a score > 12 indicating possible neuropathic pain and a score ≥ 19 indicating likely neuropathic pain.
Pain and function of the knee	Oxford Knee Score (OKS)	A 12-item questionnaire that assesses pain and function of the knee. Scores range from 0 to 48 with a lower score indicating severe knee arthritis or pain and reduced function in the knee. A higher score between 40 and 48 indicated satisfactory joint function. A minimally clinically important difference of 4 points on the scale can be used to assess the results of an intervention, for example, pain relief or TKR surgery.

OSIRIX software (University of Geneva, Geneva, Switzerland). A single trained observer measured the maximum area (cm^2) of the BMLs preoperatively and twelve months postoperatively by manually selecting the MRI slice with the greatest BML size. The MRIs at both time points were read but the observer was blinded to the questionnaire results of the patient.

6. Results

Using the 3-Tesla preoperative knee MRI, we were able to visualise a large anteromedial BML (2.21 cm^2) in a patient with painful knee osteoarthritis. There was also a corresponding smaller BML in the posterior-medial distal femur (1.17 cm^2). The preoperative MRI images with the BMLs are shown in Figure 3.

Using the MAVRIC metal artefact reduction MRI sequence 12 months postoperatively, we noted complete resection or resolution of the BMLs seen preoperatively; with the exception of a narrow band of artefact in the immediate vicinity of the implants, the subchondral marrow signal could be clearly visualised on postoperative images and was seen to have returned to normal. Of particular note, the largest preoperative BML that extended 2.6 cm caudal to the medial tibial plateau had been resected or resolved in its entirety and this was accompanied by an improvement in the patient's reported pain (Figure 4 and Table 2).

Table 2: Pre- and post-TKR questionnaire results.

Questionnaire	Pre-op score	Postoperative score
Visual Analogue Scale (VAS)	80/100	0/100
PainDetect	20 (neuropathic)	8
Beck Depression Inventory	14	8
State-Trait Anxiety	51	38
Pain Catastrophizing Scale	34	38
Oxford Knee Score	9	43

7. Discussion

This is the first reported use of the novel MAVRIC MRI sequence at 3-Tesla used in the UK after TKR surgery to report the relationship between resolving pain and the disappearance of BMLs. Our case study has reported that the resection and resolution of these nociceptive BMLs are associated with an improvement of pain and function after TKR surgery as seen with the VAS and PainDetect® score as well as the Oxford Knee Score. The patient recruited as part of this pilot work demonstrated neuropathic pain-like symptoms preoperatively as observed by her high PainDetect score. Depression and anxiety scores improved postoperatively but there was small worsening in the catastrophizing

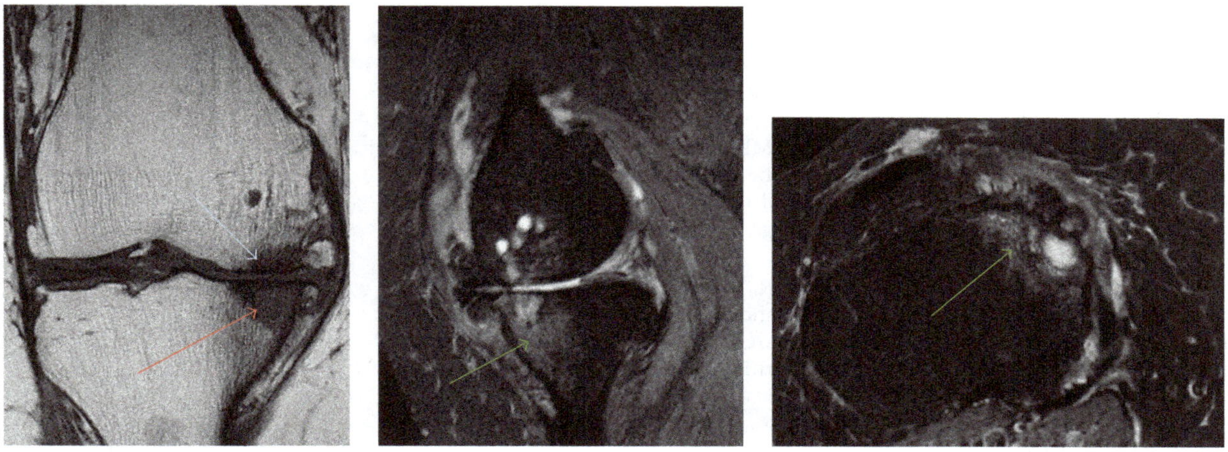

(a) (b) (c)

FIGURE 3: (a) Coronal T1 MRI with contrast image in painful knee OA patient showing large medial proximal tibial BML (red arrow) and smaller medial distal femoral BML (blue arrow). (b) Corresponding proton density weighted fat suppressed sagittal MRI sequence showing the large anteromedial BML (green arrow). (c) Axial proton density weighted fat suppressed MRI showing the tibia BML.

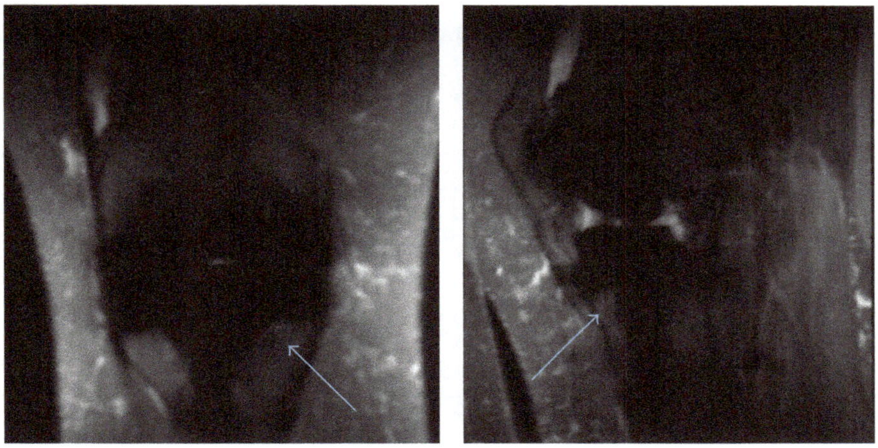

FIGURE 4: Coronal and Sagittal MAVRIC® STIR SLR MRI showing complete resection and resolution of BMLs 12 months after TKR surgery (blue arrows).

score after surgery. During TKR, approximately 10 mm of proximal femur and 10 mm of proximal tibia were resected; this included part but not all of the BMLs that had been documented. However, 12 months after arthroplasty imaging showed complete resolution of the remainder of the BML. The postoperative low PainDetect score is indicative of resolution of the neuropathic pain-like symptoms seen in central sensitization. Pain in knee osteoarthritis can originate from many sources including the subchondral bone as bone marrow lesions, synovitis, the periosteum, and osteophytes and there are many factors that can contribute to postoperative pain. However, through this important case report and future research, we hypothesise that failure to fully resect these lesions at the time of TKR surgery or the development of new BMLs within the subchondral bone after TKR surgery may act as a continued peripheral nociceptive input, maintaining pain, altered central processing, and central sensitization after TKR. This may explain some of the variance in pain relief after TKR. Further investigation into these lesions is required to understand the role of BMLs in chronic postoperative pain.

Competing Interests

The authors assert no conflict of interests. None of the authors received fees, bonuses, or other benefits for the work described in the manuscript.

Acknowledgments

Thomas Kurien is funded by the British Association for Surgery to the Knee (BASK/DePuy), the Medical Research Council (MRC), and the Royal College of Surgeons of Edinburgh on a Clinical Research Training Fellowship.

References

[1] T. Neogi, "The epidemiology and impact of pain in osteoarthritis," *Osteoarthritis and Cartilage*, vol. 21, no. 9, pp. 1145–1153, 2013.

[2] F. W. Roemer, R. Frobell, D. J. Hunter et al., "MRI-detected subchondral bone marrow signal alterations of the knee joint: terminology, imaging appearance, relevance and radiological differential diagnosis," *Osteoarthritis and Cartilage*, vol. 17, no. 9, pp. 1115–1131, 2009.

[3] A. J. Barr, T. M. Campbell, D. Hopkinson, S. R. Kingsbury, M. A. Bowes, and P. G. Conaghan, "A systematic review of the relationship between subchondral bone features, pain and structural pathology in peripheral joint osteoarthritis," *Arthritis Research & Therapy*, vol. 17, no. 1, article 228, 2015.

[4] Y. Zhang, M. Nevitt, J. Niu et al., "Fluctuation of knee pain and changes in bone marrow lesions, effusions, and synovitis on magnetic resonance imaging," *Arthritis & Rheumatism*, vol. 63, no. 3, pp. 691–699, 2011.

[5] M. J. Dunbar and F. S. Haddad, "Patient satisfaction after total knee replacement," *Bone & Joint Journal*, vol. 96, no. 10, pp. 1285–1286, 2014.

[6] J. P. Dillenseger, S. Molière, P. Choquet, C. Goetz, M. Ehlinger, and G. Bierry, "An illustrative review to understand and manage metal-induced artifacts in musculoskeletal MRI: a primer and updates," *Skeletal Radiology*, vol. 45, no. 5, pp. 677–688, 2016.

27

Treating Early Knee Osteoarthritis with the Atlas® Unicompartmental Knee System in a 26-Year-Old Ex-Professional Basketball Player: A Case Study

Konrad Slynarski[1] and Lukasz Lipinski[1,2]

[1]*Lekmed Hospital for Special Surgery, Warsaw, Poland*
[2]*Orthopedics and Pediatric Orthopedics Clinic, Medical University of Lodz, Lodz, Poland*

Correspondence should be addressed to Konrad Slynarski; konrad@slynarski.pl

Academic Editor: Werner Kolb

Knee osteoarthritis (OA) is a leading cause of disability among adults. Within the affected population, there exists a group of patients who have exhausted conservative treatment options and yet are not ideal candidates for current surgical treatments due to young age, early disease severity, or neutral mechanical knee alignment. For these patients, a new potential treatment option may be considered. We present an interesting case report of a young, ex-professional athlete treated with a minimally invasive load-altering implant (Atlas System) whose young age (26 years), disease status (tibiofemoral kissing lesions), and neutral mechanical limb alignment eliminated all traditional surgical treatment options such as high tibial osteotomy or arthroplasty. At 6 months after surgery, our patient demonstrated positive outcomes improvement in pain, function, and quality of life and had returned to high-impact athletic activity without symptoms. These initial results are promising, and longer follow-up data on the treatment will be necessary.

1. Introduction

Knee osteoarthritis (OA) is a leading cause of disability among adults [1]. Estimated mean age at knee OA diagnosis in the United States is only 53.5 years [2], with a greater number of symptomatic knee OA patients under 65 years of age than over 65 [2, 3] and an annual incidence of knee OA more than five times higher in individuals under 65 years of age than over 65 [2, 3].

The increased prevalence of knee OA in the young population is believed to be due to damage to the articular cartilage caused by repetitive impact and loading [4], biologic changes [5], and altered articular cartilage loading due to joint injuries [6–8]. Prior joint injury such as anterior cruciate ligament rupture or meniscal tear has been shown to accelerate the development of knee OA, with 50% of individuals presenting with the disease just 10 to 20 years following injury [9, 10]. As such joint injuries often occur in the young adult, they can lead to knee OA in individuals as young as 30 or 40 years of age [9].

Treatment options for the young knee OA patient initially consist of nonsurgical conservative modalities, such as activity modification, weight loss, physical therapy, and orthotics, followed by pharmacologic measures such as anti-inflammatories, analgesics, and joint injections. Patients, particularly those with earlier onset OA, often eventually fail conservative treatment [11, 12]. The procedure is considered for younger patients because it can achieve positive mid- to long-term freedom from arthroplasty and may allow a return to high activity levels [13–15]. However, HTO is contraindicated for patients with a neutral axis alignment, and the resultant load transfer may actually accelerate OA progression in the lateral compartment [16].

For these patients, a new potential treatment option may be considered. The recently introduced Atlas System (Moximed, Inc., Hayward, CA, USA) is an implantable, unicompartmental knee joint unloader. Importantly, the device is entirely extracapsular, making the procedure reversible should the patient's disease progress and require future treatment.

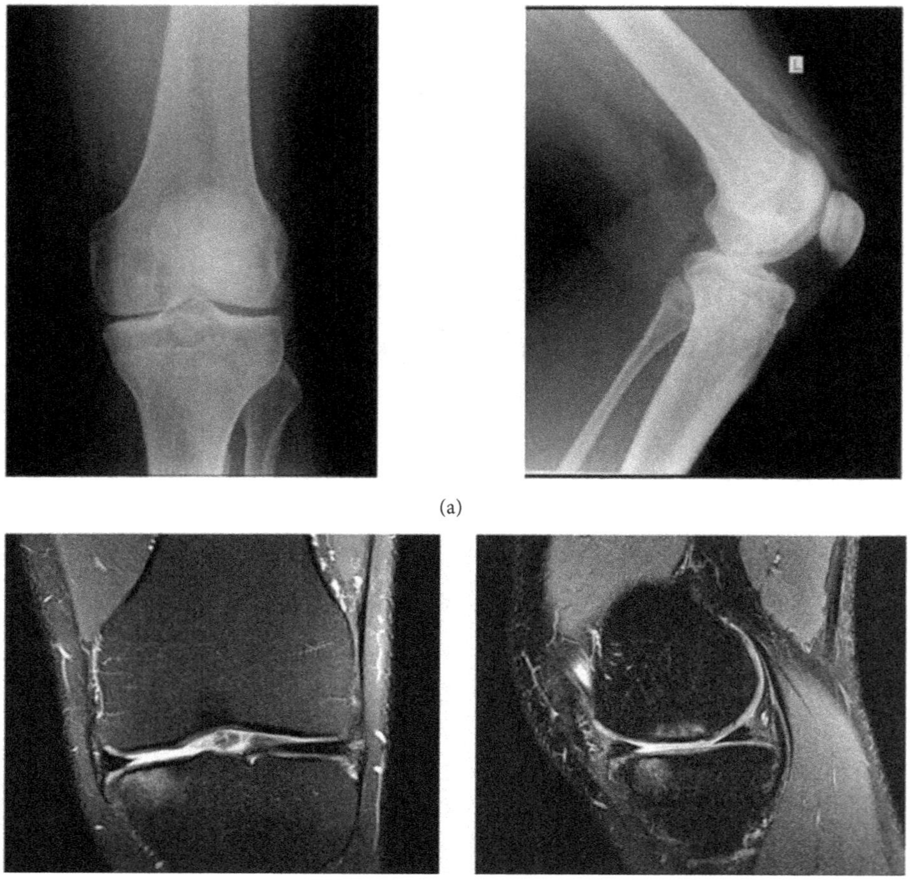

(a)

(b)

FIGURE 1: Presurgery anterior and medial radiographs (a) and coronal and sagittal MRIs (b) of the affected left knee.

We present a novel case report of the Atlas System. The case is unique and intriguing as the young age (26 years) of the patient, disease status (tibiofemoral kissing lesions), and neutral mechanical limb alignment eliminated all traditional surgical treatment options such as HTO or arthroplasty. The patient's status as an ex-professional level athlete and desire to return to high-impact activity add to the case complexity.

2. Case Report

2.1. Case Presentation. A 26-year-old male (height: 1.93 m; weight: 95 kg) presented with neutral limb alignment, painful tibiofemoral kissing lesions, and severe knee OA-related activity limitations due to pain in the left knee of one-year duration (Kellgren-Lawrence grade 2) (Figure 1). The knee OA was contained to the medial compartment, and the patient had failed lifestyle/activity modifications, physical therapy, quadriceps strengthening, and analgesics. Preoperative passive range of motion was measured to 140°, and no hyperextension or flexion deformity was recorded. During the orthopedic examination, isolated medial tibiofemoral tenderness was observed. The following symptoms were all absent: patellar tap (no joint effusion), lateral tibiofemoral tenderness, anserine bursa, patellofemoral crepitus, and patellar grind. The ligaments and meniscus were stable. The patient reported mild, continual pain during walking but distance was not limited by the knee pain.

As a former professional league basketball player, the patient indicated a strong desire to return to an active lifestyle including more strenuous activities such as jogging, racquet sports, and basketball, which he was unable to take part in due to pain. After providing written informed consent, he participated in a clinical study that received ethics committee approval and was conducted in compliance with the Ministry of Health and Declaration of Helsinki. The left knee of the patient was treated with the Atlas System, and the patient was followed for a period of six months after surgery.

2.2. Device and Surgical Technique. The Atlas System consists of a cylindrical, polycarbonate urethane (PCU) load absorber located between femoral and tibial bases (Figure 2). The device, located within the subcutaneous tissue on the medial side of the knee, is designed to reduce loading on the affected medial compartment of the knee joint, without transfer of loading to other areas of the joint. The device was inserted through a single incision, guided by direct visualization and

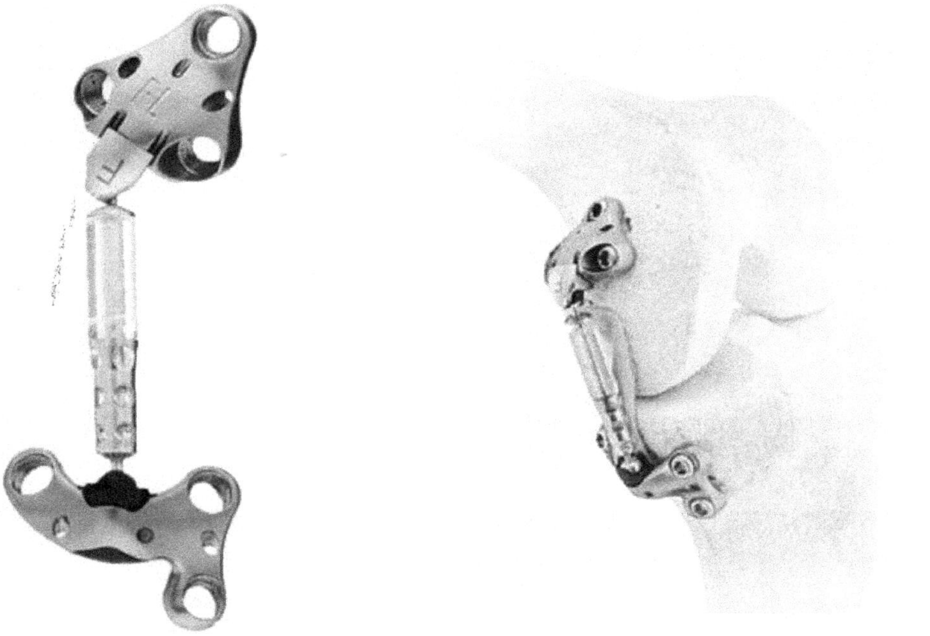

Figure 2: The assembled Atlas Knee System, designed to reduce loading on the affected medial compartment of the knee joint, consists of a load absorber located between femoral and tibial bases.

palpation of the patient's anatomy. Following identification of the femoral medial epicondyle, adductor magnus tubercle, tibial plateau, joint space, and anterior border of the superficial medial collateral ligament through visualization and palpation, the tibial and femoral fixation points were located, and an absorber length was selected based on the patient's anatomy. A trial device was introduced via two K-wires, and implant function was confirmed through direct visualization checks. Following confirmation of function of the trial device, the final implant was introduced with the femoral base placed deep to the vastus medialis obliquus muscle and the tibial base placed distal of the deep medial collateral ligament and proximal to the insertion of the pes anserine. After installation of the final device, visual confirmation of functional unloading from full extension through deep flexion was performed prior to wound closure. No concomitant intra-articular surgery was performed to ensure that any benefit was due solely to the implant. Postoperatively, the patient was given crutches and told to bear weight as tolerated and to keep the wound protected for an initial 2-week period. Following stitch removal at 2 weeks, the 2-month rehabilitation protocol focused initially on range of motion and daily living activities, followed by muscle strengthening and endurance.

3. Results

The patient experienced no device-related complications during the procedure or in follow-up (Figure 3). Six months following surgery, the patient showed clinically significant improvement (≥10-point improvement) in WOMAC pain and WOMAC function, with final scores of "0" for both domains. Importantly, the patient's KOOS quality of life score had improved by 66.7% (38 to 63). Specifically, the patient's response to the KOOS question, "in general, how much difficulty do you have with your knee?" improved from "extreme" at baseline to "mild" by six months. Physical examination at 6 months revealed full range of motion of 140° of knee flexion. When asked to rate how he was doing, considering all the ways his knee pain affected him, the patient improved from "fair" preoperatively to "very good" postoperatively. The patient's expectations were met: he indicated in an activity and satisfaction survey that he was very satisfied with the results of the procedure, in particular, as he was able to play basketball recreationally and complete his normal daily activities without pain, and would definitely undergo the surgery again for the same condition.

4. Discussion

Osteoarthritis is a common problem afflicting an increasing number of younger, active individuals. The Oxford group in the UK noted that patients with early degenerative changes to their knees should not be ignored, as they can be as symptomatic as those with end-stage disease [17]. The concept of early intervention is increasingly important as some patients with early-to-moderate symptoms of osteoarthritis are unable or unwilling to pursue more advanced surgery, such as HTO, UKA, or TKA. There exists a need for new surgical options that potentially provide symptom relief and early recovery, allow high activity, and maintain all future treatment options.

The Atlas System acts as a shock absorber to unload up to 13 kg of medial compartment joint loading, without transfer of the loading to other healthy areas of the knee

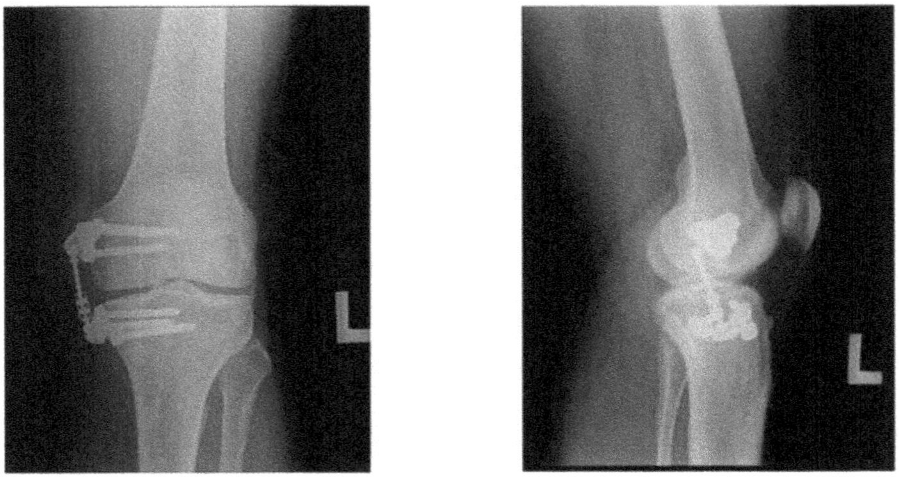

(a)

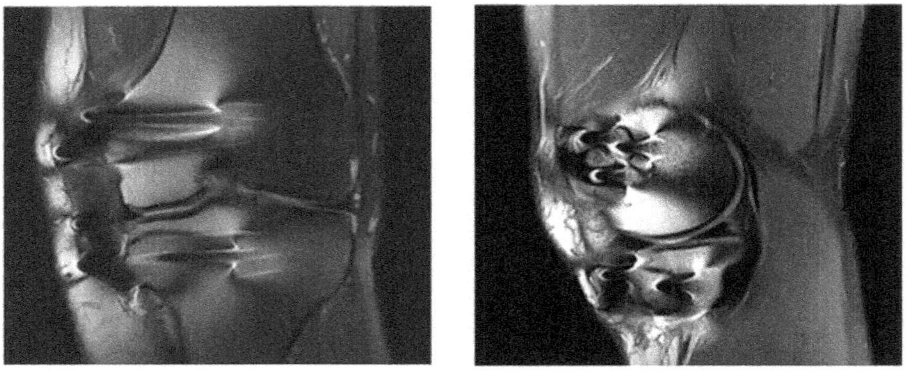

(b)

FIGURE 3: Six-month postsurgery anterior and medial radiographs (a) and coronal and sagittal MRIs (b) of the affected left knee.

joint. This amount of unloading was reported to be similar to that of HTO [18]. Without correction, increased loading on the medial compartment of the knee results in greater disease progression [19, 20] and ultimately the need for joint replacement surgery. As the Atlas System resides in the subcutaneous tissues outside of the joint capsule there is no breech of joint capsular space, nor is bone resection required, thus creating a reversible procedure and maintaining all future treatment options.

As this was a novel, early experience with the device, the rehabilitation protocol was not well-studied previously. The patient was allowed to bear full weight immediately (as tolerated) after surgery. He was discharged with crutches as a reminder to limit early activity and encourage full wound healing. Bracing was not employed after surgery, and early passive range of motion was recommended. The recovery protocol was positive, as the patient demonstrated clinically meaningful outcomes improvement and had returned to high-impact recreational sports (basketball, jogging) by six months after surgery.

Recently, authors presented improved clinical outcomes [21] in a 40-patient series of the Atlas System, with WOMAC pain and function scores improving from 52 ± 12 and 52 ± 17, respectively, at baseline to 15 ± 15 and 19 ± 17 at six months. Knee Society pain and function scores also improved, from 62 ± 15 and 71 ± 18 at baseline to 91 ± 12 and 98 ± 4 at six months. Additionally, the unicompartmental Atlas System was used in patients with cartilage defects or degenerative meniscus [22].

The results of this case study, demonstrating positive outcomes improvement in pain, function, quality of life, and activity level at an initial 6-month time period, indicate promising results in a highly unique case of a young, ex-professional athlete with early knee OA.

Competing Interests

K. Slynarski is a consultant to Moximed Inc. and Arthrex Inc.

Acknowledgments

The authors thank Jennifer Erhart-Hledik, Ph.D., for her assistance with drafting and editing of the manuscript.

References

[1] A. A. Guccione, D. T. Felson, J. J. Anderson et al., "The effects of specific medical conditions on the functional limitations of elders in the Framingham study," *American Journal of Public Health*, vol. 84, no. 3, pp. 351–358, 1994.

[2] E. Losina, A. M. Weinstein, W. M. Reichmann et al., "Lifetime risk and age at diagnosis of symptomatic knee osteoarthritis in the US," *Arthritis Care & Research*, vol. 65, no. 5, pp. 703–711, 2013.

[3] L. M. Howden and J. A. Meyer, *Age and Sex Composition: 2010*, 2011, http://www.census.gov/prod/cen2010/briefs/c2010br-03.pdf.

[4] J. A. Buckwalter and N. E. Lane, "Athletics and osteoarthritis," *American Journal of Sports Medicine*, vol. 25, no. 6, pp. 873–881, 1997.

[5] W. C. Kramer, K. J. Hendricks, and J. Wang, "Pathogenetic mechanisms of posttraumatic osteoarthritis: opportunities for early intervention," *International Journal of Clinical and Experimental Medicine*, vol. 4, no. 4, pp. 285–298, 2011.

[6] T. P. Andriacchi, S. Koo, and S. F. Scanlan, "Gait mechanics influence healthy cartilage morphology and osteoarthritis of the knee," *The Journal of Bone & Joint Surgery—American Volume*, vol. 91, supplement 1, pp. 95–101, 2009.

[7] N. M. Cattano, M. F. Barbe, V. S. Massicotte et al., "Joint trauma initiates knee osteoarthritis through biochemical and biomechanical processes and interactions," *OA Musculoskeletal Medicine*, vol. 1, no. 1, pp. 3–8, 2013.

[8] E. M. Roos, "Joint injury causes knee osteoarthritis in young adults," *Current Opinion in Rheumatology*, vol. 17, no. 2, pp. 195–200, 2005.

[9] L. S. Lohmander, A. Östenberg, M. Englund, and H. Roos, "High prevalence of knee osteoarthritis, pain, and functional limitations in female soccer players twelve years after anterior cruciate ligament injury," *Arthritis and Rheumatism*, vol. 50, no. 10, pp. 3145–3152, 2004.

[10] L. S. Lohmander, P. M. Englund, L. L. Dahl, and E. M. Roos, "The long-term consequence of anterior cruciate ligament and meniscus injuries: osteoarthritis," *American Journal of Sports Medicine*, vol. 35, no. 10, pp. 1756–1769, 2007.

[11] M. C. Hochberg, R. D. Altman, K. D. Brandt et al., "Guidelines for the medical management of osteoarthritis. Part II. osteoarthritis of the knee," *Arthritis & Rheumatism*, vol. 38, no. 11, pp. 1541–1546, 1995.

[12] D. J. Hunter and D. T. Felson, "Osteoarthritis," *British Medical Journal*, vol. 332, no. 7542, pp. 639–642, 2006.

[13] G. Bode, J. von Heyden, J. Pestka et al., "Prospective 5-year survival rate data following open-wedge valgus high tibial osteotomy," *Knee Surgery, Sports Traumatology, Arthroscopy*, vol. 23, no. 7, pp. 1949–1955, 2015.

[14] T. Saito, K. Kumagai, Y. Akamatsu, H. Kobayashi, and Y. Kusayama, "Five- to ten-year outcome following medial opening-wedge high tibial osteotomy with rigid plate fixation in combination with an artificial bone substitute," *The Bone & Joint Journal*, vol. 96, no. 3, pp. 339–344, 2014.

[15] G. M. Salzmann, P. Ahrens, F. D. Naal et al., "Sporting activity after high tibial osteotomy for the treatment of medial compartment knee osteoarthritis," *The American Journal of Sports Medicine*, vol. 37, no. 2, pp. 312–318, 2009.

[16] T. Duivenvoorden, R. W. Brouwer, A. Baan et al., "Comparison of closing-wedge and opening-wedge high tibial osteotomy for medial compartment osteoarthritis of the knee: a randomized controlled trial with a six-year follow-up," *The Journal of Bone & Joint Surgery—American Volume*, vol. 96, no. 17, pp. 1425–1432, 2014.

[17] L. D. Jones, N. Bottomley, K. Harris, W. Jackson, A. J. Price, and D. J. Beard, "The clinical symptom profile of early radiographic knee arthritis: a pain and function comparison with advanced disease," *Knee Surgery, Sports Traumatology, Arthroscopy*, vol. 24, no. 1, pp. 161–168, 2016.

[18] C. Becher, J. Huelsmann, M. Ettinger, B. Fleischer, P. Niemeyer, and G. Bode, "Comparing established and emerging surgical options for load reduction of the medial knee: a biomechanical study," *Knee Surgery, Sports Traumatology, Arthroscopy*, vol. 24, supplement 1, pp. S4–S114, 2016.

[19] E. F. Chehab, J. Favre, J. C. Erhart-Hledik, and T. P. Andriacchi, "Baseline knee adduction and flexion moments during walking are both associated with 5 year cartilage changes in patients with medial knee osteoarthritis," *Osteoarthritis and Cartilage*, vol. 22, no. 11, pp. 1833–1839, 2014.

[20] T. Miyazaki, M. Wada, H. Kawahara, M. Sato, H. Baba, and S. Shimada, "Dynamic load at baseline can predict radiographic disease progression in medial compartment knee osteoarthritis," *Annals of the Rheumatic Diseases*, vol. 61, no. 7, pp. 617–622, 2002.

[21] W. van der Merwe, K. Slynarski, J. Walawski, and R. Smigielski, "Preliminary results: 40 patient, multi-center, prospective study of an implantable, extra-capsular, polycarbonate urethane knee unloader," *Knee Surgery, Sports Traumatology, Arthroscopy*, vol. 24, supplement 1, pp. S115–S435, 2016.

[22] K. Slynarski, L. Lipinski, and A. Krzesniak, "Feasibility of joint unloading for degenerative medial meniscus, cartilage defects, and OA," *Knee Surgery, Sports Traumatology, Arthroscopy*, vol. 24, supplement 1, pp. S4–S114, 2016.

28

Lower Limb Reconstruction with Tibia Allograft after Resection of Giant Aneurysmal Bone Cyst

Joaquim Soares do Brito, Joana Teixeira, and José Portela

Orthopaedics and Trauma Department, Centro Hospitalar Lisboa Norte, EPE-Hospital de Santa Maria, 1649-036 Lisboa, Portugal

Correspondence should be addressed to Joaquim Soares do Brito; joaquimsoaresdobrito@gmail.com

Academic Editor: Byron Chalidis

Aneurysmal bone cysts (ABCs) are benign, expansible, nonneoplastic lesions of the bone, characterized by channels of blood and spaces separated by fibrous septa, which occur in young patients and, occasionally, with aggressive behavior. Giant ABC is an uncommon pathological lesion and can be challenging because of the destructive effect of the cyst on the bones and the pressure on the nearby structures, especially on weight-bearing bones. In this scenario, *en bloc* resection is the mainstay treatment and often demands complex reconstructions. This paper reports a difficult case of an unusual giant aneurysmal bone cyst, which required extensive resection and a knee fusion like reconstruction with tibia allograft.

1. Introduction

Aneurysmal bone cyst (ABC) is a rare benign bone tumor that contains blood-filled cavernous spaces separated by septa containing osteoid tissue and osteoclast giant cells [1–3]. Young patients are most often affected with tumors located in long bones metaphysis. In less frequent occasions we can find ABC in pelvis and spine, and sometimes ABC could be present with aggressive behavior [1–3].

Several treatment modalities have been described for ABC such as sole curettage, curettage with cementation or bone grafting, fibrosing agents or bone marrow injections, arterial embolization, adjuvant cryotherapy or radiotherapy, demineralized bone matrix applications, and segmental or *en bloc* resections [4]. Small lesions with minimal destruction or expansion of cortical bone can be treated with intralesional procedures with or without bone grafting; however, aggressive large-sized and expansible tumors should be treated through segmental or *en bloc* resection techniques and reconstruction with structural grafts [5]. *En bloc* resection has the additional advantage of allowing obtaining the lowest association with recurrence which is as low as 0% [6–8]. However, resection can be problematic, especially for the lesions located in functionally important segments, when the tumor is unusually large or in the presence of concomitant pathological fracture.

It is not common to find the term "giant aneurysmal bone cyst" in the literature, mainly because it is considered a benign tumor. Nonetheless, some lesions can reach remarkable sizes, particularly if not treated properly allowing their growth through time [9]. Herein we present an unusual clinical case of a giant aneurysmal bone cyst located in proximal tibia, which eventually evolved to a supracondylar femur pathological fracture. Our surgical strategy was supported on a large resection and lower limb reconstruction with knee fusion using a tibia structural allograft. One year after surgical procedure, the patient is functionally independent, without walking aid and with minimal limb length discrepancy.

2. Clinical Case

A 25-year-old black man originally from Guiney presented in the emergency department with a four-year history of a right knee slow growing mass for evaluation. The patient had a giant mass located around the right knee, which was in forced flexion and with no extension ability. There was no pain or vascular or neurological compromise despite the remarkable size of the lesion. Nonetheless, patient could not walk due to tumor size and knee fixed flexion (Figure 1). No other clinical findings or associated symptoms were disclosed.

The X-ray, CT scan, and MRI (Figures 2–5) revealed images showing an unusual large bone tumor of the proximal

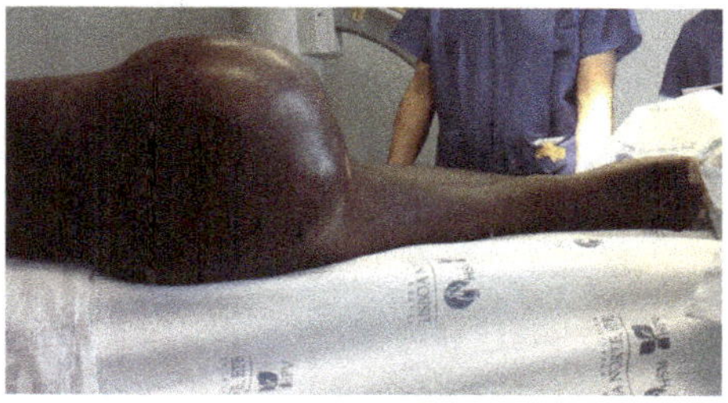

FIGURE 1

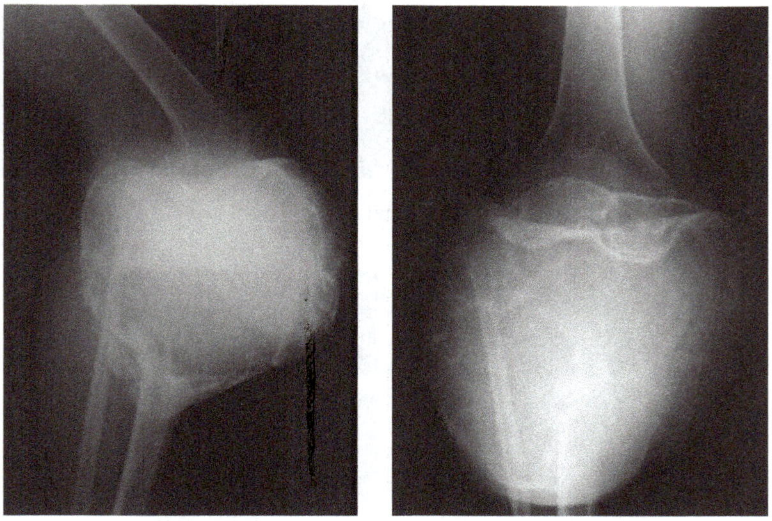

FIGURE 2

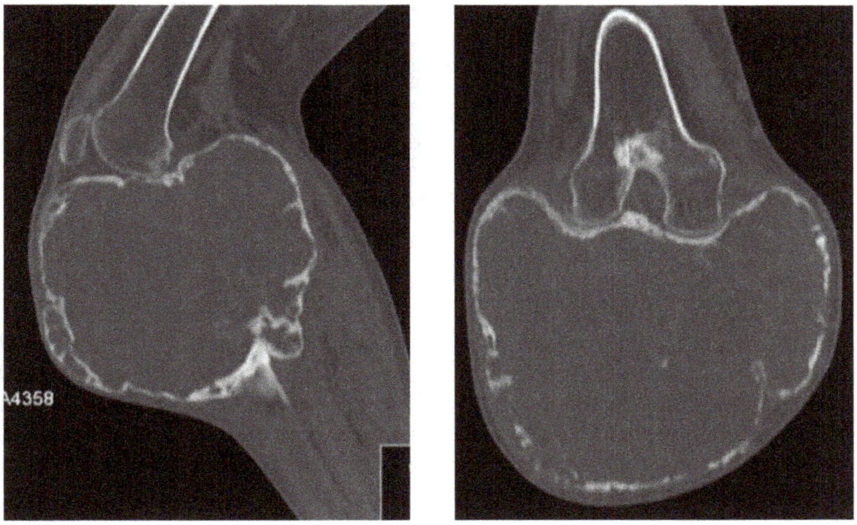

FIGURE 3

tibia. The patient underwent bone biopsy for definitive histological diagnosis, which was consistent with giant cell tumor. A radical surgical resection was proposed.

Preoperatively the patient returned to the emergency department due to a low energy fall but with an excruciating pain in the right knee. The new X-ray series disclosed a supracondylar femur fracture requiring surgery.

To obtain a most secure solution regarding a patient originally from Guiney where there is no medical assistance, we chose to perform an extensive extra-articular *en bloc*

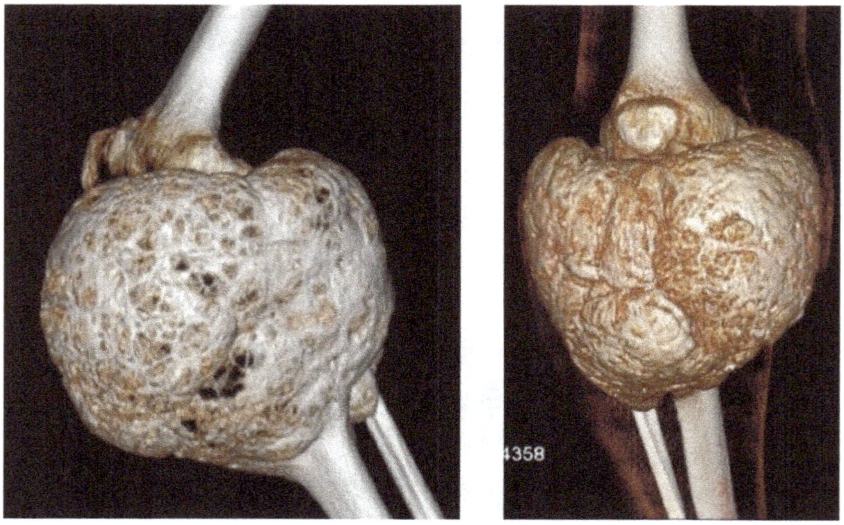

Figure 4

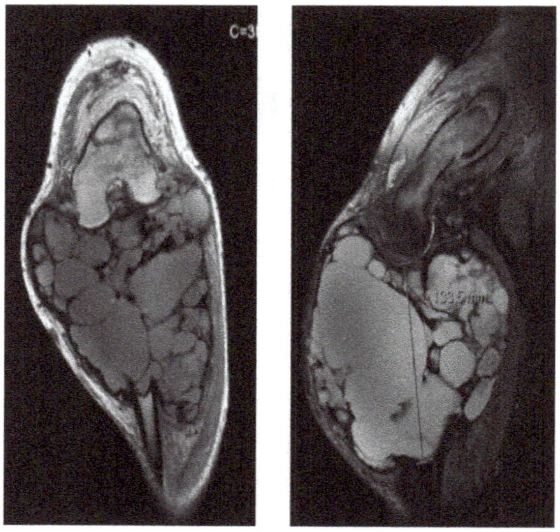

Figure 5

resection (until the supracondylar fracture site) and reconstruct the lower limb as a knee fusion, with a tibia structural allograft. Intraoperatively we performed an extra-articular resection through the supracondylar femur segment and the tibia diaphysis. All nerves and blood vessels were preserved. A tibia allograft was then interposed in the defect, and a knee arthrodesis nail was used to stabilize the construct (Figure 6). Distally, the tibia allograft received the additional support of plate and screws to increased integration probabilities within the remaining patient's tibia.

Postoperatively there were no complications, which allowed patient discharge during the first week. Partial weight bearing supported by crutches was allowed since the first day after operation. Follow-up with clinical and radiographic evaluation took place in the outpatient clinic, again without complications. The final histopathology diagnosis of the specimen (Figure 7) was an aneurysmal bone cyst.

Currently, with one year after the index operation, the patient is independent for daily live activities and only uses a walking aid occasionally. Radiographic assessment revealed no construct failure and good evolution to allograft integration (Figure 8). Limb length discrepancy is about two centimeters with no impact in function, which will allow patient to return to his home country.

3. Discussion

Aneurysmal bone cysts (ABCs) are often found in long bones metaphysis; nonetheless, they could be present in any other location, as the vertebral column and pelvis [1–5]. ABC can be present early before reaching giant size, which facilitates early diagnosis and treatment. It is well known that ABC is classified as an aggressive benign bone tumor, which means that if not treated properly, it may recur or if left untreated,

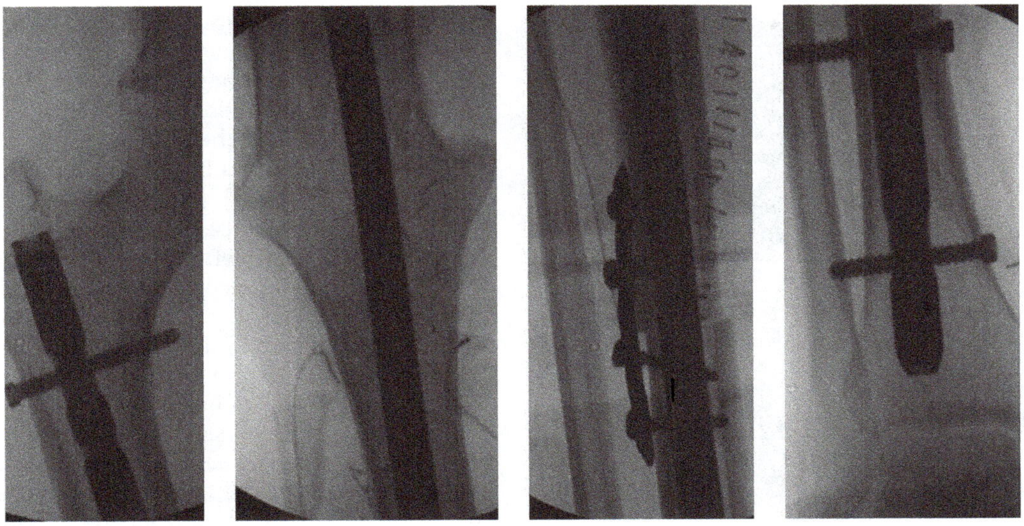

Figure 6

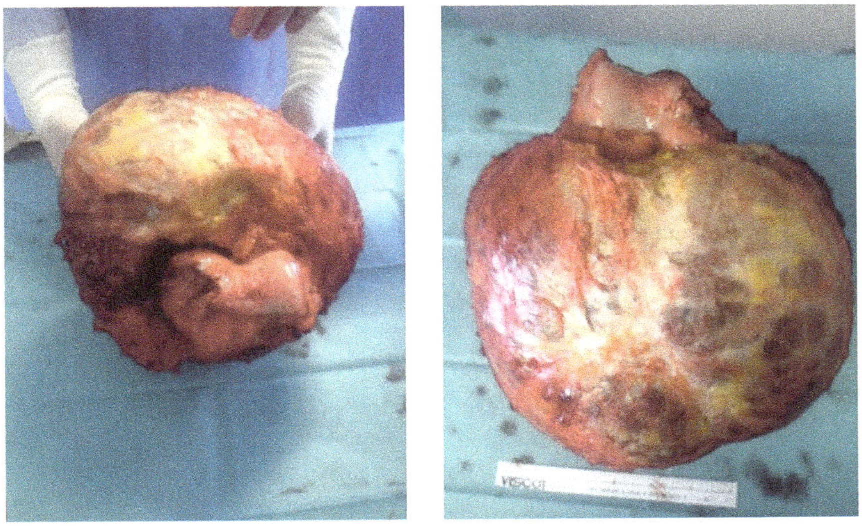

Figure 7

it may get larger and eventually grow to be a giant ABC [9]. These aggressive lesions are difficult to address and could be challenging to any orthopaedic surgeon.

Although the pathogenesis of ABCs is still unknown, they could be considered either primary (70%) or secondary (30%) [5]. Primary ABCs arise *de novo*. A secondary ABC develops in association with other neoplasms most commonly giant bone tumor (GCT) of the bone, osteoblastoma, chondroblastoma, and fibrous dysplasia [10]. Radiographically, the diagnosis of an ABC shows five classic findings [3]. First, the neoplasm is typically present as an expansile lytic lesion with a soap-bubble appearance. Second, it presents an eccentric lesion outlined by a thin layer of subperiosteal new bone. Third, it presents a centric lesion. Fourth, it reveals a metaphyseal lesion that occupies a large percentage of the bone with trabeculations at the edges. Fifth, it manifests soft tissue expansion and destruction of the cortex. Additionally, it is suggested that if the cyst's transverse diameter on radiographic examination is equal to or more than three times the diameter of the adjacent normal bone, it can be called giant ABC [5]. Our patient fits these characteristics and by doing so we could considerer this particular lesion as a giant ABC.

Curettage and/or *en bloc* resection are treatments of choice for accessible lesions; meanwhile, other treatment modalities including percutaneous intralesional injection, cryotherapy, radiation, and embolization have been used for less accessible or recurrent lesions [5]. Chemical cauterization with phenol is recommended for large primary lesion to kill any surface tumor cells of the curetted cavity [3]. Cryotherapy has also been proposed as an adjuvant therapy with surgical treatment to achieve local control [11]. Radiation is used in inaccessible sites where no surgical options are available and selective arterial embolization is recommended as a procedure for lesions whose location or size makes other treatment

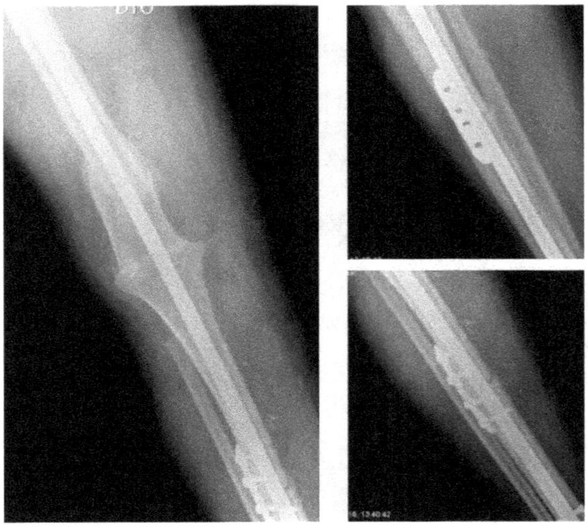

Figure 8

modalities difficult or dangerous [3, 12–17]. Additionally, in large tumors similar to this case, arterial embolization could be a definitive treatment (even with serial embolizations) or used as adjuvant to the surgical technique, which allows improving surgical safety.

This particular case had three major hazards: the size of the lesion for one side, which demanded a wide resection; the articular involvement of the knee with loss of articular function; and finally a concomitant supracondylar femur fracture, which was an adverse event that represented an additional difficulty to limb reconstruction. In this setting, it is important to focus on the patient, who was originally from Guiney, a country where medical assistance is lacking. These facts and the patient returning home were important to the final treatment decision.

Large defects after resections of aggressive and giant aneurysmal bone cysts are difficult to treat. Various reconstructive options are available to fill these defects and provide bone integrity, including allogeneic or autogenic bone grafts and many different bony substitutes [5]. Our choice was to sacrifice the knee articulation, providing a knee fusion-like construct using a tibia allograft. This option was preferred for several reasons: firstly we were looking for a definitive solution with a life span, thinking in the probable revision surgery if we had a total knee replacement; secondly there were a lack of medical assistance in Guiney and an inability to return to periodic consultation; and finally we needed a permanent solution which allows high demand performance, according to a young rural worker.

Treatments for aneurysmal bone cysts should be individualized and take into account the location, aggressiveness, and extent of the lesion [5]. Cortical strut allografts have an important role in the treatment of large benign bone lesions after resection and bring the advantage of unlimited supply without additional donor site morbidity [18]. Meanwhile, the incorporating process of allografts is slower and probably less complete than that with autografts due to a low-grade immune response or a lack of osteocytes in the graft or both [19, 20]. Vascularized bone grafts have been suggested as the best method to replace large bone defects due to the ability for faster full incorporation and remodeling. Despite these advantages, vascularized bone grafts are technically demanding procedure and with a high failure rate for those without large experience [21–24]. Nonvascularized grafts are technically much easier to use and provide excellent structural bone support at the recipient side [21]. Successful long-term results of surgical *en bloc* resection and replacement with nonvascularized, autologous fibular, or tibial graft have already been reported in the literature [25]. Abuhassan and Shannak reported the results of nonvascularized fibular graft for the reconstruction of bone defects after *en bloc* resection of giant ABC in three patients [9]. They observed insufficient graft incorporation at the distal part of the fibular graft in the humerus case at the 18th month postoperatively. They treated this patient by open reduction and internal fixation with additional bone grafting and based on this experience advised rigid fixation of fibular graft onto the normal bone as a supplemental form of internal fixation to prevent graft insufficiency [9]. In the present case, the final construct obtained was stable and allowed progressive weight bearing without graft or osteosynthesis material failure. One year after surgery, the patient is independent and ready to return home.

Competing Interests

The authors declare that they have no competing interests.

References

[1] M. Campanacci, F. Bertoni, and P. Bacchini, "Aneurysmal bone cyst," in *Bone and Soft Tissue Tumors*, pp. 725–751, Springer, Berlin, Germany, 1990.

[2] A. M. Vergel de Dios, J. R. Bond, T. C. Shives, R. A. McLeod, and K. K. Unni, "Aneurysmal bone cyst. A clinicopathologic study of 238 cases," *Cancer*, vol. 69, no. 12, pp. 2921–2931, 1992.

[3] M. Campanacci, R. Capanna, and P. Picci, "Unicameral and aneurysmal bone cysts," *Clinical Orthopaedics and Related Research*, vol. 204, pp. 26–36, 1986.

[4] R. Kaila, M. Ropars, T. W. Briggs, and S. R. Cannon, "Aneurysmal bone cyst of the paediatric shoulder girdle: a case series and literature review," *Journal of Pediatric Orthopaedics Part B*, vol. 16, no. 6, pp. 429–436, 2007.

[5] M. Güven, M. Demirel, T. Özler, I. C. Başsorgun, S. Ipek, and S. Kara, "An aggressive aneurysmal bone cyst of the proximal humerus and related complications in a pediatric patient," *Strategies in Trauma and Limb Reconstruction*, vol. 7, no. 1, pp. 51–56, 2012.

[6] K. Başarir, A. Pişkin, B. Güçlü, Y. Yildiz, and Y. Sağlik, "Aneurysmal bone cyst recurrence in children: a review of 56 patients," *Journal of Pediatric Orthopaedics*, vol. 27, no. 8, pp. 938–943, 2007.

[7] M. Szendröi, I. Cser, A. Kónya, and A. Rényi-Vámos, "Aneurysmal bone cyst. A review of 52 primary and 16 secondary cases," *Archives of Orthopaedic and Trauma Surgery*, vol. 111, no. 6, pp. 318–322, 1992.

[8] W. G. Cole, "Treatment of aneurysmal bone cysts in childhood," *Journal of Pediatric Orthopaedics*, vol. 6, no. 3, pp. 326–329, 1986.

[9] F. O. Abuhassan and A. Shannak, "Non-vascularized fibular graft reconstruction after resection of giant aneurysmal bone cyst (ABC)," *Strategies in Trauma and Limb Reconstruction*, vol. 5, no. 3, pp. 149–154, 2010.

[10] A. Bonakdarpour, W. M. Levy, and E. Aegerter, "Primary and secondary aneurysmal bone cyst: a radiological study of 75 cases," *Radiology*, vol. 126, no. 1, pp. 75–83, 1978.

[11] H. W. B. Schreuder, R. P. H. Veth, M. Pruszczynski, J. A. M. Lemmens, H. Schraffordt Koops, and W. M. Molenaar, "Aneurysmal bone cysts treated by curettage, cryotherapy and bone grafting," *The Journal of Bone & Joint Surgery—British Volume*, vol. 79, no. 1, pp. 20–25, 1997.

[12] E. Yildirim, S. Ersözlü, I. Kirbaş, A. F. Özgür, T. Akkaya, and E. Karadeli, "Treatment of pelvic aneurysmal bone cysts in two children: selective arterial embolization as an adjunct to curettage and bone grafting," *Diagnostic and Interventional Radiology*, vol. 13, no. 1, pp. 49–52, 2007.

[13] G. Rossi, A. F. Mavrogenis, E. Rimondi et al., "Selective arterial embolisation for bone tumours: experience of 454 cases," *La Radiologia Medica*, vol. 116, no. 5, pp. 793–808, 2011.

[14] G. Rossi, E. Rimondi, T. Bartalena et al., "Selective arterial embolization of 36 aneurysmal bone cysts of the skeleton with N-2-butyl cyanoacrylate," *Skeletal Radiology*, vol. 39, no. 2, pp. 161–167, 2010.

[15] A. F. Mavrogenis, G. Rossi, E. Rimondi, P. J. Papagelopoulos, and P. Ruggieri, "Embolization of bone tumors," *Orthopedics*, vol. 34, no. 4, pp. 303–310, 2011.

[16] J. A. Green, M. C. Bellemore, and F. W. Marsden, "Embolization in the treatment of aneurysmal bone cysts," *Journal of Pediatric Orthopaedics*, vol. 17, no. 4, pp. 440–443, 1997.

[17] J. Soares Do Brito and J. Portela, "Selective arterial embolization for a large pelvic aneurysmal bone cyst treatment," *Acta Medica Portuguesa*, vol. 28, no. 6, pp. 780–783, 2015.

[18] H.-N. Shih, J.-Y. Su, K.-Y. Hsu, and R. W.-W. Hsu, "Allogeneic cortical strut for benign lesions of the humerus in adolescents," *Journal of Pediatric Orthopaedics*, vol. 17, no. 4, pp. 433–436, 1997.

[19] H.-N. Shih, Y.-J. Chen, T.-J. Huang, K.-Y. Hsu, and R. W.-W. Hsu, "Semistructural allografting in bone defects after curettage," *Journal of Surgical Oncology*, vol. 68, no. 3, pp. 159–165, 1998.

[20] G. L. Glancy, D. J. Brugioni, R. E. Eilert, and F. M. Chang, "Autograft versus allograft for benign lesions in children," *Clinical Orthopaedics and Related Research*, vol. 262, pp. 28–33, 1991.

[21] C. G. Finkemeier, "Bone-grafting and bone-graft substitutes," *The Journal of Bone & Joint Surgery—American Volume*, vol. 84, no. 3, pp. 454–464, 2002.

[22] M. Ghert, N. Colterjohn, and M. Manfrini, "The use of free vascularized fibular grafts in skeletal reconstruction for bone tumors in children," *Journal of the American Academy of Orthopaedic Surgeons*, vol. 15, no. 10, pp. 577–587, 2007.

[23] K. Arai, S. Toh, K. Tsubo, S. Nishikawa, S. Narita, and H. Miura, "Complications of vascularized fibula graft for reconstruction of long bones," *Plastic and Reconstructive Surgery*, vol. 109, no. 7, pp. 2301–2306, 2002.

[24] A. Minami, T. Kasashima, N. Iwasaki, H. Kato, and K. Kaneda, "Vascularised fibular grafts," *Journal of Bone and Joint Surgery B*, vol. 82, no. 7, pp. 1022–1025, 2000.

[25] A. Grzegorzewski, E. Pogonowicz, M. Sibinski, M. Marciniak, and M. Synder, "Treatment of benign lesions of humerus with resection and non-vascularised, autologous fibular graft," *International Orthopaedics*, vol. 34, no. 8, pp. 1267–1272, 2010.

29

Osteolysis of the Greater Trochanter Caused by a Foreign Body Granuloma Associated with the Ethibond® Suture after Total Hip Arthroplasty

Keiji Kamo,[1,2] Hiroaki Kijima,[2,3] Koichiro Okuyama,[1] Nobutoshi Seki,[1] Shin Yamada,[2,3] Naohisa Miyakoshi,[3] and Yoichi Shimada[2,3]

[1] *Department of Orthopedic Surgery, Akita Rosai Hospital, Odate, Japan*
[2] *Akita Hip Research Group (AHRG), Akita, Japan*
[3] *Department of Orthopedic Surgery, Akita University Graduate School of Medicine, Akita, Japan*

Correspondence should be addressed to Keiji Kamo; keiji-kamo@par.odn.ne.jp

Academic Editor: John Nyland

The present case shows a case of progression of osteolysis of the greater trochanter caused by a foreign body granuloma associated with the number 5 Ethibond suture in cementless THA with the direct lateral approach that was completely healed by removal of the Ethibond suture. A 55-year-old Japanese woman with secondary osteoarthritis caused by acetabular dysplasia underwent left cementless THA with the direct lateral approach. After setting of the total hip prosthesis, the gluteus medius muscle and vastus lateralis muscle were reattached to the greater trochanter through two bone tunnels using number 5 Ethibond EXCEL sutures. The left hip pain disappeared after surgery, but the bone tunnels enlarged gradually and developed osteolysis at 10 weeks. The removal of the Ethibond sutures and debridement improved the osteolysis. Histological examination showed the granuloma reaction to a foreign body with giant cell formation. The Ethibond suture has the lowest inflammatory tissue reaction and relatively high tension strength among nonabsorbable suture materials. However, number 5 Ethibond has the potential to cause osteolysis due to a foreign body granuloma, as in the present case.

1. Introduction

The direct lateral approach to the hip was described by Hardinge in 1982. With this approach, the anterior half of the gluteus medius muscle and the vastus lateralis muscles are detached from the greater trochanter [1]. In this case, the gluteus medius should be reattached to the greater trochanter to prevent a positive Trendelenburg sign after surgery. Several techniques of soft tissues reattachment in total hip arthroplasty (THA) have been reported [2–5]. The technique of soft tissues reattachment by nonabsorbable suture through bone tunnels is often used in THA with the direct lateral approach and posterior approach [2–4]. Ethibond suture has characteristics of both the lowest inflammatory tissue reaction and relatively high tension strength among nonabsorbable suture materials. Therefore, Ethibond suture is preferably used for reattachment of the abductor muscles, the capsule, and the external rotators in THA. Osteolysis of the greater trochanter associated with the Ethibond suture after THA is very rare. A case of osteolysis of the greater trochanter caused by a foreign body granuloma associated with number 5 Ethibond suture, which was used to reattach the gluteus medius to the greater trochanter through bone tunnels in THA, is presented. Written informed consent was obtained from the patient for publication of this case report.

2. Case Presentation

A 55-year-old Japanese woman with secondary osteoarthritis caused by acetabular dysplasia underwent left cementless THA with the direct lateral approach. The operation was performed in the lateral position. The anterior half of the gluteus medius muscle and the vastus lateralis muscle were detached from the greater trochanter. After setting of the

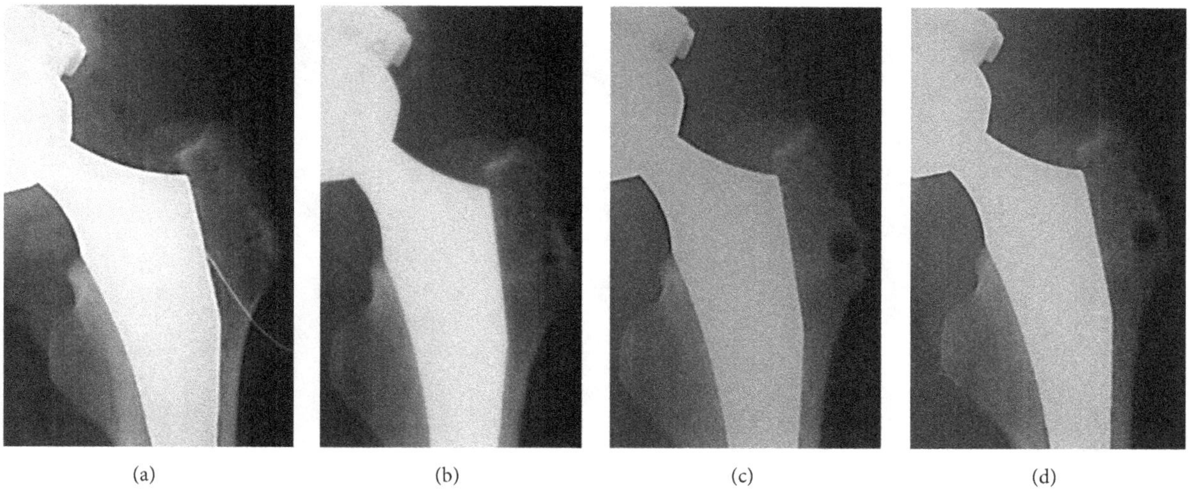

FIGURE 1: Radiographs of the left hip joint after THA. (a) The initial radiograph after THA. (b) At 4 weeks after THA. (c) At 8 weeks. (d) At 10 weeks.

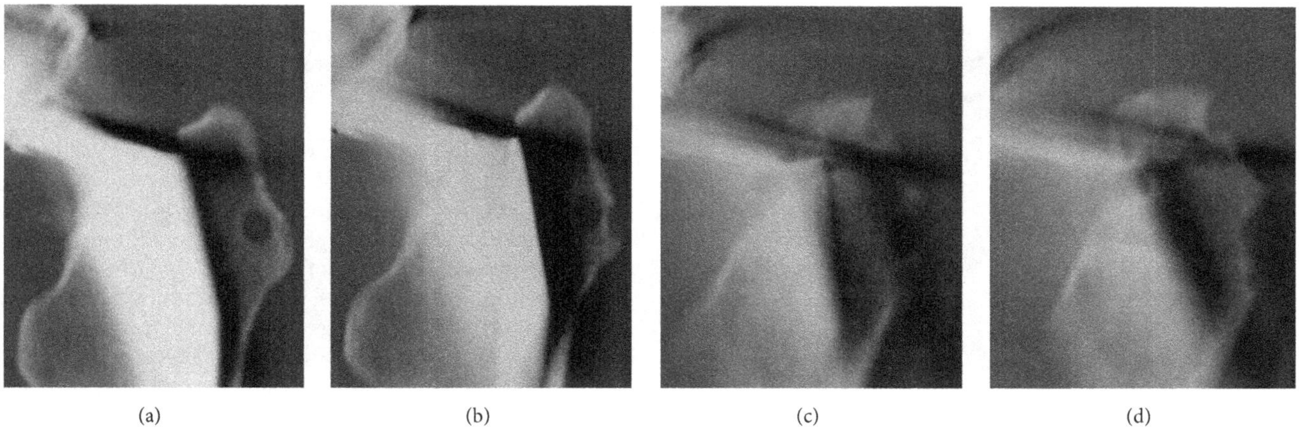

FIGURE 2: Coronal view of computed tomography showing osteolysis clearly ((a)–(d)).

total hip prosthesis, the gluteus medius muscle and vastus lateralis muscle were reattached to the greater trochanter through two bone tunnels using number 5 Ethibond EXCEL (ETHICON, Johnson & Johnson, Tokyo, Japan) sutures. The left hip pain disappeared after surgery, but the bone tunnels were slightly enlarged on the radiograph 4 weeks after operation. They enlarged gradually and developed osteolysis of 10 mm in diameter at 10 weeks in the radiographs (Figure 1). Computed tomography (CT) showed the osteolysis clearly (Figure 2). Magnetic resonance imaging (MRI, 1.5 T Magnetom Symphony a Tim System, Siemens, Germany) showed the mass at the greater trochanter as low intensities on both T1-weighted images and T2 star-weighted images. The area surrounding the mass had low intensities on T1-weighted images and high intensities on T2 star-weighted images (Figure 3). The patient had no pain, and inflammatory sign was not observed on the operated site. There was no sign of infection on blood biochemical examinations. The removal of the Ethibond sutures and debridement were performed to prevent progressive osteolysis and a pathological fracture of the greater trochanter. At the time of the surgery, granulation tissue was seen surrounding the Ethibond sutures in the greater trochanter. The Ethibond sutures and the granulation tissues were completely removed. The gluteus medius muscle was repaired using absorbable number 2 Vicryl Plus® (ETHICON, Johnson & Johnson, Tokyo, Japan) sutures. Histological examination showed the granuloma reaction to a foreign body with giant cell formation and proliferation of small blood vessels (Figure 4).

After the second surgery, the bone tunnels gradually decreased and disappeared. There was no evidence of osteolysis of the greater trochanter in the radiograph at 10 months after the second operation (Figure 5). The patient can walk without pain and without a Trendelenburg sign.

3. Discussion

The present case is the first report of progression of osteolysis of the greater trochanter caused by a foreign body granuloma associated with the Ethibond suture in cementless THA that

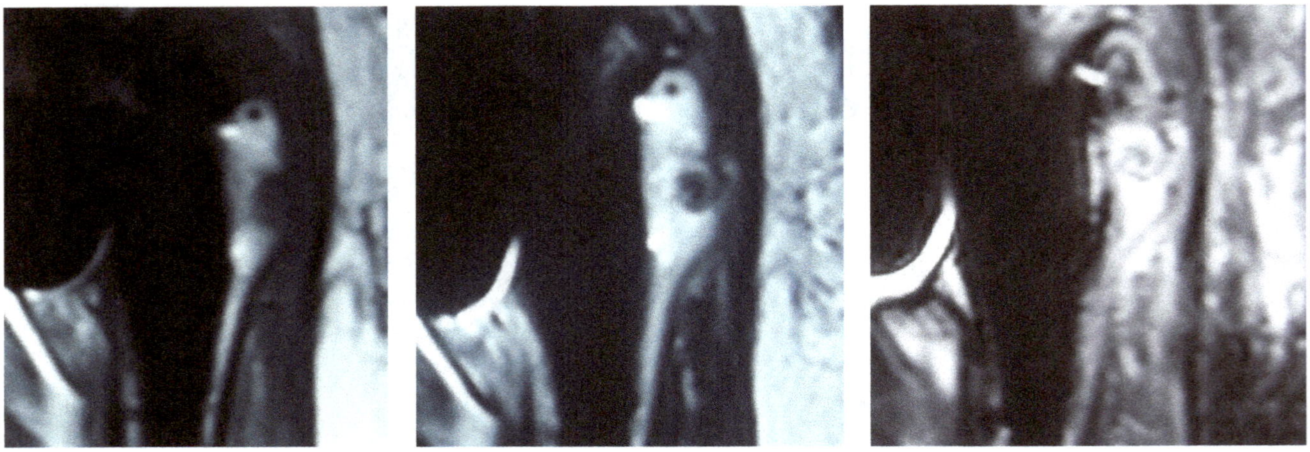

(a) (b) (c)

FIGURE 3: Magnetic resonance imaging at 10 weeks after THA. (a) T1-weighted image. (b) T2 star-weighted image. (c) T2 Short-TI Inversion Recovery (STIR) image.

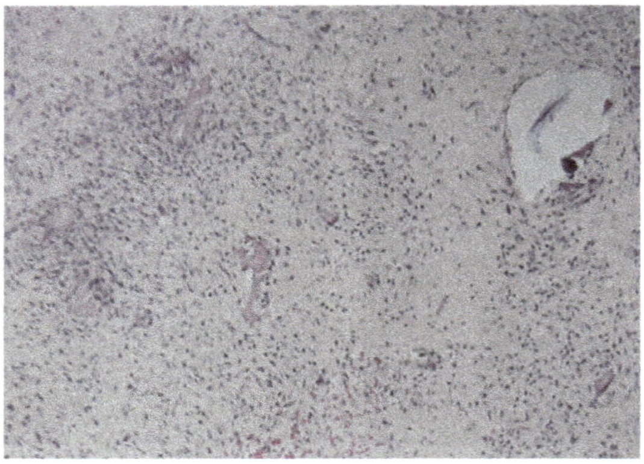

FIGURE 4: Histological examination showing the foreign body reaction granuloma with giant cell formation and proliferation of small blood vessels (hematoxylin and eosin stain; magnification: 100x).

was completely healed by removal of the Ethibond suture. The technique of repairing muscle tendon units and ligaments by nonabsorbable suture through bone tunnels is widely used in orthopedic surgery. In THA, this technique is useful when reattaching abductor muscles to the greater trochanter in the direct lateral approach and for repairing the capsule and external rotator muscles in the posterior approach.

Ethibond is a nonabsorbable, braided surgical suture. It consists of high molecular weight, long chain, and linear polyesters with recurrent aromatic rings as an integral component and is covered with polybutylate [6]. Because of its coverage, it causes less tissue reaction and has better mechanical properties compared with the uncovered braided polyesters [7]. Therefore, Ethibond is often used for reattachment of the abductor muscles, the capsule, and the external rotators in THA [3, 4].

In the present case, the second surgery and debridement were performed to prevent progressive osteolysis of the greater trochanter caused by the granuloma associated with the number 5 Ethibond suture. There have been few reports of osteolysis caused by the Ethibond suture. Kundra et al. reported 27 cases of cemented THA that had osteolysis of the greater trochanter following reattachment of hip abductors using number 5 Ethibond sutures through bone tunnels [4]. These patients displayed a predominantly osteolytic pattern of bone reaction around the greater trochanter bone tunnels. Histological examination of the specimen showed chronic inflammation with a giant cell foreign body reaction that was similar to the present findings around the suture material.

The use of bone suture anchors was reported as another method of abductor muscle reattachment to the greater trochanter in THA. Harwin reported the results of bone anchors used for abductor reattachment in cementless THA of 214 cases with the direct lateral approach [5]. There were several complications, such as anchor migration from the bone, progressive osteolysis of the greater trochanter, and pathological fracture of the greater trochanter. Because of these complications and the associated significantly increased cost, they did not recommend the use of bone anchors to repair the abductors in THA with the direct lateral approach.

Esenyel et al. reported that the Ethibond suture showed the lowest inflammatory reaction among three nonabsorbable suture materials at 6 weeks after operation in a rabbit model [6]. Ollivere et al. reported a case of foreign body granulomatous reaction associated with Fiberwire® which is braided blend of polyester and polyethylene suture used in Achilles tendon repair. The tissue reaction in the case was similar to the finding of polyethylene wear debris associated with osteolysis [8]. Therefore, the Ethibond suture has the lowest inflammatory tissue reaction and relatively high tension strength among nonabsorbable suture materials at the present time. However, number 5 Ethibond has the potential to cause osteolysis due to a foreign body granuloma, as in the present case. Therefore, Kundra et al. suggested that the use of a thinner polyester suture or a different material be recommended for abductor reattachment in THA to

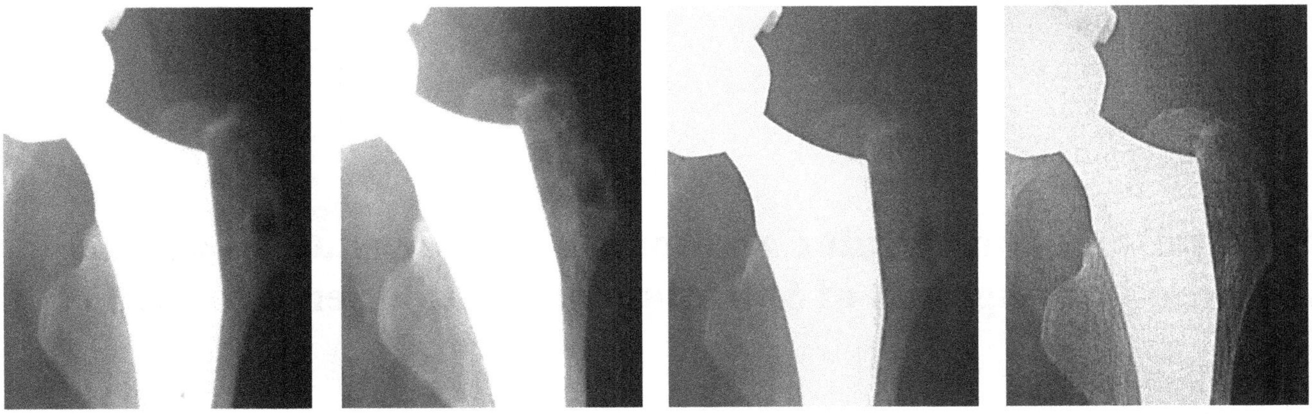

(a) (b) (c) (d)

Figure 5: Radiographs of the left hip joint after the removal of the Ethibond suture and the granulation tissue. Bone tunnels gradually decrease and disappear. There is no evidence of osteolysis of the greater trochanter at 10 months after the second surgery. (a) At 1 month after the second surgery. (b) At 2 months. (c) At 3 months. (d) At 10 months.

prevent the osteolysis of the greater trochanter [4]. Another nonabsorbable suture should not be challengingly used in reattachment of the hip abductors in THA as the long term result of its usage has not been reported. At the present, in terms of low inflammatory tissue reaction, the absorbable suture is recommended for the procedure although it has less mechanical properties than nonabsorbable ones. The osteolysis caused by number 5 Ethibond suture has to be kept in mind as a complication when it was used for repairing abductors through bone tunnels in THA.

4. Conclusion

A case of osteolysis of the greater trochanter caused by a foreign body granuloma associated with the number 5 Ethibond suture after THA with the direct lateral approach was presented. Although Ethibond suture has the lowest inflammatory tissue reaction among the nonabsorbable sutures, the number 5 Ethibond may cause osteolysis due to granuloma formation. The osteolysis caused by number 5 Ethibond suture has to be kept in mind as a complication when it was used for repairing abductors through bone tunnels in THA.

Competing Interests

The authors declare that they have no conflict of interests.

References

[1] K. Hardinge, "The direct lateral approach to the hip," *The Journal of Bone & Joint Surgery—British Volume*, vol. 64, no. 1, pp. 17–19, 1982.

[2] J. A. Browne and M. W. Pagnano, "Surgical technique: a simple soft-tissue-only repair of the capsule and external rotators in posterior-approach THA," *Clinical Orthopaedics and Related Research*, vol. 470, no. 2, pp. 511–515, 2012.

[3] R. E. White Jr., T. J. Forness, J. K. Allman, and D. W. Junick, "Effect of posterior capsular repair on early dislocation in primary total hip replacement," *Clinical Orthopaedics and Related Research*, no. 393, pp. 163–167, 2001.

[4] R. K. Kundra, S. N. Karim, and T. Lawrence, "Osteolysis of the greater trochanter following reattachment of hip abductors using polyester suture in total hip arthroplasty," *HIP International*, vol. 19, no. 3, pp. 274–278, 2009.

[5] S. F. Harwin, "Osteolysis of the greater trochanter: a result of bone anchors used for abductor reattachment at total hip arthroplasty," *Journal of Arthroplasty*, vol. 21, no. 1, pp. 97–101, 2006.

[6] C. Z. Esenyel, M. Demirhan, O. Kilicoglu et al., "Evaluation of soft tissue reactions to three nonabsorbable suture materials in a rabbit model," *Acta Orthopaedica et Traumatologica Turcica*, vol. 43, no. 4, pp. 366–372, 2009.

[7] I. Capperauld, "Suture materials: a review," *Clinical Materials*, vol. 4, no. 1, pp. 3–12, 1989.

[8] B. J. Ollivere, H. A. Bosman, P. W. P. Bearcroft, and A. H. N. Robinson, "Foreign body granulomatous reaction associated with polyethelene 'Fiberwire®' suture material used in Achilles tendon repair," *Foot and Ankle Surgery*, vol. 20, no. 2, pp. e27–e29, 2014.

30

Perforation of an Occult Carcinoma of the Prostate as a Rare Differential Diagnosis of Subcutaneous Emphysema of the Leg

Mirko Velickovic and Thomas Hockertz

Department of Orthopedic Surgery, Sports Traumatology and Trauma Surgery, Städtisches Klinikum Wolfenbüttel (Wolfenbüttel Municipal Hospital), Alter Weg 80, 38302 Wolfenbüttel, Germany

Correspondence should be addressed to Mirko Velickovic; mirko.velickovic@klinikum-wolfenbuettel.de

Academic Editor: Akio Sakamoto

We report a case of subcutaneous emphysema caused by perforation of the rectum due to a carcinoma of the prostate. Although rare, an abdominal cause must always be considered as a rare differential diagnosis of subcutaneous emphysema. As a matter of fact adequate diagnostic with rapid treatment is essential for the outcome.

1. Introduction

Carcinoma of the prostate is a frequent malignancy in men. In Germany the incidence is about 25,4%. The average patient is 69 years old when getting the diagnosis. Due to determination of the PSA (prostate specific antigen) early diagnosis is possible. Subcutaneous emphysema of the lower extremities is usually caused by an infection with aerogenic bacteria's which is often seen after major traumas like open fractures. A perforation of an abdominal organ is quite rare. We report a case of a 98-year-old patient with an occult carcinoma of the prostate with perforation of the rectum and development of subcutaneous emphysema mimicking gas edema.

2. Case Report

A 98-year-old patient was admitted to the emergency department with a history of pain and swelling of the left thigh of 5-day duration after minor trauma. The patient suffered from dementia so an adequate communication was impossible. On admission, the vital parameters were normal, no fever. The physical examination revealed extensive subcutaneous crepitus in the whole left leg. There was no external wound. Other signs of inflammation were absent. Laboratory studies showed a WBC count of 11,400/μL, CRP 146,2 mg/L, and procalcitonin 0,59 ng/mL. There were although signs of chronic renal failure as well as hypothyreosis. X-ray of the left leg showed massive gas shadows in the left thigh, knee, and lower leg. Furthermore there was a tenderness of the abdomen with pain in the lower abdomen during palpation. The further examination revealed a perianal abscess. We performed a CT of the abdomen/pelvis and the complete left leg. CT revealed a 9 cm large carcinoma of the prostate gland necrotizing into the rectum and into the subcutaneous tissue causing a perianal abscess formation. Additionally metastatic lesions in the right lower lung and in 4 vertebral bodies in the thoracic and lumbar spine could be found (Figures 1–4). Contrast agent showed free air spreading from the rectum and the perforation as its origin into the gluteal region passing the adductor muscle going deep in the lower leg. An explorative laparotomy was performed. The complete exploration of the pelvic cavity was due to the extensive tumor mass not possible but an obvious perforation of the bowel was not found. There were no signs of peritonitis. The general condition of the patient was pure so we created a permanent artificial bowel outlet and collected specimen for microbiologic examination. During the digital rectal examination the tumor was clearly palpable and a biopsy sample was taken with a biopsy forceps. In a second step a fasciotomy of the left leg from the thigh to the calf was performed. Additional specimens for the microbiologic examination were collected (Figure 5). The pathologic examination of the specimen verified an adenocarcinoma of the prostate (Gleason 4 + 4).

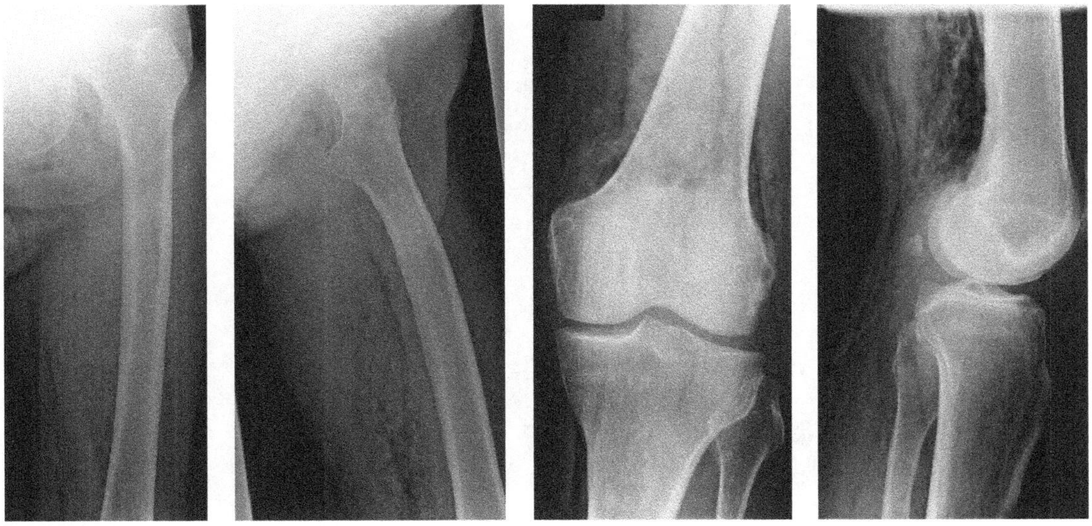

FIGURE 1: X ray of the left proximal femur and knee with demonstration of free air.

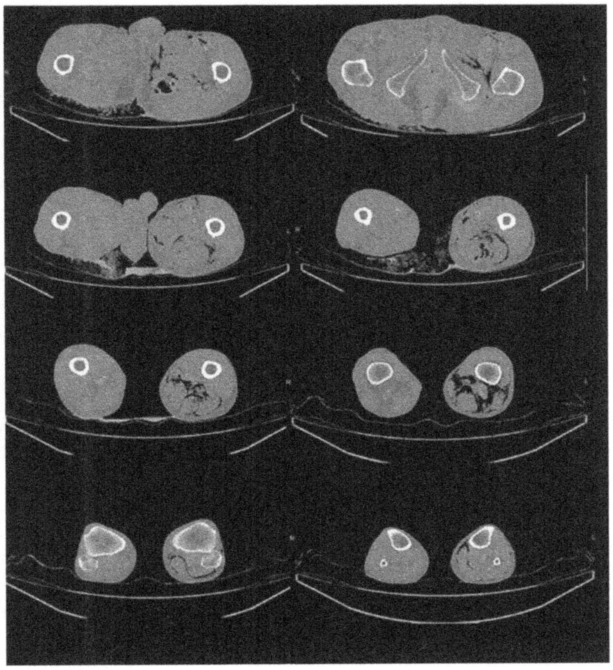

FIGURE 2: Axial CT scan of the lower leg starting from the hip to the knee with sharply demarcated free air in the soft tissue.

The microbiologic samples of the leg were sterile so a gas gangrene as a causative agent could be excluded. The swabs from the gut showed the presence of bacteria of the normal intestinal flora so a systemic antibiotic therapy was not necessary. Four days after the first laparotomy wound healing disturbances developed after the fasciotomy of the leg and of the abdomen so secondary wound closure was performed. During the course the patient suffered from a paralytic ileus so a third laparotomy with decompression of the small bowel and a VAC therapy was started. Finally the wound dehiscence was closed using a Vicryl mesh in a forth operation (Figures 6 and 7).

Later on the patient developed urinary tract infection which was treated with Sulfamethoxazole/Trimethoprim (Cotrim) for 19 days. Additionally the patient suffered from shingles which appeared as reddening of the skin with fluid-filled pustules on the abdomen, for which he received conservative treatment. The MRSA screening was negative. During the in-patient stay the CRP showed a declining trend with 26 mg/L; the leucocytes were already normal. Due to the

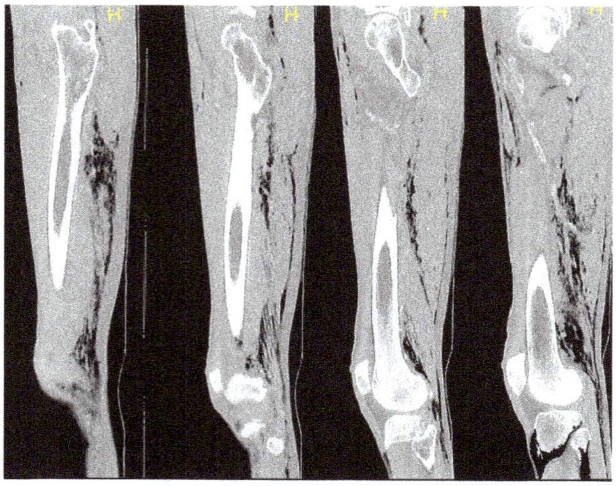

FIGURE 3: Sagittal sequence of the same CT scan.

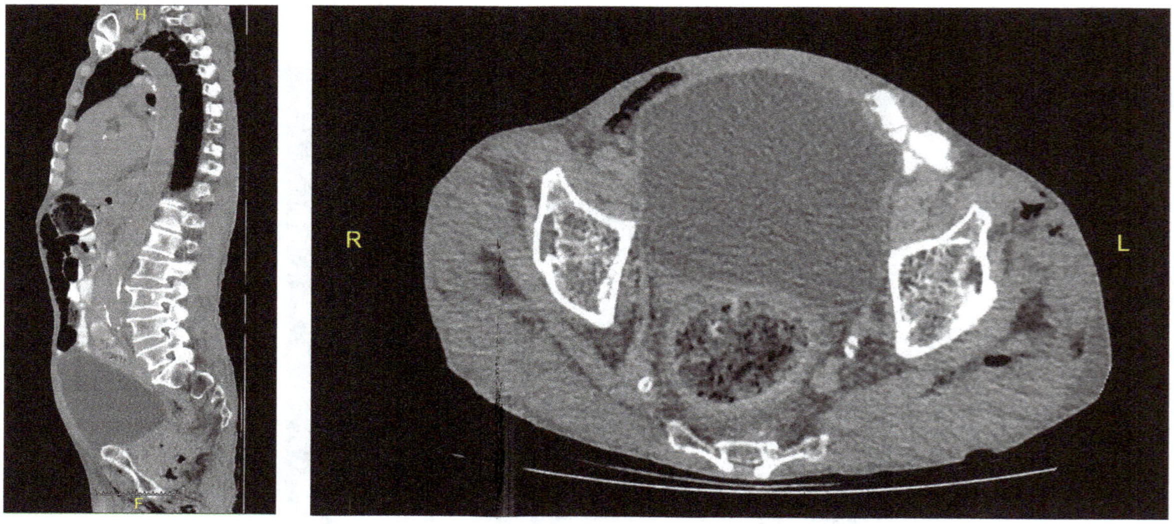

FIGURE 4: An image of tumor of the prostate.

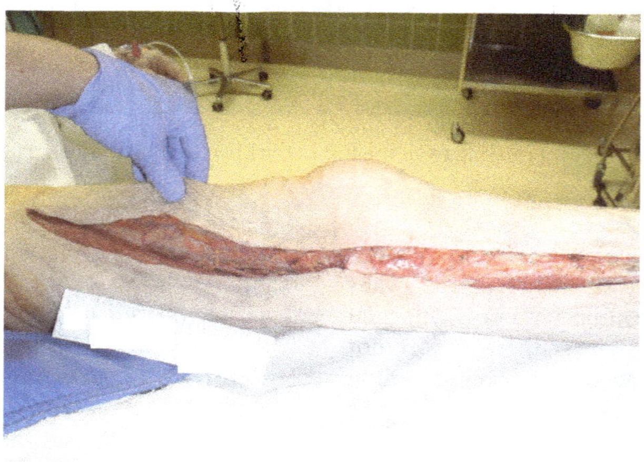

FIGURE 5: Intraoperative site with incision of the left leg.

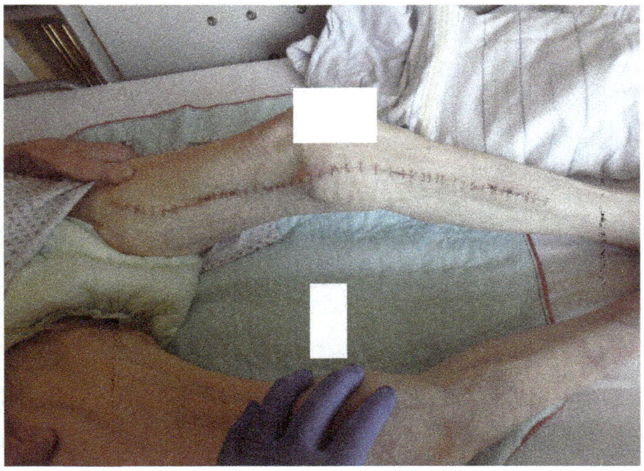

FIGURE 6: Left leg after operation with good healing process.

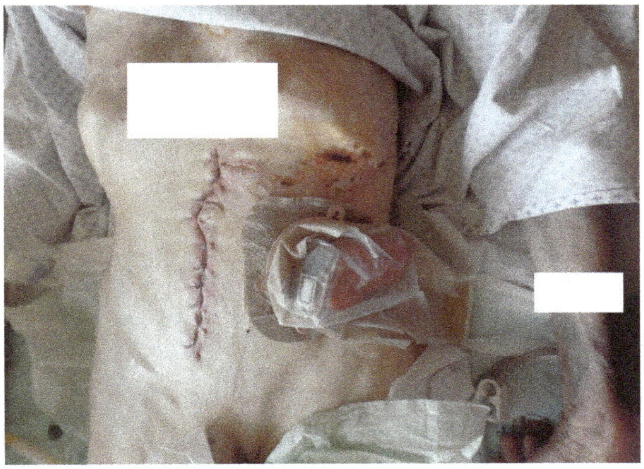

FIGURE 7: Operation site after operation with laparotomy scar and artificial anus (anus praeter).

advanced findings an adequate surgical treatment of the local focus was not likely to be successful anymore and prognosis becomes infaust. We started a hormone withdrawal therapy with Flutamide for 5 days as well as Enantone every 4 weeks. The patient stayed 28 days in hospital.

3. Discussion

The presence of subcutaneous emphysema caused by the perforation of an abdominal organ is quite rare, so that misdiagnosis of this condition is presumably quite higher [1]. Nevertheless, in the presence of free air the physician should keep the possibility of an abdominal cause in mind [2]. The classic gas gangrene is an acute illness with devastating outcome. Due to the high mortality rate early diagnosis is essential [3] and requires immediate radical therapy of the soft tissue infection as well as searching of the tumor [4]. The diagnostic standards include the medical history, the physical examination, X-ray to detect free air, and laboratory investigations. The determination of the procalcitonin might be helpful. Usually the physician can find small wounds which serve as the entry portal for the organisms. In most cases the medical history is pathbreaking. What makes our case quite rare is that despite the advanced finding the patient was asymptomatic over a long period of time and the disease was unidentified. Due to the pronounced findings only a palliative care was possible. Four months after admission the patient underwent X-rays of the left leg and of the pelvis after a fall to exclude a fracture. There was no free air in the soft tissue detectible anymore (Figure 8).

Reference Values

CRP < 5 mg/L

Leukocytes 4–11 × $10^3/\mu$L

Procalcitonin 0,05–0,5 ng/mL

Prostate specific antigen < 4 ng/mL.

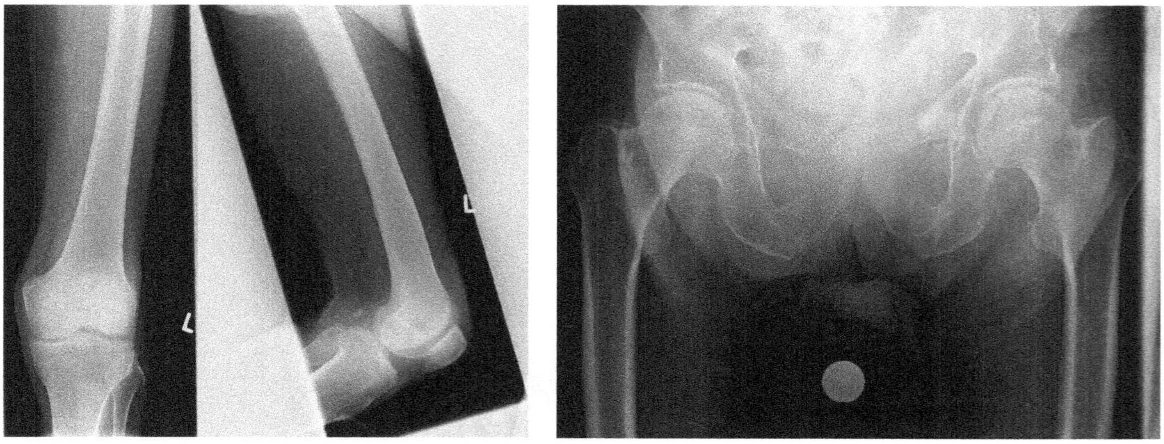

(a) (b)

FIGURE 8: X rays of the left proximal lower leg as well of the pelvis 4 months after admission.

Competing Interests

The authors declare that they have no competing interests.

References

[1] G. G. Hallock, "Delayed antemortem diagnosis of adenocarcinoma of the cecum presenting as lower extremity gas gangrene," *Diseases of the Colon & Rectum*, vol. 27, no. 2, pp. 131–133, 1984.

[2] K.-B. Lee, E.-S. Moon, S.-T. Jung, and H.-Y. Seo, "Subcutaneous emphysema mimicking gas gangrene following perforation of the rectum: a case report," *Journal of Korean Medical Science*, vol. 19, no. 5, pp. 756–758, 2004.

[3] T. A. Fox Jr., J. Gomez, and J. Bravo, "Subcutaneous emphysema of the lower extremity of gastrointestinal origin," *Diseases of the Colon & Rectum*, vol. 21, no. 5, pp. 357–360, 1978.

[4] O. Assadin, A. Assadin, C. Senekowitsch, A. Makristhathis, and G. Hagmüller, "Gasbrand durch Clostridium perfringens in zwei intravenös Drogenabhängigen in Wien," *Wiener Klinische Wochenschrift*, vol. 7-8, pp. 264–267, 2004.

31

Cartilage Delamination Flap Mimicking a Torn Medial Meniscus

Gan Zhi-Wei Jonathan, Hamid Rahmatullah Bin Abd Razak, and Mitra Amit Kanta

Singapore General Hospital, Outram Road, Singapore 169608

Correspondence should be addressed to Gan Zhi-Wei Jonathan; j.ganzw@gmail.com

Academic Editor: John Nyland

We report a case of a chondral delamination lesion due to medial parapatellar plica friction syndrome involving the medial femoral condyle. This mimicked a torn medial meniscus in clinical and radiological presentation. Arthroscopy revealed a chondral delamination flap, which was debrided. Diagnosis of chondral lesions in the knee can be challenging. Clinical examination and MRI have good accuracy for diagnosis and should be used in tandem. Early diagnosis and treatment of chondral lesions are important to prevent progression to early osteoarthritis.

1. Introduction

We report a case of a chondral delamination lesion due to medial parapatellar plica friction syndrome involving the medial femoral condyle. This mimicked a torn medial meniscus in clinical and radiological presentation.

2. Case Report

A 39-year-old gentleman presented to us in clinic with a primary complaint of right knee pain for 3 years, on a background history of previous right medial meniscus tear 3 years priorly. The pain was localized to the posteromedial aspect of the knee and was worse when squatting, kneeling, or walking down the stairs. His regular sporting activities involved cycling, which did not cause significant discomfort. There was no history of specific injury or trauma to the knee and no effusion. He reported crepitus from the knee. He had no previous operations of the knee.

On examination, the posterior one-third of the medial joint line was tender. No synovial swelling or effusion was detected. There was a palpable click when performing the patella grinding test, suggestive of injury to the patella or a medial parapatellar plica. The range of motion of the knee was normal.

The patient reported having a previous magnetic resonance imaging (MRI) scan of the right knee approximately 3 years and 9 months prior to the consult, which showed an intrasubstance medial meniscus tear. The pain had been constant since then.

A repeat MRI scan of the knee was performed (using a GE Healthcare Optima MR430s 1.5T machine). The following sequences were performed and reviewed: Proton Density (PD) sequences in coronal, sagittal, and axial cuts, Proton Density (PD) Fast Spin Echo (FSE) sequence in coronal cuts, and T2-weighted Fast Spin Echo (FSE) with fat suppression (FS) in sagittal cuts. The scan was reported as showing a horizontal tear of the posterior horn of the medial meniscus with superior articular surface contact, extending into the posterior root attachment (Figures 3 and 4). The anterior cruciate ligament was intact.

The patient underwent arthroscopy for treatment of the symptoms. During arthroscopy, a stiff medial parapatellar plica was noted, which was contacting and impinging on the medial femoral condyle (MFC) during knee flexion (Figures 5 and 6). Outerbridge grade 3 changes were noted of the cartilage in this area. A 2 × 2 cm cartilage flap was noted, attached anteriorly to the MFC (Figures 3 and 4). The flap was circular, approximately 2-3 mm thick, and attached along its anterior third to the anterior part of the medial femoral condyle (Figure 1). Its posterior two-thirds were free. There was no medial meniscus tear. Although not reported as showing a thickened medial parapatellar plica, review of the MRI showed a prominent medial parapatellar plica (Figure 2).

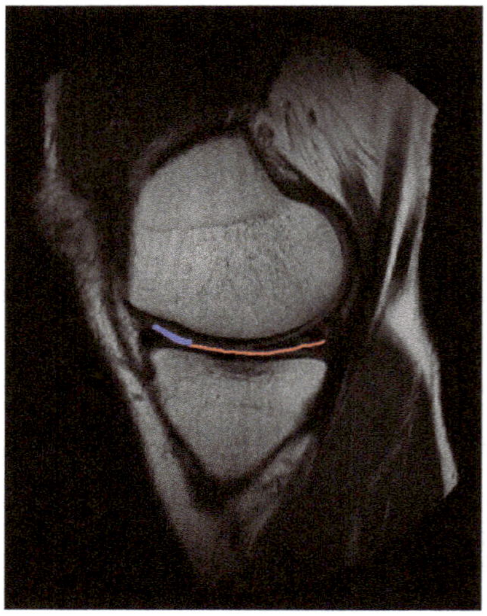

FIGURE 1: Cartilage flap indicated by red and blue line. The red line indicates the unattached, posterior two-thirds of the flap, and the blue line indicates the attached anterior third of the flap.

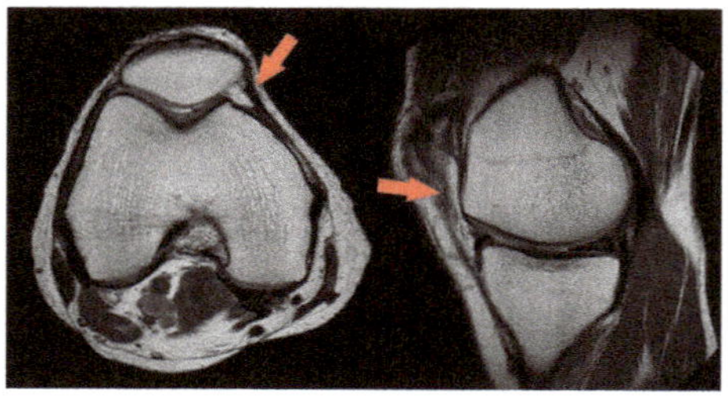

FIGURE 2: Prominent medial parapatellar plica indicated by arrowheads.

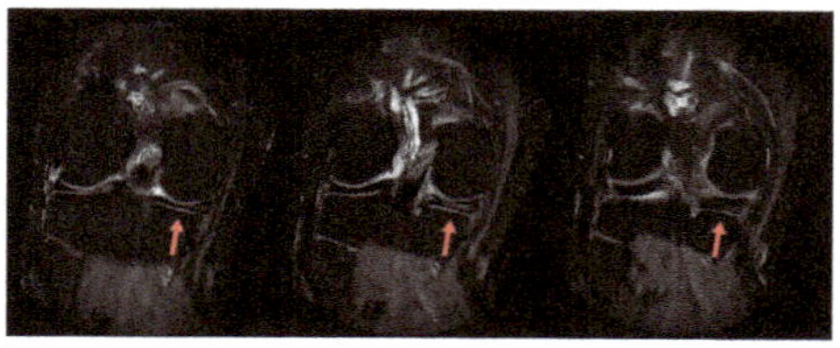

FIGURE 3: Coronal Proton Density (PD) fat suppression (FS) magnetic resonance imaging showing the chondral flap with an appearance similar to that of a torn medial meniscus (arrow). No underlying bone edema is seen.

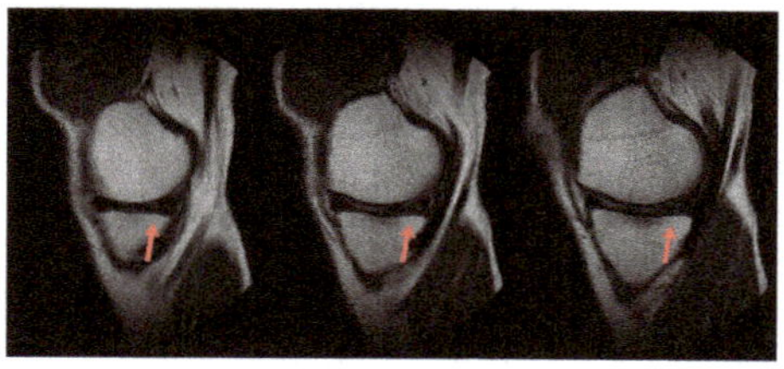

FIGURE 4: Sagittal Proton Density (PD) magnetic resonance imaging showing the chondral flap (arrow). It appears flap-like and is attached at its anterior aspect.

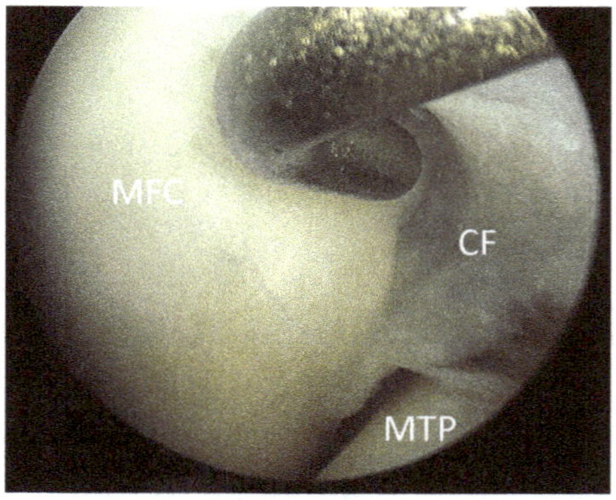

FIGURE 5: Arthroscopic view of the chondral flap. MFC: medial femoral condyle. CF: chondral flap. MTP: medial tibial plateau.

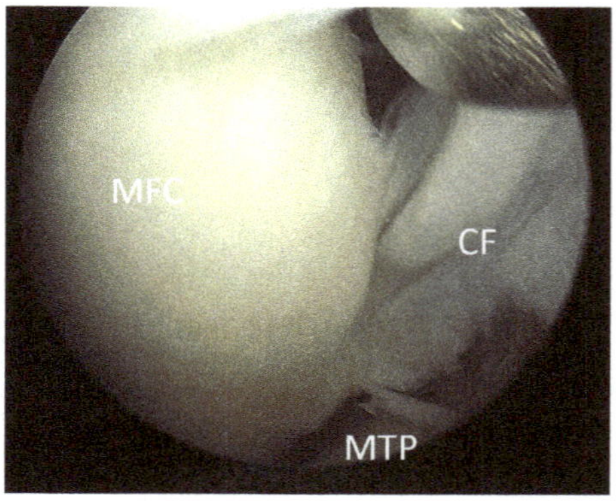

FIGURE 6: Arthroscopic view of the chondral flap. MFC: medial femoral condyle. CF: chondral flap. MTP: medial tibial plateau.

The lesion was debrided using a shaver until the remaining cartilage was stable with no loose edges. The cartilage underlying the flap showed Outerbridge grade 3 changes. The medial parapatellar plica was debrided, and no further impingement was noted during subsequent flexion/extension.

The patient's symptoms greatly improved after the operation. He was discharged the day after the operation, attended outpatient physiotherapy, and was able to resume normal work and activities after 2 week. He was sent for physiotherapy. During review at 3 months postoperatively, he was noted to have residual anterior knee pain, with some pain when squatting. Subsequently, during review 7 months after operation, the knee pain had resolved, with minimal pain when squatting, and he noted that his knee felt normal and he had recovered his strength. Knee examination was unremarkable.

3. Discussion

3.1. Common Clinical Presentation of Meniscal and Articular Cartilage Injuries. Meniscal injuries may present with pain, locking, catching, giving way, or pain when kneeling or squatting. Clinically, an effusion may be present. The Thessaly test, Mcmurray's test, and Apley's test may be positive, and joint line tenderness may be present. However, these tests have limited diagnostic accuracy [1–3], and further investigations are often required, such as magnetic resonance imaging (MRI) studies.

Articular cartilage injuries may present with pain, swelling, and locking. A history of injury, such as that of acute trauma, or twisting, may be present [4, 5]. Symptoms mimic a meniscal tear [6], and diagnosis may be challenging.

Parapatellar plica syndrome may present as anterior knee pain after prolonged sitting or when using the stairs. Retropatellar pain or medial knee pain may also be present. Other nonspecific symptoms such as intermittent clicking or locking or swelling may also occur [7]. A symptomatic medial parapatellar plica may be palpable on examination, especially if significantly thickened. During knee flexion between 30° and 60°, a snap or pop may be present. Palpation may also reveal retropatellar pain, clicking, or crepitations [8].

3.2. Structure of Cartilage. The structure of articular hyaline cartilage can be said to contain two large zones, a calcified and noncalcified zone. The noncalcified zone may be further subdivided into a superficial zone of thickness, in which collagen fibres are arranged parallel to the surface and offer good resistance to shear force, a transitional zone, in which collagen fibres run obliquely, and a deep zone, where collagen fibres are oriented perpendicularly to the surface and resist compression well. The calcified zone of cartilage contains cartilage fibres, anchored by hydroxyapatite crystals to the subchondral bone. The junction between the calcified and noncalcified zone is the tidemark [4, 9].

3.3. Clinical Presentation and Investigation of Injury. Partial-thickness separation or delamination injuries of articular cartilage similar to the one observed in our case (with the formation of a cartilage flap attached at one edge) have previously been described in the literature [5, 10, 11]. The delamination typically occurs at the tidemark, with the calcified zone of cartilage remaining attached to the subchondral bone.

The cartilage delamination in our patient was likely due to repeated injury and impingement from the stiff medial parapatellar plica; increasing Young's modulus of the plica is associated with greater contact pressures on the underlying cartilage [12]. Synovial plicae may cause injuries to the underlying cartilage through a combination of compression, friction, and shear forces [13] and are associated with an increase in underlying articular cartilage lesions when present in a joint [7, 14, 15].

In our case, the history and physical examination suggested a meniscal tear. The previous MRI scan findings of a torn medial meniscus in the context of pain since the time of diagnosis pointed to a torn medial meniscus as the cause of pain. This appeared to be borne out by the current MRI, which showed what we expected to see: a tear of the posterior horn of the medial meniscus.

History and clinical examination are an important step in the diagnosis of knee injuries. On its own, clinical examination can diagnose meniscal lesions with significant accuracy. Mohan et al. reported diagnostic accuracy of 88% for medial meniscus injuries and 92% for lateral meniscus injuries when compared to arthroscopy [16].

Clinical examination for meniscal injury has diagnostic accuracy similar to that of MRI [17–19] and when performed by an experienced surgeon may even surpass MRI [20]. Although other authors have noted less success (Sharma et al. found clinical accuracy of 73–78% compared to MRI accuracy of 92–95%, [21]); on the whole the accuracy of clinical examination remains high and should not be neglected in favour of MRI.

MRI is a good choice of imaging modality and has good sensitivity and specificity for diagnosis of meniscus tears. Sensitivities and specificities of over 80% have been described for detection of meniscal tears when compared with arthroscopy as a gold standard [22–24].

In contrast, MRI sensitivity for detection of articular cartilage injury is significantly lower than that for meniscal injury. A meta-analysis by Zhang et al. in 2013 found that sensitivity for detection of chondral injury was 75% (62%–84%) and overall specificity was 94% (89%–97%).

MRI features of chondral delamination after acute injury were described by Kendell et al. [25], who reported that all 5 of their cases showed increased T2-weighted (fast spin-echo) signal in subchondral bone underlying the cartilage injury, indicating oedema. Other authors have also described similar findings [26, 27].

It can be difficult to determine the exact Outerbridge grade of the chondral lesion on MRI. In addition, MRI has higher sensitivity for more severe lesions (Outerbridge grades 3 and 4), with a progressive decrease in sensitivity with lower Outerbridge grades [28]. Low-grade early lesions of the articular cartilage are less likely to be detected.

In our case, atypically, there was minimal subchondral oedema underlying the chondral flap, possibly due to a long interval between injury and diagnosis and the mechanism of injury. The mechanism of injury was likely to have been nontraumatic in nature or as a result of repetitive microtrauma (i.e., friction and/or shear force resulting from medial plica syndrome) rather than a typical cause of chondral injury (such as acute trauma or twisting injury). These factors might have contributed to the unusual features of the lesion.

Location of the lesion in the posterior aspect of the knee may have been another contributing factor. Imaging at or around the posterior meniscal horn can be challenging. Sharifah et al. described significantly lower sensitivities when the meniscal tears were located in the posterior horn [22]. In the same vein, Naranje et al. reviewed the accuracy of MRI for diagnosis of meniscal lesions [23]. Four out of 6 of their false-positive meniscal tears were in the posterior horn, which the authors felt could have been related to complex anatomy in this area.

MRI is a useful tool for diagnosis of plicae in the knee. Nakanishi et al. found the sensitivity of MRI (when compared to arthroscopy) to be 93.1% and specificity to be 81.8% [29]. Plicae have low intensity on T1-weighted and T2-weighted MR sequences. Presence of a knee effusion may improve visualization of plicae on MR imaging sequences [30].

3.4. Areas for Improvement of Diagnostic Accuracy with Magnetic Resonance Imaging: Magnet Strength. Identification and characterization of lesions may improve with use of a 3T magnet instead of a 1.5T magnet. The MRI in our study used a 1.5T magnet. Van dyck and Kenis et al. showed that sensitivity of detection of all grades of cartilage lesions in the knee joint improved with use of a 3T magnet [31].

3.5. Areas for Improvement of Diagnostic Accuracy with Magnetic Resonance Imaging: Use of Specific Sequences. Use of specific MR imaging sequences may improve diagnosis of articular cartilage lesions. Gustas et al. [32] reported in 2015 that use of a 3D FSE sequence with use of both radial and conventional reformatted images had improved sensitivity and similar specificity to use of 2D FSE sequences alone. Similarly, Kijowski et al. reported improvements in sensitivity with a small reduction in specificity with addition of a T2 mapping sequence when a 3T magnet was used [33]. Kohl et al. reported good results for Outerbridge grade III and IV lesions with a 3T magnet and 3D-DESS cartilage specific sequences [28].

3.6. Importance of Early Recognition of Articular Cartilage Injury. Early diagnosis of injury to the articular cartilage is important, because undiagnosed lesions represent an opportunity for further cartilage injury and early osteoarthritis. In particular, lesions larger than 9 mm result in increased pressure on the rims of the defects and will likely result in further chondrocyte insult and progression of cartilage injury [34]. The size of the defect in our case was approximately 20 mm by 20 mm and as such would likely see progressive worsening.

4. Conclusion

Pain from intra-articular knee injury may result from injury to various structures in the knee, including articular cartilage and menisci. Clinical presentation of chondral injury and meniscal injury may present similarly, and in some cases, accurate diagnosis may be challenging.

We recommend a focused history and clinical examination for complaints of knee pain, followed by magnetic resonance imaging with a 3T magnet if available, with relevant specific MR imaging sequences. Atypical cases such as ours are rare, but we should remain on high alert for chondral injury, as timely diagnosis and expeditious treatment may prevent worsening of defects and progression to early osteoarthritis.

Competing Interests

The authors declare that there is no conflict of interests regarding the publication of this paper.

Authors' Contributions

Hamid Rahmatullah Bin Abd Razak and Mitra Amit Kanta are contributing authors

References

[1] M. Blyth, I. Anthony, B. Francq et al., "Diagnostic accuracy of the thessaly test, standardised clinical history and other clinical examination tests (Apley's, mcmurray's and joint line tenderness) for meniscal tears in comparison with magnetic resonance imaging diagnosis," *Health Technology Assessment*, vol. 19, no. 62, pp. 5–61, 2015.

[2] S.-J. Kim, B.-Y. Hwang, D.-H. Choi, and Y. Mei, "The paradoxical McMurray test for the detection of meniscal tears: an arthroscopic study of mechanisms, types, and accuracy," *The Journal of Bone and Joint Surgery. American*, vol. 94, no. 16, pp. e1181–e1187, 2012.

[3] T. Moya, J. Javaloy, R. Montés-Micó, J. Beltrán, G. Muñoz, and R. Montalbán, "More than a decade of experience with implantable collamer lens," *Journal of Refractive Surgery*, vol. 31, no. 12, pp. 854–855, 2015.

[4] A. J. Sophia Fox, A. Bedi, and S. A. Rodeo, "The basic science of articular cartilage: structure, composition, and function," *Sports Health*, vol. 1, no. 6, pp. 461–468, 2009.

[5] C. Johnson-Nurse and D. J. Dandy, "Fracture-separation of articular cartilage in the adult knee," *The Journal of Bone & Joint Surgery—British Volume*, vol. 67, no. 1, pp. 42–43, 1985.

[6] J. S. Gilley, M. I. Gelman, D. M. Edson, and R. W. Metcalf, "Chondral fractures of the knee. Arthrographic, arthroscopic, and clinical manifestations," *Radiology*, vol. 138, no. 1, pp. 51–54, 1981.

[7] T. Vaughan-Lane and D. J. Dandy, "The synovial shelf syndrome," *The Journal of Bone & Joint Surgery—British Volume*, vol. 64, no. 4, pp. 475–476, 1982.

[8] O. S. Schindler, "'The Sneaky Plica' revisited: morphology, pathophysiology and treatment of synovial plicae of the knee," *Knee Surgery, Sports Traumatology, Arthroscopy*, vol. 22, no. 2, pp. 247–262, 2014.

[9] J. Mollenhauer and K. E. Kuettner, "Articular cartilage," in *Principles of Orthopaedic Practice*, R. Dee, L. C. Hurst, M. A. Gruber, and S. A. Kottmeier, Eds., McGraw Hill, New York, NY, USA, 2nd edition, 1997.

[10] A. S. Levy, J. Lohnes, S. Sculley, M. Lecroy, and W. Garrett, "Chondral delamination of the knee in soccer players," *The American Journal of Sports Medicine*, vol. 24, no. 5, pp. 634–639, 1996.

[11] W. J. Hopkinson, W. A. Mitchell, and W. W. Curl, "Chondral fractures of the knee. Cause for confusion," *American Journal of Sports Medicine*, vol. 13, no. 5, pp. 309–312, 1985.

[12] D. S. Liu, Z. W. Zhuang, and S. R. Lyu, "Relationship between medial plica and medial femoral condyle—a three-dimensional dynamic finite element model," *Clinical Biomechanics*, vol. 28, no. 9-10, pp. 1000–1005, 2013.

[13] M. Ozcan, C. Copuroğlu, M. Ciftdemir, F. N. Turan, and O. U. Calpur, "Does an abnormal infrapatellar plica increase the risk of chondral damage in the knee," *Knee Surgery, Sports Traumatology, Arthroscopy*, vol. 19, no. 2, pp. 218–221, 2011.

[14] J. J. Christoforakis, J. Sanchez-Ballester, N. Hunt, R. Thomas, and R. K. Strachan, "Synovial shelves of the knee: association with chondral lesions," *Knee Surgery, Sports Traumatology, Arthroscopy*, vol. 14, no. 12, pp. 1292–1298, 2006.

[15] S.-R. Lyu and C.-C. Hsu, "Medial plicae and degeneration of the medial femoral condyle," *Arthroscopy*, vol. 22, no. 1, pp. 17–26, 2006.

[16] B. R. Mohan and H. S. Gosal, "Reliability of clinical diagnosis in meniscal tears," *International Orthopaedics*, vol. 31, no. 1, pp. 57–60, 2007.

[17] T. Sladjan, V. Zoran, and B. Zoran, "Correlation of clinical examination, ultrasound sonography, and magnetic resonance imaging findings with arthroscopic findings in relation to acute and chronic lateral meniscus injuries," *Journal of Orthopaedic Science*, vol. 19, no. 1, pp. 71–76, 2014.

[18] F. Rayan, S. Bhonsle, and D. D. Shukla, "Clinical, MRI, and arthroscopic correlation in meniscal and anterior cruciate ligament injuries," *International Orthopaedics*, vol. 33, no. 1, pp. 129–132, 2009.

[19] A. M. Navali, M. Bazavar, M. A. Mohseni, B. Safari, and A. Tabrizi, "Arthroscopic evaluation of the accuracy of clinical examination versus MRI in diagnosing meniscus tears and cruciate ligament ruptures," *Archives of Iranian Medicine*, vol. 16, no. 4, pp. 229–232, 2013.

[20] E. Ercin, I. Kaya, I. Sungur, E. Demirbas, A. A. Ugras, and E. M. Cetinus, "History, clinical findings, magnetic resonance imaging, and arthroscopic correlation in meniscal lesions," *Knee Surgery, Sports Traumatology, Arthroscopy*, vol. 20, no. 5, pp. 851–856, 2012.

[21] U. K. Sharma, B. K. Shrestha, S. Rijal et al., "Clinical, MRI and arthroscopic correlation in internal derangement of knee," *Kathmandu University Medical Journal*, vol. 9, no. 35, pp. 174–178, 2011.

[22] M. I. A. Sharifah, C. L. Lee, A. Suraya, A. Johan, A. F. S. K. Syed, and S. P. Tan, "Accuracy of MRI in the diagnosis of meniscal tears in patients with chronic ACL tears," *Knee Surgery, Sports Traumatology, Arthroscopy*, vol. 23, no. 3, pp. 826–830, 2015.

[23] S. Naranje, R. Mittal, H. Nag, and R. Sharma, "Arthroscopic and magnetic resonance imaging evaluation of meniscus lesions in the chronic anterior cruciate ligament-deficient knee," *Arthroscopy*, vol. 24, no. 9, pp. 1045–1051, 2008.

[24] M. K. Gupta, M. K. Rauniyar, N. K. Karn, P. L. Sah, K. Dhungel, and K. Ahmad, "MRI evaluation of knee injury with arthroscopic correlation," *Journal of Nepal Health Research Council*, vol. 12, no. 26, pp. 63–67, 2014.

[25] S. D. Kendell, C. A. Helms, J. W. Rampton, W. E. Garrett, and L. D. Higgins, "MRI appearance of chondral delamination injuries of the knee," *American Journal of Roentgenology*, vol. 184, no. 5, pp. 1486–1489, 2005.

[26] D. A. Rubin, "Magnetic resonance imaging of chondral and osteochondral injuries," *Topics in Magnetic Resonance Imaging*, vol. 9, no. 6, pp. 348–359, 1998.

[27] D. A. Rubin, C. D. Harner, and J. M. Costello, "Treatable chondral injuries in the knee: frequency of associated focal subchondral edema," *American Journal of Roentgenology*, vol. 174, no. 4, pp. 1099–1106, 2000.

[28] S. Kohl, S. Meier, S. S. Ahmad et al., "Accuracy of cartilage-specific 3-Tesla 3D-DESS magnetic resonance imaging in the diagnosis of chondral lesions: comparison with knee arthroscopy," *Journal of Orthopaedic Surgery and Research*, vol. 10, no. 1, article 191, 2015.

[29] K. Nakanishi, M. Inoue, T. Ishida et al., "MR evaluation of mediopatellar plica," *Acta Radiologica*, vol. 37, no. 4, pp. 567–571, 1996.

[30] R. García-Valtuille, F. Abascal, L. Cerezal et al., "Anatomy and MR imaging appearances of synovial plicae of the knee," *Radiographics*, vol. 22, no. 4, pp. 775–784, 2002.

[31] P. Van Dyck, C. Kenis, F. M. Vanhoenacker et al., "Comparison of 1.5- and 3-T MR imaging for evaluating the articular cartilage of the knee," *Knee Surgery, Sports Traumatology, Arthroscopy*, vol. 22, no. 6, pp. 1376–1384, 2014.

[32] C. N. Gustas, D. G. Blankenbaker, A. M. Del Rio, C. S. Winalski, and R. Kijowski, "Evaluation of the articular cartilage of the knee joint using an isotropic resolution 3D fast spin-echo sequence with conventional and radial reformatted images," *American Journal of Roentgenology*, vol. 205, no. 2, pp. 371–379, 2015.

[33] R. Kijowski, D. G. Blankenbaker, A. Munoz del Rio, G. S. Baer, and B. K. Graf, "Evaluation of the articular cartilage of the knee joint: value of adding a T2 mapping sequence to a routine mr imaging protocol," *Radiology*, vol. 267, no. 2, pp. 503–513, 2013.

[34] G. Papaioannou, C. K. Demetropoulos, and Y. H. King, "Predicting the effects of knee focal articular surface injury with a patient-specific finite element model," *The Knee*, vol. 17, pp. 61–68, 2010.

32

A Case of Bilateral Permanent Subluxation of the Lateral Meniscus

Jun Suganuma, Tadashi Sugiki, and Yutaka Inoue

Department of Orthopaedic Surgery, Hiratsuka City Hospital, 1-19-1 Minamihara, Hiratsuka, Kanagawa 254-0065, Japan

Correspondence should be addressed to Jun Suganuma; junsugar@wa2.so-net.ne.jp

Academic Editor: John Nyland

We report a case of bilateral, permanent subluxation of the lateral meniscus. To our knowledge, the present case is the first reported description of bilateral irreducible anterior dislocation of the posterior segment of the lateral meniscus. This disorder is characterized by a flipped meniscus sign of the lateral meniscus on sagittal magnetic resonance images of the knee joint, with no history of trauma or locking symptoms. A detailed examination of serial magnetic resonance images of the lateral meniscus can help differentiate this condition from malformation of the lateral meniscus, that is, a double-layered meniscus. We recommend two-stage treatment for this disorder. First, the knee joint is kept in straight position for 3 weeks after the lateral meniscus is reduced to the normal position. Second, if subluxation of the lateral meniscus recurs, meniscocapsular suture is then performed. Although subluxation of the lateral meniscus without locking symptoms is rare, it is important to be familiar with this condition to diagnose and treat it correctly.

1. Introduction

We present a case in which the bilateral posterior segments of the lateral menisci were dislocated anteriorly and irreducibly. To our knowledge, this is the first reported description of permanent subluxation of the lateral menisci. However, there is a previously reported case of bilateral malformation of the lateral menisci, in which the pathological characteristics resemble those of the current case [1]. The aim of this report is to differentiate permanent subluxation of the lateral meniscus from meniscal malformation, especially the double-layered lateral meniscus [2], and recommend a treatment for this pathology.

2. Case Report

This case report was approved by the Institutional Review Board of our hospital. A 37-year-old housewife was referred to our knee joint clinic in January 2011 with a complaint of bilateral knee pain. In August 2010, she had been practicing a dance that involved hopping alternately on her right and left legs when she suddenly experienced severe pain in her right knee joint. She was unable to move her knee joint or walk. Before the incident, she had not engaged in athletic activities or experienced any problems with her knee joints. She consulted an orthopaedist, had a radiograph taken, and was diagnosed as having no serious problems. However, the pain and swelling of the right knee joint persisted, despite treatment with ointment and analgesics. In December 2010, she started suffering from slight left knee pain during daily activity.

The clinical examination revealed slight swelling, quadriceps muscle atrophy, and pain during the McMurray test manoeuvre for the lateral meniscus in the right knee joint; there were no other abnormal findings. The range of motion of both knee joints was 0 to 155°. Laboratory examination showed no abnormalities. On anteroposterior radiographs of both knee joints, a suspicious osteophyte was seen on the lateral tibial plateau (LTP) (Grade 1 according to the Kellgren-Lawrence grading system). On coronal views from magnetic resonance images (MRI) of both knee joints, the posterior segment of the lateral meniscus was seen in the intercondylar space, and there was only a small space for the lateral meniscus in its normal location between the articular surfaces of the lateral femoral condyle (LFC) and the LTP (Figure 1(a)). On sagittal views, a dislocated meniscus was

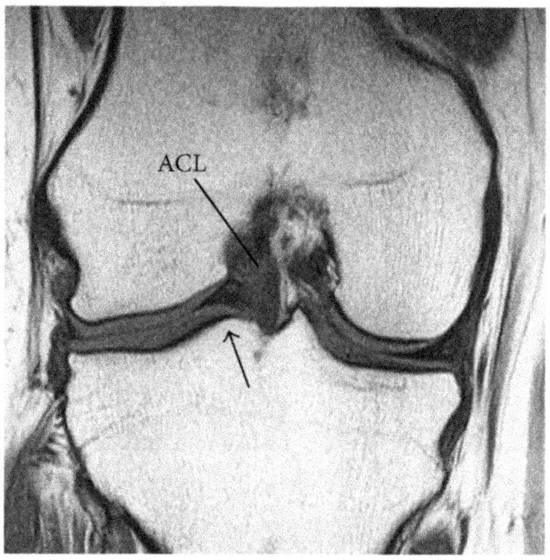

(a)

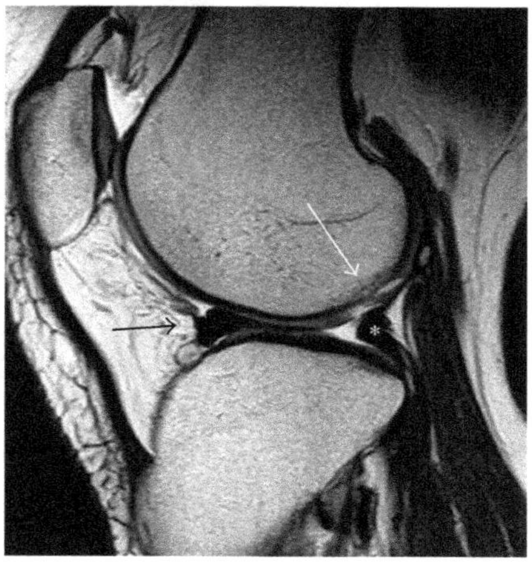

(b)

FIGURE 1: Magnetic resonance imaging of the right knee joint. (a) T1-weighted coronal image showing the posterior segment of the lateral meniscus dislocated into the intercondylar space. The arrow indicates the dislocated posterior segment, which is adjacent to the anterior cruciate ligament (ACL). (b) T2-weighted sagittal image of the lateral compartment depicting the middle segment of the lateral meniscus flipped onto the anterior segment, producing the flipped meniscus sign (black arrow). The popliteus tendon is located on the tibial plateau (asterisk) and displays a similar appearance to the posterior segment of the lateral meniscus. The white arrow indicates an osteochondral defect on the lateral femoral condyle.

seen on the anterior segment of the lateral meniscus, depicting the flipped meniscus sign (Figure 1(b)) [3]. The popliteus tendon ran from the LFC into the articular space between the LFC and LTP instead of running distally around the LFC and LTP. Consequently, the popliteus tendon initially looked like the posterior segment of the lateral meniscus, although the popliteus tendon was not located on the articular surfaces as closely as the posterior segment of the lateral meniscus normally is. An osteochondral defect was detected on the LFC in the right knee joint.

Arthroscopy of both knee joints was performed through anteromedial and anterolateral portals using a 30° angled arthroscope in February 2011. On arthroscopic examination of the right knee joint, the middle segment of the lateral meniscus was dislocated anteriorly on the anterior segment of the lateral meniscus (Figure 2(a)), and the posterior segment was located in the intercondylar space adjacent to the anterior cruciate ligament. An oval osteochondral defect (International Cartilage Repair Society (ICRS) Grade 4) measuring about 15 × 20 mm was detected on the LFC (Figure 2(b)). As the dislocated meniscus had adhered to tissue inside the intercondylar space, it could not be reduced to its normal position using a probe, although some of the dislocated part was barely reduced to the centre of the LTP. The popliteus tendon was running on the articular surface of the LTP and had a similar appearance to the posterior segment of the lateral meniscus (Figure 2(c)). There was a fibrous band connecting the popliteus tendon to the dislocated posterior horn of the lateral meniscus. The articular cartilage of the LTP was slightly frayed (ICRS Grade 2). There were no abnormal findings in the medial or patellofemoral compartments or in the cruciate ligaments. The arthroscopic findings of the left knee joint were almost identical to those of the right knee joint, except for the osteochondral defect of the LFC in the right knee joint.

The patient has not requested any further surgical treatment after symptoms in bilateral knee joints were alleviated with rehabilitation.

3. Discussion

The pathoanatomic features of this case are similar to those in recurrent subluxation of the lateral meniscus (RSLM) [4]. In most cases of RSLM, the first locking symptoms occur with severe pain when patients extend their knee joint from deep flexion [4–6]; the youngest reported age at which the first locking symptoms have occurred is 6 years [4]. Both disorders show subluxation of the lateral meniscus without tears or anomalies. The only difference between RSLM and this case is that the lateral meniscus is subluxated repeatedly in the former [4, 6], while the subluxated lateral meniscus cannot be reduced in the latter. Therefore, we have named this disorder permanent subluxation of the lateral meniscus (PSLM).

The cause of dislocation of the posterior segment of the lateral meniscus without tears or anomalies or instability of the knee joint has yet to be elucidated. However, the onset of locking symptoms seems to be related to several factors, including insufficiency of the popliteomeniscal fascicles [7] and internal rotation of the knee joint [4]. The developmental mechanism of PSLM seems to be even more complicated and appears to be related to both congenital and environmental factors, as the dislocated lateral meniscus needs to be adhered to the surrounding tissue.

As the present case involved irreducible anterior dislocation of the posterior segment of the lateral menisci in

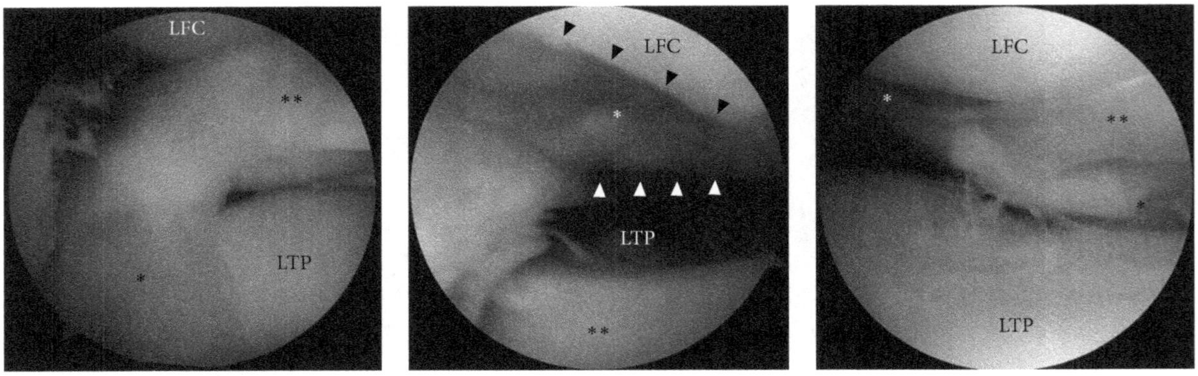

(a) (b) (c)

FIGURE 2: Arthroscopic findings of the right knee joint. (a) The anteriorly dislocated middle segment of the lateral meniscus (double asterisks). The asterisk indicates the anterior horn of the lateral meniscus, which is located in the normal position. (b) An osteochondral defect (asterisk) on the lateral femoral condyle (LFC). The black arrowheads indicate the anterior margin of the defect, and the white arrowheads indicate the posterior margin. The double asterisks indicate the anteriorly dislocated middle segment of the lateral meniscus. (c) The popliteus tendon (white asterisk) originating from the LFC, running on the articular surface of the lateral tibial plateau (LTP), and continuing to the popliteus muscle (black asterisk). A fibrous band (double asterisks) connects the popliteus tendon to the dislocated posterior horn of the lateral meniscus.

bilateral knee joints without history of evident trauma or locking symptoms, these subluxations must have occurred in an early stage of the patient's life. In embryological studies of the human knee joint, knee extension decreases gradually from 33 weeks owing to the lack of space in the uterus, and the knee joints are kept in a deeply flexed position from 38 weeks [8]. Therefore, late gestation can be a vulnerable period for the lateral menisci of foetuses because locking symptoms of RSLM usually occur related to deep flexion of the knee joint [4–6]. It seems that anterior dislocation of the posterior segment of the lateral meniscus can occur when risk factors such as insufficiency of the popliteomeniscal fascicles and internal rotation of the knee joint are present; this dislocation could lead to irreducible subluxation of the lateral meniscus if the dislocated meniscus is not reduced spontaneously during extension of the knee joint.

There is a previously reported case in which the pathological characteristics had a distinct resemblance to the present case. Fujikawa et al. reported the case of a 37-year-old man with bilateral lateral meniscal malformation consisting of a duplicated anterior horn and the absence of the lateral portion of the menisci [1]. They did not think that the condition was caused by a displaced bucket-handle tear, because they could not move the duplicated smooth-surfaced menisci. They also did not observe mobile unstable fragments or a ragged free margin, which are expected in displaced bucket-handle tears. The significant difference between the previous case and our present case is that their case involved marked osteoarthritic changes in the LFC on the MRI; this osteoarthritis was probably due to the higher level of activity of their patient.

There have been multiple reports on meniscal malformations, which are categorized into three groups: hyperplastic (discoid, double-layered [2], abnormal band [9], accessory [10], and ring-shaped [11]), hypoplastic (absence [12], partial deficiency [13], and separation [14]), and insertional anomalies. It does not seem difficult to differentiate PSLM from meniscal malformations, because PSLM does not involve any malformation. However, PSLM can be seen as a combination of two malformations: double-layered and partially deficient meniscus. A meniscus whose posterior segment is dislocated anteriorly can look like a double-layered anterior horn. Furthermore, the popliteus tendon in PSLM looks like the posterior segment of the lateral meniscus, as the popliteus tendon runs on the articular surface of the LTP. Consequently, only the middle segment of the lateral meniscus might look deficient. However, a detailed examination of serial MRI of the lateral meniscus and the popliteus tendon reveals that there is neither duplication nor deficiency in the lateral meniscus, and the structure that appears to be the posterior segment of the lateral meniscus is actually the popliteus tendon. Arthroscopy revealed a fibrous band that connected the popliteus tendon to the posterior horn of the lateral meniscus (Figure 2(c)). As the posterior horn of the lateral meniscus was dislocated anteriorly, the popliteus tendon might be pulled anteriorly onto the articular surface of the LTP by the fibrous band, which was considered to be the posteroinferior (or third) popliteomeniscal fascicle [15, 16].

The reason why we did not perform any interventions for the subluxated lateral menisci during arthroscopic examination is that the patient declined intensive treatment, because she was busy with child rearing and her job at that time. However, if the patient had wanted to undergo thorough treatment, we would have released the adhesion between the lateral meniscus and tissue inside the intercondylar space and reduced the subluxated meniscus to the normal position after making sure that the size of the lateral meniscus is large enough. Based on our experience with other patients in whom the lateral meniscus had been kept subluxated for more than 1 month and had then been reduced to the normal position arthroscopically, such a meniscus is liable to undergo redislocation to the same position during even slight flexion of the knee joint. To break this predisposition, we recommend two-stage treatment. First, the knee joint is kept in a straight position with a plaster cast for 3 weeks after reduction of the lateral meniscus to the normal position. The patient is then encouraged to walk with full weight bearing on the knee joint after the correct position of the lateral meniscus is verified on MRI. Reposition of the posterior segment of the lateral meniscus can push the popliteus tendon off the LTP to the normal position, which makes meniscocapsular suture [5, 6] possible. Active flexion exercise of the knee joint is started after the plaster cast is removed. Second, if subluxation of the lateral meniscus recurs, immediate repositioning of the meniscus and meniscocapsular suture, which would be much easier compared to at first repositioning of the meniscus, are performed simultaneously.

As PSLM seems to remain clinically silent until the occurrence of an osteochondral fracture or osteoarthritis caused by the loss of meniscal function, there would be little chance of detecting PSLM while patients are young. However, if a flipped meniscus sign of the lateral meniscus is detected on MRI in a knee joint without a history of trauma or locking symptoms, PSLM should be considered.

4. Conclusion

Permanent subluxation of the lateral meniscus without tears or anomalies or a history of locking symptoms is a rare disorder. We recommend two-stage treatment for this pathology. First, the knee joint is kept straight for 3 weeks after reduction of the lateral meniscus to the normal position. Second, if subluxation of the lateral meniscus subsequently recurs, meniscocapsular suture is performed. We believe that this may pose a challenge clinically and radiologically; hence, preliminary knowledge of this condition is important.

Competing Interests

The authors have no conflict of interests to declare.

References

[1] A. Fujikawa, H. Amma, Y. Ukegawa, T. Tamura, and Y. Naoi, "MR imaging of meniscal malformations of the knee mimicking displaced bucket-handle tear," *Skeletal Radiology*, vol. 31, no. 5, pp. 292–295, 2002.

[2] K. Takayama, R. Kuroda, T. Matsumoto et al., "Bilateral double-layered lateral meniscus: a report of two cases," *Knee Surgery, Sports Traumatology, Arthroscopy*, vol. 17, no. 11, pp. 1336–1339, 2009.

[3] N. Haramati, R. B. Staron, S. Rubin, E. H. Shreck, F. Feldman, and H. Kiernan, "The flipped meniscus sign," *Skeletal Radiology*, vol. 22, no. 4, pp. 273–277, 1993.

[4] J. Suganuma and T. Ohkoshi, "Association of internal rotation of the knee joint with recurrent subluxation of the lateral meniscus," *Arthroscopy*, vol. 27, no. 8, pp. 1071–e129, 2011.

[5] R. Garofalo, C. Kombot, O. Borens, A. Djahangiri, and E. Mouhsine, "Locking knee caused by subluxation of the posterior horn of the lateral meniscus," *Knee Surgery, Sports Traumatology, Arthroscopy*, vol. 13, no. 7, pp. 569–571, 2005.

[6] M. Kimura, K. Shirakura, A. Hasegawa, Y. Kobayashi, and E. Udagawa, "Anatomy and pathophysiology of the popliteal tendon area in the lateral meniscus: 2. Clinical investigation," *Arthroscopy*, vol. 8, no. 4, pp. 424–427, 1992.

[7] P. T. Simonian, P. S. Sussmann, M. van Trommel, T. L. Wickiewicz, and R. F. Warren, "Popliteomeniscal fasciculi and lateral meniscal stability," *The American Journal of Sports Medicine*, vol. 25, no. 6, pp. 849–853, 1997.

[8] K. Katz, R. Mashiach, A. Bar On, P. Merlob, M. Soudry, and I. Meizner, "Normal range of fetal knee movements," *Journal of Pediatric Orthopaedics*, vol. 19, no. 6, pp. 739–741, 1999.

[9] B. Giordano and J. Goldblatt, "Abnormal band of lateral meniscus," *Orthopedics*, vol. 32, no. 1, article 51, 2009.

[10] M. Karahan and B. Erol, "Accessory lateral meniscus: a case report," *American Journal of Sports Medicine*, vol. 32, no. 8, pp. 1973–1976, 2004.

[11] C. Esteves, R. Castro, R. Cadilha, F. Raposo, and L. Melão, "Ring-shaped lateral meniscus with hypoplasic anterior cruciate ligament," *Skeletal Radiology*, vol. 44, no. 12, pp. 1813–1818, 2015.

[12] V. T. Tolo, "Congenital absence of the menisci and cruciate ligaments of the knee: a case report," *The Journal of Bone & Joint Surgery—American Volume*, vol. 63, no. 6, pp. 1022–1024, 1981.

[13] O. Tetik, M. N. Doral, Ö. A. Atay, G. Leblebicioğlu, and S. Türker, "Partial deficiency of the lateral meniscus," *Arthroscopy*, vol. 19, no. 5, article E42, 2003.

[14] N. Komatsu, K. Yamamoto, and E. Chosa, "Bilateral congenital separation of the lateral meniscus: a case report," *Knee*, vol. 15, no. 4, pp. 330–332, 2008.

[15] A. J. Peduto, A. Nguyen, D. J. Trudell, and D. L. Resnick, "Popliteomeniscal fascicles: anatomic considerations using MR arthrography in cadavers," *American Journal of Roentgenology*, vol. 190, no. 2, pp. 442–448, 2008.

[16] G. C. Terry and R. F. LaPrade, "The posterolateral aspect of the knee. Anatomy and surgical approach," *The American Journal of Sports Medicine*, vol. 24, no. 6, pp. 732–739, 1996.

33

Latissimus Dorsi Tendon Transfer with GraftJacket® Augmentation to Increase Tendon Length for an Irreparable Rotator Cuff Tear

John G. Skedros[1,2,3] and Tanner R. Henrie[2]

[1]*Department of Orthopaedic Surgery, The University of Utah, Salt Lake City, UT, USA*
[2]*Utah Orthopaedic Specialists, Salt Lake City, UT, USA*
[3]*Intermountain Medical Center, Salt Lake City, UT, USA*

Correspondence should be addressed to John G. Skedros; jskedrosmd@uosmd.com

Academic Editor: Dimitrios S. Karataglis

Massive irreparable rotator cuff tears can be reconstructed with latissimus dorsi tendon transfers (LDTT). Although uncommon, the natural length of the latissimus dorsi tendon (LDT) could be insufficient for transfer even after adequate soft tissue releases. Descriptions of cases where grafts were needed to lengthen the LDT are therefore rare. We located only two reports of the use of an acellular dermal matrix to increase effective tendon length in tendon transfers about the shoulder: (1) GraftJacket patch for a pectoralis major tendon reconstruction and (2) ArthroFlex® patch for LDTT. Both of these brands of allograft patches are obtained from human cadavers. These products are usually used to cover soft tissue repairs and offer supplemental support rather than for increasing tendon length. Extending the LDTT with GraftJacket to achieve adequate length, to our knowledge, has not been reported in the literature. We report the case of a 50-year-old male who had a massive, irreparable left shoulder rotator cuff tear that was reconstructed with a LDTT. The natural length of his LDT was insufficient for transfer. This unexpected situation was rectified by sewing two patches of GraftJacket to the LDT. The patient had greatly improved shoulder function at two-year follow-up.

1. Introduction

Massive irreparable rotator cuff tears can be reconstructed with latissimus dorsi tendon transfers (LDTT) (Figures 1(a) and 1(b)). LDTT for irreparable rotator cuff tears was described nearly three decades ago and has since become a viable treatment option in these cases [1, 2]. LDTT is indicated in younger patients that lack significant glenohumeral arthritis [3]. Sometimes the teres major tendon is transferred in addition to the latissimus dorsi tendon (LDT) in order to obtain better external rotation of the shoulder [4, 5]. Additionally, removal of some humeral bone along with the LDT enables direct transosseous fixation of the LDTT, achieving higher integrity of the transfer [6, 7].

Preoperative active range of motion and sex are important predictors of outcome in LDTT (females have worse outcomes) [8]. Additionally, inadequate subscapularis and deltoid function and fatty infiltration of the teres minor can adversely affect the results of LDTT [8–10]. Additional challenges in LDTT include obtaining an adequate view to release the LDT and achieving sufficient length to reach the eventual attachment point [11, 12]. Adequate tendon length can be reliably achieved by releasing soft tissue attachments along the LDT at its muscle belly [11]. But it is known that the natural length of the LDT, even after adequate soft tissue releases, could be insufficient [11, 12]. A similar problem can occur during pectoralis major tendon reconstruction. In these cases, hamstring and patellar tendon-bone autografts and fascia lata and Achilles tendon allografts have been used to bridge the defect between the damaged muscle and its insertion point on the humerus [13]. Joseph et al. [14] describe the case of a pectoralis tendon rupture that was lengthened with an Achilles tendon allograft to provide additional length in order to repair the defect. The use of acellular dermal matrix allograft patches to extend rotator cuff tears that had insufficient length for repair is well described [15–17].

Descriptions of cases where grafts were needed to extend (i.e., lengthen) the LDT are rare, showing that this situation is very uncommon. For example, we only found one case where an acellular dermal matrix patch was used to increase the natural length of the LDT [12]. The patch used in that case was a 3 mm ArthroFlex patch (a brand of human acellular dermal matrix). This product is usually used to cover soft tissue repairs and offer supplemental support rather than for increasing their length [16, 18, 19].

Extending the LDTT with an alternative common acellular dermal matrix (GraftJacket) to achieve adequate length, to our knowledge, has not been reported in the literature. We report the case of a 50-year-old male who had a massive, irreparable left shoulder rotator cuff tear that was reconstructed with a LDTT. The main novel aspect of our case is that the patient's LDT was found to be inadequate during surgery. This unexpected situation was rectified by sewing two patches of GraftJacket to the free end of his LDT. This yielded greatly improved shoulder function at two-year follow-up.

2. Case Report

This left-hand-dominant 50-year-old male (weight: 112 kg; height: 185 cm; BMI: 33 kg/m^2) fell off of his porch on 31 August 2014 and sustained a massive rotator cuff tear (both the supraspinatus and infraspinatus were torn). The subscapularis and teres minor were deemed to be of good quality. Three months later, he had an attempt at repair, but the surgeon found the tendon tear irreparable. It was likely that the patient had a previous but smaller chronic rotator cuff tear from a sports-related injury many years previously. The patient understood that nothing other than a reverse total shoulder arthroplasty could be done to adequately restore shoulder function.

The patient came to our clinic one month after this unsuccessful attempt at repair. Physical examination at that time showed pseudoparalysis as exhibited by active forward flexion and abduction at 60–65° and superior-posterior shoulder subluxations (Table 1). We recommended a LDTT. If active range of motion was not achieved to his satisfaction but the graft healed, then he would likely achieve a tenodesis effect. This in turn would help reduce subluxations of his glenohumeral joint and thereby reduce pain while likely increasing active motion to a moderate amount [21].

The patient then had an arthroscopic evaluation followed by an open acromioplasty with partial repair of the torn infraspinatus and an open LDTT. The surgery was performed by JGS in accordance with the technique described by Dr. Iannotti and colleagues [8]. A superior approach to the rotator cuff was made by detaching the deltoid origin from the anterior aspect of the acromion and with splitting of the middle deltoid fibers for 3.5 cm. The coracoacromial ligament was released with the deltoid and reattached at the conclusion of the operation. The bursa was excised, and the rotator cuff was inspected. A second incision was made along the lateral border of the latissimus dorsi muscle, extending to the posterior axillary crease. The LDT insertion was identified with the arm abducted and internally rotated, and it was detached sharply from the humerus. The neurovascular pedicle was identified and protected, and the muscle was released from its deep fascia attachments. A number 2 nonabsorbable suture was passed with use of a Krakow suture technique along each side of the tendon from the musculotendinous junction to the end of the tendon (Figure 1(a)). Blunt dissection was performed to construct a tunnel deep to the deltoid and superficial to the posterior rotator cuff musculature.

In the conventional surgical technique, the latissimus dorsi muscle and tendon are routinely brought over the top of the humeral head and repaired anterior to the subscapularis, lateral to the greater tuberosity, and medial to the torn edges of the rotator cuff (Figure 1(b)). However, during surgery, our patient's LDT was found to be only 5 cm long, less than the mean LDT length reported by Goldberg et al. [22] (mean: 7.3 cm; range: 6.6–7.8 cm; SD: 0.38 cm) and nearly 5.5 cm shorter than what was needed for an adequate reconstruction. The patient was consented for use of an acellular dermal matrix graft (GraftJacket) but not for other allograft or autograft tissues. The anticipated use of GraftJacket was for augmentation at the repair site. However, GraftJacket has been mechanically tested and was found to be superior in strength to comparable xenografts and allografts (CuffPatch™, Restore, Permacol™, and TissueMend®) [23]. Additionally, an added layer of thickness from folding the GraftJacket allograft was deemed sufficiently strong to extend the length of the LDT.

Two 4 × 7 cm patches of GraftJacket were used to extend the LDT. The thickness of each patch was 2.0 mm (GraftJacket Maximum Force Extreme; Wright Medical Technologies, Inc.; http://documents.wright.com/Document/Get/010660). Each patch was folded in half along its short dimension, which resulted in 4 × 3.5 cm patches that were 4.0 mm thick each. The folded margins of the patches were sewn together with number 2 nonabsorbable sutures (Figure 1(c)). The "biologically resorbable" surface of the GraftJacket was exposed so that it would be in direct contact to the bone at the insertion site for the tendon reconstruction. This surface represents the anatomically deeper part of the graft and it is placed facing the bone in order to allow incorporation of the graft [24].

The first patch was overlapped on the free end of the LDT by 12.5 mm and was then sutured with two rows of nonabsorbable number 2 sutures (Figure 1(c)). The second GraftJacket patch was overlapped by 12.5 mm to the first patch and was sewn with two rows of nonabsorbable number 2 sutures. The total extension of the LDT was then 5.5 cm. A Krakow suture technique with number 2 suture was then passed along the sides of the latissimus tendon to the free end of the graft extension as shown in Figure 1(a). As described below, the extended LDT was then attached directly to the "footprint" that was created for the supraspinatus, upper infraspinatus, and upper subscapularis (Figure 1(b)).

Before attaching the extended LDT to the footprint, residual infraspinatus tendon at the lower portion of the natural insertion site was mobilized by sharp dissection and moved

Table 1: Shoulder motion and function of left shoulder.

(a)

Date	Action	Range of motion	Strength
1 month preop*	Forward flexion	65	2/5
	Abduction	60	
	External rotation	50	3/5
	Internal rotation	30	
	Extension	35	
	Adduction	35	
18 months postop†	Forward flexion	180	4/5
	Abduction	170	
	External rotation	60	4/5
	Internal rotation	70	
	Extension	45	
	Adduction	45	

*Preop, preoperatively.
†Postop, postoperatively.

(b) Shoulder survey scores

	Preop*	Postop†	
10 cm VAS score for pain	6.5	2	
ASES score	26.6	68.3	(Best is 100)
WORC score		923 (56.1%)	(Best is 0 (100%))
Simple shoulder test		10 out of 12	(12 is best)
DASH score			(Best is 0; worst is 100)
Total		14.17	
Work module		0	
Sports/performing arts module		37.5	
Short-Form 36 (SF-36)			(Best is 100 for all)
Physical functioning		95	
Physical role		100	
Bodily pain		61	
General health		82	
Vitality		60	
Social functioning		75	
Emotional role		100	
Mental health		68	

*Preop, preoperatively.
†Postop, postoperatively.

15 mm upward and sutured to the upper natural insertion site for this muscle. This was done with number 2 FiberWire sutures through drill holes posteriorly and also with the sutures from a Mitek Healix™ anchor that was placed at the location where the supraspinatus and upper infraspinatus naturally merge. This anchor was double-loaded with number Orthocord® sutures.

The LDT with the GraftJacket extension was then pulled upward beneath the posterior deltoid and anteriorly across the defect in the rotator cuff. Along the lateral portion of the footprint, four pairs of horizontal mattress sutures (number 2 FiberWire) were passed through drill holes. The GraftJacket extension was then fastened in place with these number 2 FiberWire sutures and with the two sutures from the aforementioned Mitek Healix anchor. Additional fixation included a series of separate number 2 FiberWire sutures passing through the upper subscapularis and also a series of separate sutures passing medially through the residual supraspinatus tendon near the glenoid. The shoulder was then passively tested for stability and motion; elimination of the posterior-superior subluxations showed that a tenodesis effect was clearly achieved.

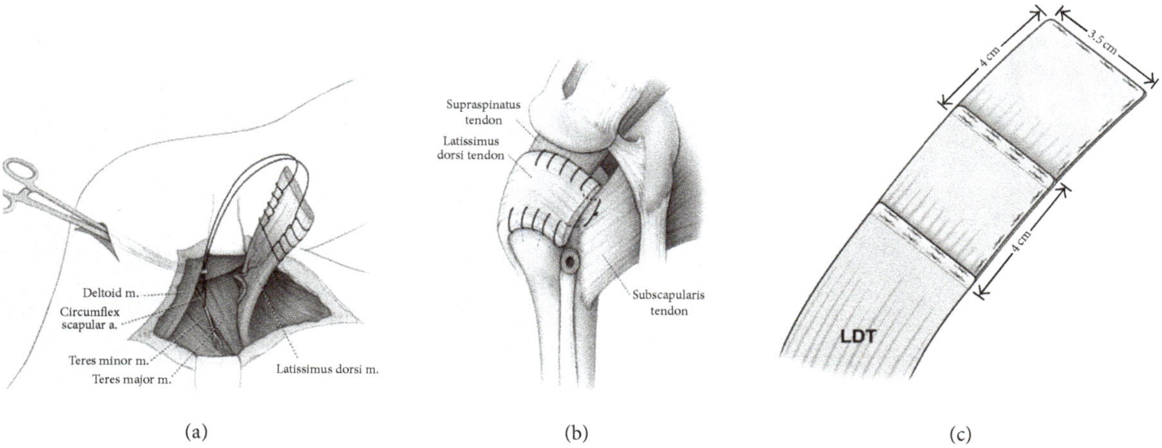

FIGURE 1: Drawings (a) and (b) show how a LDT is typically transferred and sewn to the defect where the rotator cuff would normally insert. Drawing (c) shows how we extended the tendon with two allograft patches. The running stitches along the margins of the LDT shown in (a) were also done, but this is not shown in (c) (images (a) and (b) are reproduced from [20] with permission of the Journal of Bone and Joint Surgery, Inc.).

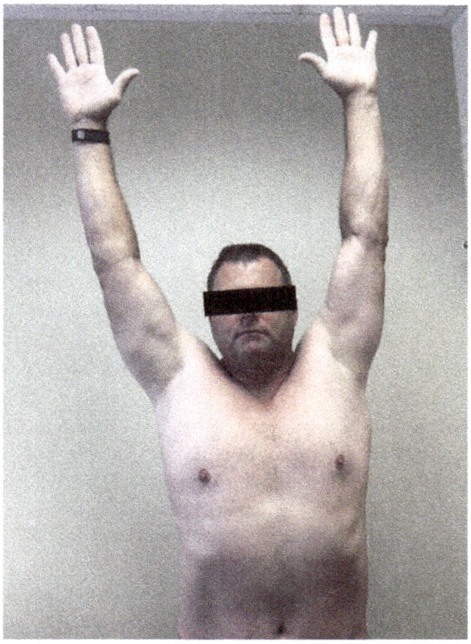

FIGURE 2: Photograph showing the patient's left shoulder motion at 18-month follow-up (active forward flexion is 165°). Preoperative photographs were not available, but active forward flexion was only 65°.

After wound closure, the patient was placed in a rigid shoulder orthosis in neutral rotation and 45° abduction for two months, following Gerber et al.'s [9] postoperative treatment. Gentle passive shoulder motion was allowed only after 6 weeks. Active overhead motion was not allowed until four months after surgery. Weight bearing exercise at the shoulder was allowed at nine months after surgery but no lifting over 20 lbs (9 kg) overhead until one year after surgery.

At follow-up 18 months later, the patient had regained significant strength and range of motion in his left shoulder (Table 1 and Figure 2). He reported being very satisfied with the overall results achieved from his surgery. However, he avoided sleeping on his left side because his shoulder "aches really bad" and he reported shoulder fatigue with repetitive overhead reach. He was not taking regular pain medication besides occasional over-the-counter NSAIDs.

At 18 months after his LDTT, magnetic resonance (MR) scanning was done solely for the purpose of examining integrity of the graft. The graft was found to be intact and without evidence of thinning (Figure 3). Mild glenohumeral arthritis was noted in the MR images, which likely contributed to some of his continuing low-level pain. At final follow-up at two years after surgery, the pain had improved to only trace and his function was maintained.

3. Discussion

At the time of our patient's tendon reconstruction surgery, there was no anticipation that the length of the LDT would be inadequate after releasing it sharply from its insertion and mobilizing the latissimus dorsi muscle belly of the various soft tissue attachments that could restrict the transfer. Although removing some humeral bone along with the LDT would have increased LDT length, it would not have provided the additional 5.5 cm needed for the LDTT. For this reason, we used GraftJacket allograft acellular dermal matrix to extend the LDT. This material has been mechanically tested and was found to have superior resistance in tension loading compared to comparable allografts and xenografts like CuffPatch, Restore, Permacol, and TissueMend [23]. GraftJacket has been used in augmentation of rotator cuff repairs and has been shown to have superior results to nonaugmented repairs [19].

When GraftJacket is used in the context of LDTT for irreparable rotator cuff tear, it would be expected that it would be for augmenting the new attachment site. To our knowledge, the use of GraftJacket to extend the LDT has not

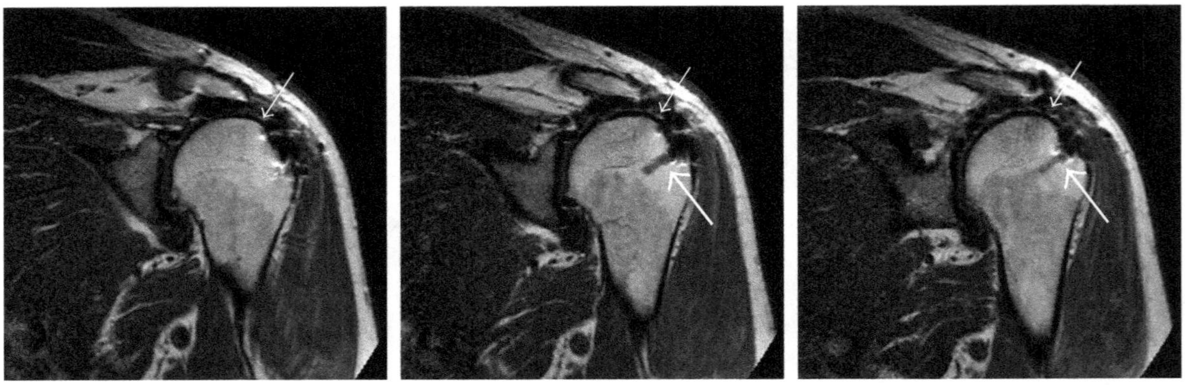

FIGURE 3: A series of adjacent coronal MR images taken at 18 months after surgery showing the graft (thin white arrow) and suture anchor (thicker white arrow). Mild arthritic changes are also seen.

been reported. Similar to our case, Petri et al. [12] described lengthening of a LDT using another brand of acellular dermal matrix (ArthroFlex patch) [18].

Additionally, our patient's increased function after the LDTT could be attributed to the latissimus dorsi acting as an active rotator and elevator or because the LDTT simply provided a tenodesis effect that stabilized the shoulder joint. Henseler et al. [25] evaluated eight patients at one year after LDTT. Although they found that the latissimus dorsi has activity after LDTT, they observed a passive tenodesis effect. The tenodesis effect that is achieved resembles that described by Mihata and colleagues [26] as a "superior capsular reconstruction." One potential problem that could occur in our patient's future is thinning of the graft to the point that the tenodesis effect is lost [21]. Loss of the tenodesis effect of the LDTT can start at approximately six months following the operation, which could also be attributed to elongation of the muscle [21]. There was no evidence that this was occurring in our patient at his 2-year follow-up.

4. Conclusion

Our patient had marked improvement in his shoulder range of motion after LDTT with GraftJacket extension of the LDT. Thus, the use of GraftJacket acellular dermal matrix to increase LDT length may be indicated in LDTT cases, where sufficient LDT length is unobtainable. However, studies with much longer follow-up are needed to determine if these good results are maintained.

Ethical Approval

Each author certifies that his institution has approved the reporting of this case, that all investigations were conducted in conformity with ethical principles of research, and that informed consent for participation in the study was obtained.

Competing Interests

The authors declare that there are no competing interests regarding the publication of this paper.

References

[1] C. Gerber, T. S. Vinh, R. Hertel, and C. W. Hess, "Latissimus dorsi transfer for the treatment of massive tears of the rotator cuff. A preliminary report," *Clinical Orthopaedics and Related Research*, no. 232, pp. 51–61, 1988.

[2] J. Grimberg and J. Kany, "Latissimus dorsi tendon transfer for irreparable postero-superior cuff tears: current concepts, indications, and recent advances," *Current Reviews in Musculoskeletal Medicine*, vol. 7, no. 1, pp. 22–32, 2014.

[3] R. Omid and B. Lee, "Tendon transfers for irreparable rotator cuff tears," *Journal of the American Academy of Orthopaedic Surgeons*, vol. 21, no. 8, pp. 492–501, 2013.

[4] P. Boileau, C. Chuinard, Y. Roussanne, L. Neyton, and C. Trojani, "Modified latissimus dorsi and teres major transfer through a single delto-pectoral approach for external rotation deficit of the shoulder: as an isolated procedure or with a reverse arthroplasty," *Journal of Shoulder and Elbow Surgery*, vol. 16, no. 6, pp. 671–682, 2007.

[5] L. L. Shi, K. E. Cahill, E. T. Ek, J. D. Tompson, L. D. Higgins, and J. J. P. Warner, "Latissimus dorsi and teres major transfer with reverse shoulder arthroplasty restores active motion and reduces pain for posterosuperior cuff dysfunction," *Clinical Orthopaedics and Related Research*, vol. 473, no. 10, pp. 3212–3217, 2015.

[6] M. Moursy, R. Forstner, H. Koller, H. Resch, and M. Tauber, "Latissimus dorsi tendon transfer for irreparable rotator cuff tears: a modified technique to improve tendon transfer integrity," *Journal of Bone and Joint Surgery—Series A*, vol. 91, no. 8, pp. 1924–1931, 2009.

[7] M. Tauber, M. Moursy, R. Forstner, H. Koller, and H. Resch, "Latissimus Dorsi tendon transfer for irreparable rotator cuff tears: a modified technique to improve tendon transfer integrity: surgical techniquee," *Journal of Bone & Joint Surgery*, vol. 92, no. 1, pp. 226–239, 2010.

[8] J. P. Iannotti, S. Hennigan, R. Herzog et al., "Latissimus dorsi tendon transfer for irreparable posterosuperior rotator cuff tears: factors affecting outcome," *Journal of Bone and Joint Surgery - Series A*, vol. 88, no. 2, pp. 342–348, 2006.

[9] C. Gerber, S. A. Rahm, S. Catanzaro, M. Farshad, and B. K. Moor, "Latissimus dorsi tendon transfer for treatment of irreparable posterosuperior rotator cuff tears: long-term results at a minimum follow-up of ten years," *Journal of Bone and Joint Surgery—Series A*, vol. 95, no. 21, pp. 1920–1926, 2013.

[10] J. J. P. Warner and I. M. Parsons IV, "Latissimus dorsi tendon transfer: a comparative analysis of primary and salvage reconstruction of massive, irreparable rotator cuff tears," *Journal of Shoulder and Elbow Surgery*, vol. 10, no. 6, pp. 514–521, 2001.

[11] P. D. G. Henry, T. Dwyer, M. D. McKee, and E. H. Schemitsch, "Latissimus dorsi tendon transfer for irreparable tears of the rotator cuff: an anatomical study to assess the neurovascular hazards and ways of improving tendon excursion," *The Bone & Joint Journal*, vol. 95, no. 4, pp. 517–522, 2013.

[12] M. Petri, J. A. Greenspoon, S. Bhatia, and P. J. Millett, "Patch-augmented latissimus dorsi transfer and open reduction-internal fixation of unstable os acromiale for irreparable massive posterosuperior rotator cuff tear," *Arthroscopy Techniques*, vol. 4, no. 5, pp. e487–e492, 2015.

[13] T. Dehler, A. L. Pennings, and A. W. ElMaraghy, "Dermal allograft reconstruction of a chronic pectoralis major tear," *Journal of Shoulder and Elbow Surgery*, vol. 22, no. 10, pp. e18–e22, 2013.

[14] T. A. Joseph, M. J. Defranco, and G. G. Weiker, "Delayed repair of a pectoralis major tendon rupture with allograft: a case report," *Journal of Shoulder and Elbow Surgery*, vol. 12, no. 1, pp. 101–104, 2003.

[15] D. P. Ferguson, M. R. Lewington, T. D. Smith, and I. H. Wong, "Graft utilization in the augmentation of large-to-massive rotator cuff repairs: a systematic review," *The American Journal of Sports Medicine*, vol. 44, no. 11, pp. 2984–2992, 2016.

[16] C. R. Jones and S. J. Snyder, "Massive irreparable rotator cuff tears: a solution that bridges the gap," *Sports Medicine and Arthroscopy Review*, vol. 23, no. 3, pp. 130–138, 2015.

[17] M. Petri, R. J. Warth, M. P. Horan, J. A. Greenspoon, and P. J. Millett, "Outcomes after open revision repair of massive rotator cuff tears with biologic patch augmentation," *Arthroscopy*, vol. 32, no. 9, pp. 1752–1760, 2016.

[18] D. C. Acevedo, B. Shore, and R. Mirzayan, "Orthopedic applications of acellular human dermal allograft for shoulder and elbow surgery," *Orthopedic Clinics of North America*, vol. 46, no. 3, pp. 377–388, 2015.

[19] F. A. Barber, J. P. Burns, A. Deutsch, M. R. Labbé, and R. B. Litchfield, "A prospective, randomized evaluation of acellular human dermal matrix augmentation for arthroscopic rotator cuff repair," *Arthroscopy*, vol. 28, no. 1, pp. 8–15, 2012.

[20] M. J. Codsi, S. Hennigan, R. Herzog et al., "Latissimus dorsi tendon transfer for irreparable posterosuperior rotator cuff tears. Surgical technique," *The Journal of Bone and Joint Surgery*, vol. 89, supplement 2, part 1, pp. 1–9, 2007.

[21] A. Erşen, H. Ozben, M. Demirhan, A. C. Atalar, and M. Kapıcıoğlu, "Time-dependent changes after latissimus dorsi transfer: tenodesis or tendon transfer?" *Clinical Orthopaedics and Related Research*, vol. 472, no. 12, pp. 3880–3888, 2014.

[22] B. A. Goldberg, B. Elhassan, S. Marciniak, and J. H. Dunn, "Surgical anatomy of latissimus dorsi muscle in transfers about the shoulder," *American Journal of Orthopedics*, vol. 38, no. 3, pp. E64–E67, 2009.

[23] F. A. Barber, M. A. Herbert, and D. A. Coons, "Tendon augmentation grafts: biomechanical failure loads and failure patterns," *Arthroscopy—Journal of Arthroscopic and Related Surgery*, vol. 22, no. 5, pp. 534–538, 2006.

[24] S. J. Snyder, S. P. Arnoczky, J. L. Bond, and R. Dopirak, "Histologic evaluation of a biopsy specimen obtained 3 months after rotator cuff augmentation with GraftJacket Matrix," *Arthroscopy*, vol. 25, no. 3, pp. 329–333, 2009.

[25] J. F. Henseler, J. Nagels, R. G. H. H. Nelissen, and J. H. de Groot, "Does the latissimus dorsi tendon transfer for massive rotator cuff tears remain active postoperatively and restore active external rotation?" *Journal of Shoulder and Elbow Surgery*, vol. 23, no. 4, pp. 553–560, 2014.

[26] T. Mihata, T. Q. Lee, Y. Itami, A. Hasegawa, M. Ohue, and M. Neo, "Arthroscopic superior capsule reconstruction for irreparable rotator cuff tears: a prospective clinical study in 100 consecutive patients with 1 to 8 years of follow-up," *Orthopaedic Journal of Sports Medicine*, vol. 4, no. 3, 2016.

34

Metatarsal Shaft Fracture with Associated Metatarsophalangeal Joint Dislocation

Taranjit Singh Tung

Division of Orthopaedic Surgery, Boundary Trails Health Centre, P.O. Box 2000, Station Main, Winkler, MB, Canada R6W 1H8

Correspondence should be addressed to Taranjit Singh Tung; taranjittung@hotmail.com

Academic Editor: Stamatios A. Papadakis

Metatarsophalangeal joint dislocations of lesser toes are often seen in the setting of severe claw toes. Traumatic irreducible dislocations have been reported in rare cases following both low-energy and high-energy injuries to the forefoot. In this case report, I present a previously unreported association of a metatarsal shaft fracture with metatarsophalangeal joint dislocation of a lesser toe.

1. Introduction

Irreducible traumatic metatarsophalangeal (MTP) joint dislocations have been reported in various case reports following both low-energy and high-energy injuries. Often these dislocations are dorsal in direction and associated with plantar plate injuries [1–4].

I report a case of traumatic lesser metatarsal (MT) fracture and MTP joint dislocation in an adult male after a motor vehicle accident. This case illustrates a previously unreported association between MT shaft fracture and MTP joint stability and failure of early recognition of radiographic subluxation at the MTP joint and offers a systematic approach to a symptomatic patient with a semiacute MTP dislocation with MT malunion.

2. Case Report

This is the case of a 56-year-old man who was involved in a motor vehicle accident resulting in a right ulna fracture and multiple fractures in his left foot. The fractures in his left foot included a second-metatarsal (MT) neck fracture, proximal third-MT fracture, and a comminuted fracture of the fourth MT (Figure 1). Subluxation of the fourth metatarsophalangeal (MTP) joint was not recognized by the treating physician; hence between the patient and his treating physician nonoperative treatment for his injuries was decided upon.

His past medical history was significant for West Nile encephalopathy resulting in residual right upper extremity weakness and spasms.

The patient was referred to my fracture clinic nine weeks after his injury with ongoing pain in the left foot at the known fracture sites but also at the level of his fourth MTP joint. Radiographs and CT scan imaging of his foot revealed healing fractures of the 2nd and 3rd MTs in acceptable position, a partial malunion of the 4th MT, and a dorsal dislocation of the 4th MTP joint (Figures 2 and 3). On careful evaluation of his images it was evident that he had disrupted the normal lateral descending cascade of the lesser metatarsals [5]—with his 4th metatarsal having been lengthened via the malunion site to almost the same length as his 3rd metatarsal. An in-depth discussion regarding treatment options was held with the patient, and he opted for surgical intervention. An informed consent for the procedure and publication of this case report was obtained from the patient.

Patient received a general anesthetic. He was positioned supinely on the operating table and a thigh tourniquet was used. Attempt at closed reduction of the 4th MTP joint was unsuccessful. Dorsal longitudinal incision centered over the 4th MT was utilized to get to the fracture site. Three main fragments were noted. Some healing in extension was noted on the dorsal surface between a couple of the fragments, but a free floating plantar fragment was also seen. Even after the fragments were mobilized, closed reduction of the 4th MTP joint was not possible. The incision was thus extended distally,

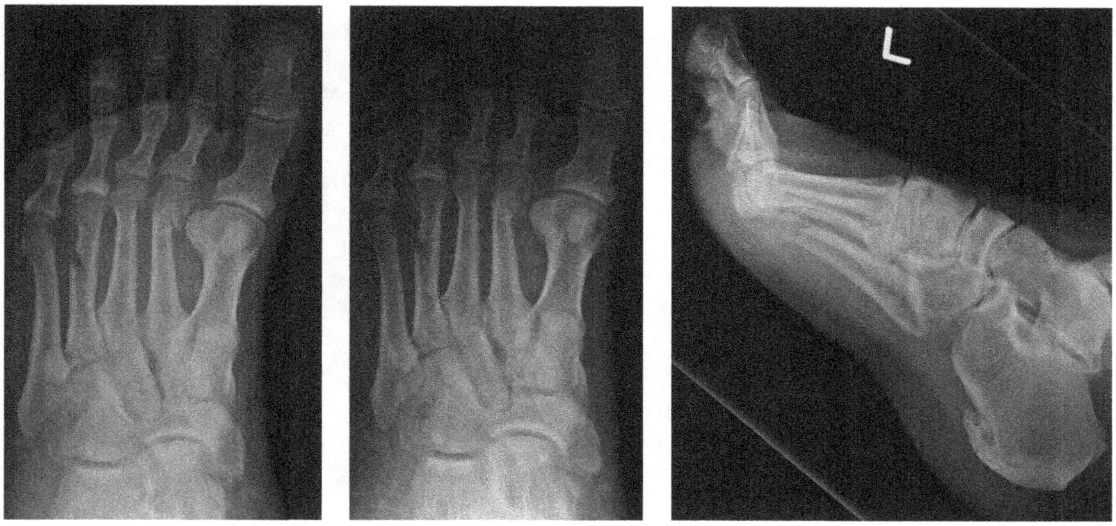

(a) (b) (c)

FIGURE 1: Dorsoplantar (a), oblique (b), and lateral (c) radiographs of the left foot at initial presentation.

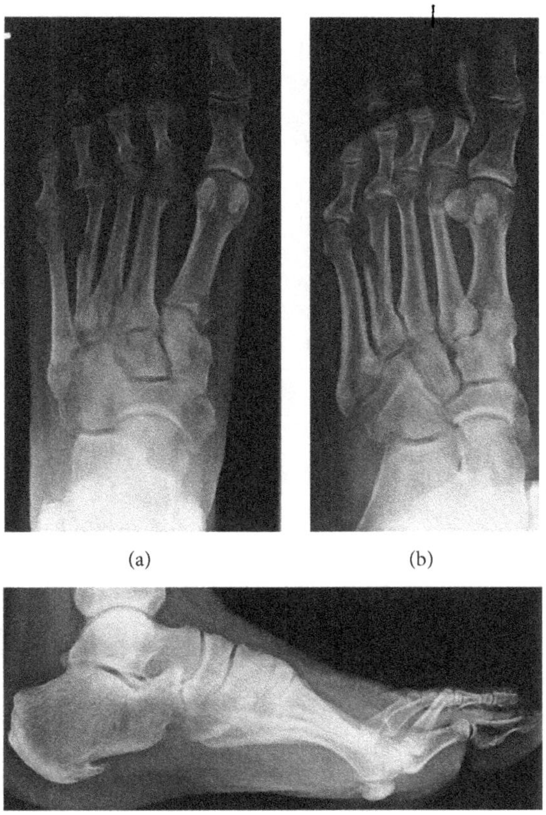

(a) (b)

(c)

FIGURE 2: Preoperative dorsoplantar (a), oblique (b), and lateral (c) radiographs of the left foot showing malunion at fracture site, resulting in a lengthened fourth MT, and a dorsal dislocation at the fourth MTP joint.

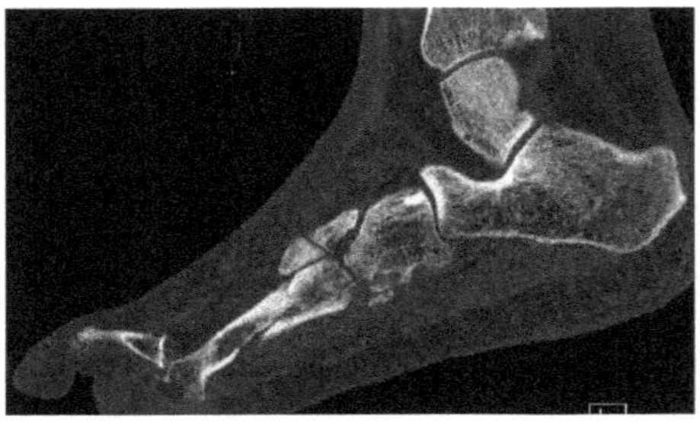

FIGURE 3: CT scan at the level of the left 4th toe illustrating fracture malunion and dorsal dislocation at the MTP joint.

the extensor tendons were mobilized, a dorsal capsulotomy was performed, and the collateral ligaments were released off the MT head. Even with that, a reduction of the dislocated joint was not possible. So at this point I decided to shorten the MT through the fracture site and secure it with a minifragment locking plate (Synthes, Mississauga, Ontario). A lag screw through the plate was utilized to secure the plantar fragment, which was sculptured to fit in. The 4th MTP joint was then reduced. The plantar plate was inspected and noted to be intact. The position of the reduced MTP joint was maintained with a 1.6 mm Kirschner wire. Layered closure of the incision was performed prior to immobilizing the foot in a cast boot. Three doses of antibiotics were administered postoperatively, and the patient was discharged home the following day. Stitches were taken out about three weeks later, and the pin was removed about 6 weeks postoperatively. Heel weight-bearing was allowed at 6 weeks and full-weight-bearing was allowed at 12 weeks. Patient did have delayed wound healing but made excellent recovery, and, at final follow-up eight months after surgery, his 4th MT was fully healed, 4th MTP joint maintained a reduced position, there was some evidence of disuse osteopenia but no evidence of avascular necrosis (AVN) of the MT head, and he was back to his preinjury level of activity (Figure 4).

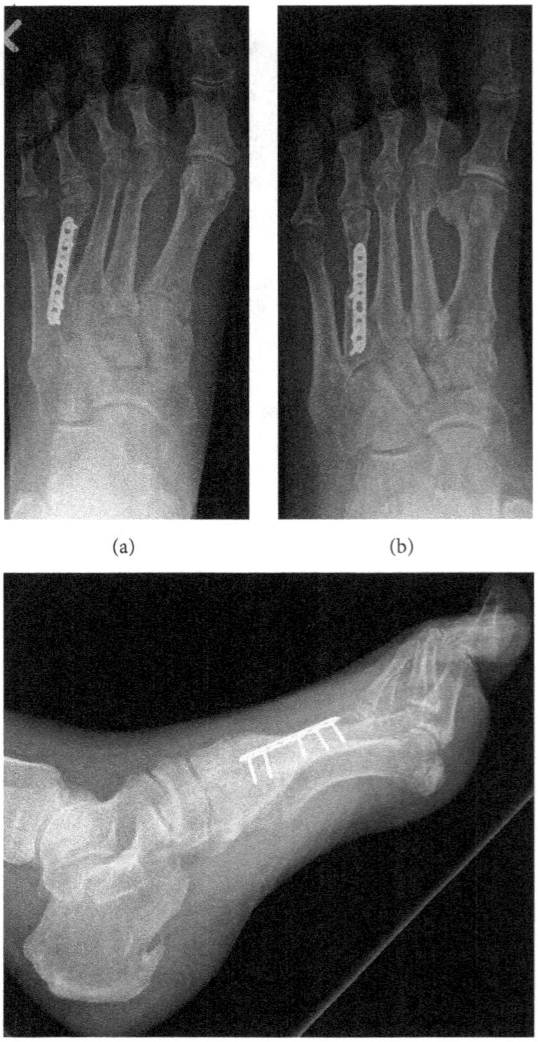

(a) (b)

(c)

FIGURE 4: Final dorsoplantar (a), oblique (b), and lateral (c) radiographs showing fusion at fracture site, shortening of fourth MT, and maintained reduction at the fourth MTP joint.

3. Discussion

MTP dislocations are often noted in 2nd toes in association with hallux valgus deformities, especially in patients with a long second MT relative to the 1st MT [6, 7]. In rheumatoid feet multiple claw toe deformities and associated MTP dislocations are common [8]. Irreducible traumatic MTP dislocations have been reported in various case reports. These are usually dorsal in direction and often a result of axial load applied to hyperextended toes [1–4]. Plantar dislocations are rare and usually due to dorsally directed force on the plantar aspect of metatarsal heads [9]. This paper presents a previously undescribed injury comprising both MT shaft fracture and MTP joint subluxation and ultimately dislocation of a lesser toe. Due to the initial displacement, the fracture partially healed, nonanatomically, with lengthening through the fracture site—effectively increasing the length of the 4th MT and thus disrupting the normal metatarsal parabola. Failure of early recognition and management of the subtle subluxation gradually caused the subluxed 4th proximal phalanx to ultimately dislocate dorsally on the MT head. Attempt at closed reduction of the MTP joint at nine weeks proved to be futile without first addressing the MT length. Weil's osteotomy is commonly used to shorten the MT length to aid in correction of severe claw toe deformities, allowing reduction of the MTP joint [10]. Similar shortening osteotomies can also be performed through the shaft of the MT [11]. Using this latter principle in this case of irreducible MTP joint following traumatic lengthening of the MT, shortening through the fracture site offered an attractive option to address the MT length and thereby facilitate reduction at the MTP joint. Unlike most of the other reported cases of traumatic MTP dislocation, a tear of the plantar plate was not noted, likely due to force dissipation through not just the MTP joint but also the MT shaft. It is possible that the MT fractured first, and as it was displaced it resulted in lengthening of the MT, which, in turn, disrupted the normal metatarsal parabola, causing the MTP joint to initially sublux and then be ultimately dislocated dorsally. Thus correction of MT length was integral in achieving reduction of this lesser toe MTP dislocation. Immobilization of the reduced joint with a K-wire to allow for soft tissue scarring proved to be beneficial. To avoid pin breakage and minimize motion at the fracture/osteotomy site the patient was kept non-weight-bearing in a cast boot for 6 weeks, prior to progressing his weight-bearing.

4. Conclusion

This case illustrates an unusual injury, MT shaft fracture with associated MTP subluxation—ultimately resulting into MTP joint dislocation, the need for early recognition of such an injury, and a practical, systematic approach to management of a semiacute MTP dislocation following MT malunion—with shortening of the MT, dorsal capsulotomy, collateral ligament release, reduction of MTP joint, maintenance of reduction with K-wire fixation, and immobilization till soft tissues scar in, to achieve an excellent clinical outcome.

Competing Interests

The author declares no competing interests.

References

[1] H. W. Hey, G. Chang, C. C. Hong, and W. S. Kuan, "Irreducible dislocation of the fourth metatarsophalangeal joint—a case report," *The American Journal of Emergency Medicine*, vol. 31, no. 1, pp. 265.e1–265.e3, 2013.

[2] J. P. Rao and M. T. Banzon, "Irreducible dislocation of the metatarsophalangeal joints of the foot," *Clinical Orthopaedics and Related Research*, vol. 145, pp. 224–226, 1979.

[3] F. Turkmensoy, S. Erinc, O. N. Ergin, K. Ozkan, and B. Kemah, "Irreducible fifth metatarsophalangeal joint after car crush injury," *Case Reports in Orthopedics*, vol. 2015, Article ID 894057, 3 pages, 2015.

[4] M. Boussouga, J. Boukhriss, A. Jaafar, and K. H. Lazrak, "Irreducible dorsal metatarsophalangeal joint dislocation of the fifth toe: a case report," *The Journal of Foot and Ankle Surgery*, vol. 49, no. 3, pp. 298.e17–298.e20, 2010.

[5] M. Maestro, J.-L. Besse, M. Ragusa, and E. Berthonnaud, "Forefoot morphotype study and planning method for forefoot osteotomy," *Foot and Ankle Clinics*, vol. 8, no. 4, pp. 695–710, 2003.

[6] K. Shirzad, C. D. Kiesau, J. K. DeOrio, and S. G. Parekh, "Lesser toe deformities," *Journal of the American Academy of Orthopaedic Surgeons*, vol. 19, no. 8, pp. 505–514, 2011.

[7] J. R. Weber, P. M. Aubin, W. R. Ledoux, and B. J. Sangeorzan, "Second metatarsal length is positively correlated with increased pressure and medial deviation of the second toe in a robotic cadaveric simulation of gait," *Foot and Ankle International*, vol. 33, no. 4, pp. 312–319, 2012.

[8] R. V. Abdo and L. J. Iorio, "Rheumatoid arthritis of the foot and ankle," *Journal of the American Academy of Orthopaedic Surgeons*, vol. 2, no. 6, pp. 326–332, 1994.

[9] L. De Palma, A. Santucci, and M. Marinelli, "Traumatic dislocation of metatarsophalangeal joints: report of three different cases," *Foot and Ankle Surgery*, vol. 7, no. 4, pp. 229–234, 2001.

[10] L. S. Barouk, *Forefoot Reconstruction*, Springer, Paris, France, 2nd edition, 2005.

[11] N. J. Giannestras, "Shortening of the metatarsal shaft in the treatment of plantar keratosis; an end-result study," *The Journal of Bone and Joint Surgery. American Volume*, vol. 40, no. 1, pp. 61–71, 1958.

35

Symptomatic Bilateral Torn Discoid Medial Meniscus Treated with Saucerization and Suture

Enrique Sevillano-Perez,[1,2] Alejandro Espejo-Reina,[2,3] and María Josefa Espejo-Reina[2]

[1] *Department of Orthopaedic Surgery, Regional University Hospital of Málaga, 29010 Málaga, Spain*
[2] *Hospital Vithas Parque San Antonio, 29016 Málaga, Spain*
[3] *Department of Orthopaedic Surgery, Virgen de la Victoria University Hospital, 29010 Málaga, Spain*

Correspondence should be addressed to Enrique Sevillano-Perez; enriquesevillanocot@yahoo.com

Academic Editor: Akio Sakamoto

Discoid meniscus is an anatomical congenital anomaly more often found in the lateral meniscus. A discoid medial meniscus is a very rare anomaly, and even more rare is to diagnose a bilateral discoid medial meniscus although the real prevalence of this situation is unknown because not all the discoid medial menisci are symptomatic and if the contralateral knee is not symptomatic then it is not usually studied. The standard treatment of this kind of pathology is partial meniscectomy. Currently the tendency is to be very conservative so suture and saucerization of a torn discoid meniscus when possible are gaining support. We present the case of a 13-year-old patient who was diagnosed with symptomatic torn bilateral discoid medial meniscus treated by suturing the tear and saucerization. To the best of our knowledge this is the first case reported of bilateral torn discoid medial meniscus treated in this manner in the same patient.

1. Introduction

Discoid meniscus is a type of meniscus with an atypical shape, thicker, covering a bigger surface of tibial plateau than a normal meniscus but more fragile which explains the higher frequency of lesions.

The reported incidence rates for discoid lateral meniscus range from 1,2% to 5,2% being the incidence much lower for discoid medial meniscus (0,12–0,3%) [1, 2]. However, in Asian population the reported incidence for discoid menisci ranges from 30% to 50% [3]. There are few reports of medial bilateral discoid menisci in the literature although the real incidence is difficult to determine because an unknown percentage of discoid menisci may be asymptomatic [4].

There are different classifications for discoid meniscus being Watanabe, the most accepted, in which discoid meniscus is classified into three different types according to the arthroscopic aspect: type I or complete, type II or incomplete, and type III or Wrisberg-ligament type in which the posterior meniscofemoral attachment is absent resulting in an unstable meniscus with hypermobility [5]. Jordan classified discoid meniscus depending on its peripheral rim stability as stable type (includes both complete and incomplete types, further divided by the presence of symptoms and tears or not) and unstable type (includes unstable normal and unstable discoid meniscus since both have the same symptoms and treatment) [6].

2. Case Presentation

2.1. Right Knee. The patient is a 13-year-old male, recreational football player, who presented with pain and is unable to fully extend the knee fully after a low energy impact on his right knee, without episodes of locking or instability.

On physical examination the patient had normal alignment of the right lower limb, full flexion with pain on the medial side on the last degrees of flexion and the last 15° degrees of extension; tenderness on the medial joint line, painful click with McMurray test with no effusion, and no ligamentous laxity. Patellar tracking was normal. Simple X-ray of the knee showed no abnormalities and a discoid medial meniscus with peripheral and horizontal tear and the upper side of the meniscus folded in the intercondylar notch was

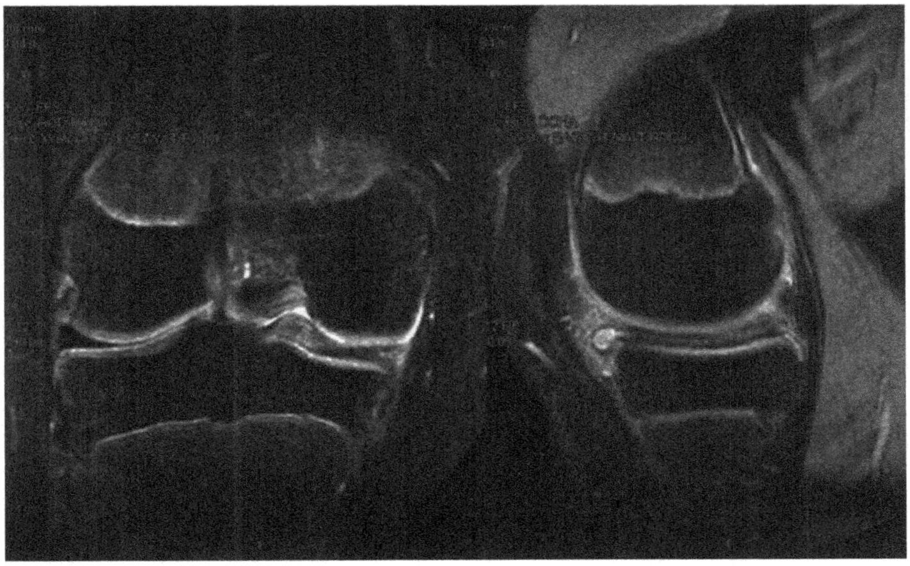

(a) (b)

FIGURE 1: MRI of the right knee. (a) Coronal view showing the upper side of the medial meniscus folded in the intercondylar notch. (b) Sagittal view demonstrating the horizontal tear.

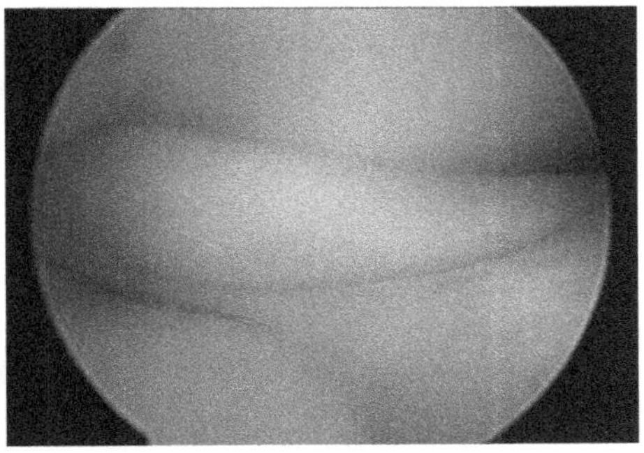

FIGURE 2: Arthroscopic image of the medial femorotibial compartment of the right knee from the anterolateral portal showing the upper side of the medial meniscus folded in the intercondylar notch.

found on magnetic resonance imaging (MRI) scan with no other abnormalities associated (Figure 1).

2.1.1. Surgical Technique. An arthroscopy of the right knee was performed with the thigh in a leg holder using standard anterolateral and anteromedial portals under general anesthesia. A complete medial discoid meniscus with a partial longitudinal tear in red zone of the body and posterior horn was found. Its upper side was folded to the intercondylar notch behaving as a bucket handle tear (Figure 2). The tear was found to be reducible with a probe. It was refreshed with a shaver (Figure 3(a)) and the meniscus was repaired using an inside-out technique with a specific suturing device (Figure 3(b)) [7] and number 2 Force-Fiber suture (Stryker Endoscopy, San Jose CA). Once the tear was sutured and its stability tested with a probe the body of the meniscus was saucerized with a shaver and radiofrequency at the lowest intensity allowed by the device, to avoid damage to the auricular cartilage, reproducing the shape of a normal meniscus (Figure 4).

Postoperatively the knee was immobilized with a knee orthotic in extension during two weeks and partial weight bearing and limiting flexion to 90° during two more weeks. At three months sport was gradually resumed.

2.2. Left Knee. Six months after the surgery the patient started with pain and incapacity to fully extend the left knee with no trauma associated (and asymptomatic right knee). On physical examination the patient had complete flexion and pain on the last 10° of extension, with tenderness on the medial joint line with no effusion or ligamentous laxity. Patellar tracking was normal. No abnormalities were found on X-ray and MRI showed a tear very similar to the contralateral knee (Figure 5).

2.2.1. Surgical Technique. An arthroscopy was performed on the left knee in the same manner as the right one. A complete medial discoid meniscus was found with a longitudinal tear in red zone affecting the body and posterior horn, very similar to the right knee except the upper part of the tear was not folded on the intercondylar notch although it was easily displaced to the notch with the probe (Figure 6). The meniscus was sutured with an inside-out technique using the same specific device and suture used on the right knee. Once the stability of the suture was tested the body of the meniscus was saucerized using a technique similar to that described above (Figure 7). Postoperative care was the same as the right knee.

The patient was reviewed at 6 months, one year, and two years after surgery being asymptomatic and with same preinjury activity level.

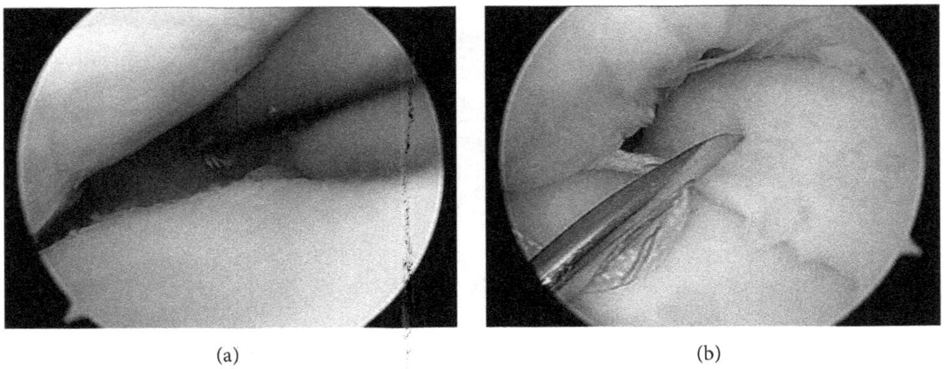

FIGURE 3: Arthroscopic image of the medial femorotibial compartment of the right knee from the anterolateral portal. (a) Refreshment of the tear with a shaver. (b) Inside-out suture technique of the tear with a specific device.

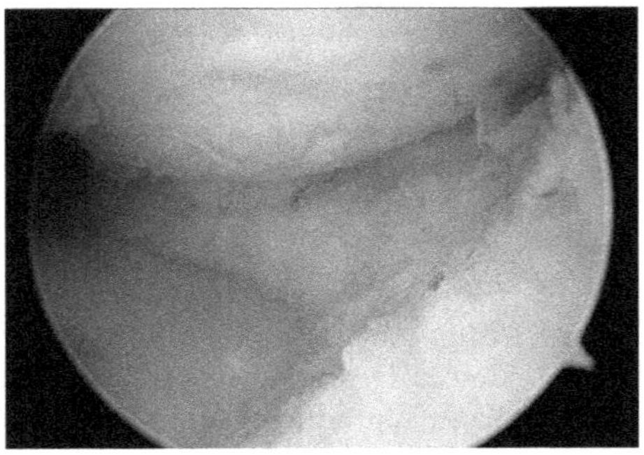

FIGURE 4: Arthroscopic image of the medial femorotibial compartment of the right knee from the anterolateral portal. Saucerization after the suture.

MRI was performed two years after the surgery and a reduction of the size and intensity in T2 signal of both repaired menisci was found (Figure 8).

3. Discussion

To the best of our knowledge this is the first case published of bilateral medial discoid menisci tear treated with arthroscopic repair and saucerization.

There are different reports of bilateral discoid menisci [8] being very scarce the ones about bilateral medial discoid meniscus [2, 9].

The symptoms of a torn discoid meniscus are usually the same of those caused by a tear of a normal one. In the lateral discoid menisci common finding of "snapping knee" syndrome may help in the diagnosis whereas in the medial menisci it is less specific [10]. In our case the main complaint was knee extension limitation.

Medial discoid meniscus may be asymptomatic and found incidentally after MRI requested for other reasons. In plain radiographs, some abnormalities such as widening of the medial joint margin and cupping of the medial tibia plateau or proximal medial physeal collapse can be found associated with discoid medial meniscus [11]. There are other several abnormalities associated with medial discoid meniscus found on MRI including anomalous insertion of the anterior horn of the medial meniscus into the anterior cruciate ligament, discoid lateral meniscus in the same knee, pathologic medial patella plica, or meniscal cyst [12]. None of these were present in our patient.

The treatment of symptomatic torn discoid meniscus has classically been meniscectomy. Total meniscectomy increases the probability of osteoarthritis compared with partial meniscectomy with a stable peripheral rim [13–15]. Management of torn discoid meniscus has evolved to more conservative surgery. Partial meniscectomy using the saucerization technique resecting the central portion of the meniscus in order to recreate the shape of a normal meniscus has obtained better results in medial and long-term follow-up for torn discoid meniscus than total meniscectomy [12, 16]. Currently, tears in medial discoid menisci are treated with saucerization and suture when the type of lesion allows so [15]. Partial meniscectomy and suture of a torn medial meniscus are more conservative than subtotal meniscectomy but it has not shown better results in the midterm, being subtotal meniscectomy an appropriate choice of treatment for unrepairable tears in a medial discoid meniscus. Results depend on the age at the time of surgery, being worse in children over ten years [17].

Postoperatively the knees were immobilized with a knee orthotic in extension during two weeks allowing partial weight bearing with flexion of the knee limited to 90° the following two weeks. At three months sport was gradually resumed. A generalized rehabilitation protocol has not been established for these kinds of lesions. In sutured bucket handle tears flexion of the knee is from 0° to 90° while bearing weight increases compressive and shear loads in the posterior horn of the meniscus by a factor of 4 [18]. With flexion of the knee the meniscus is displaced posteriorly. The amount of displacement of the meniscus depends on the flexion angle but also on the weight bearing condition [19].

In the case presented the patient had an excellent result, without symptoms at two-year follow-up with the same preinjury level although the patient was 13 years old at the time of surgery.

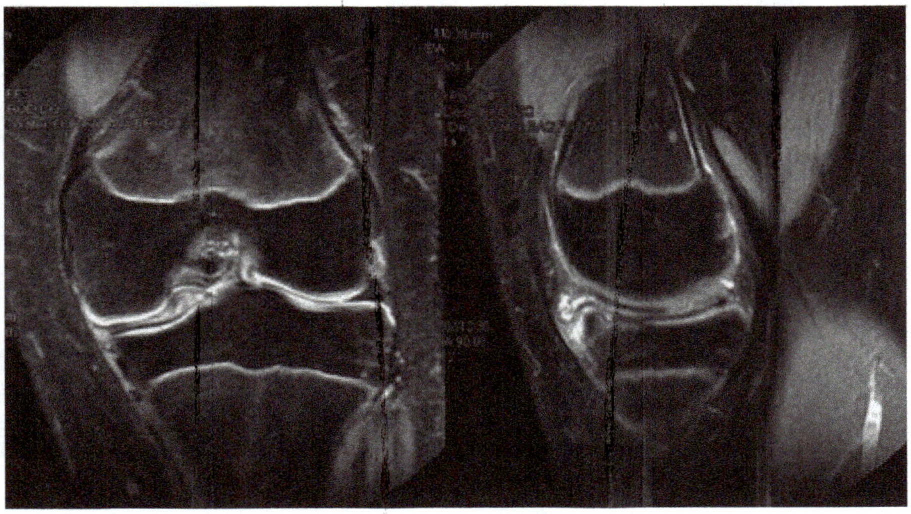

(a) (b)

FIGURE 5: MRI of the left knee. (a) Coronal view showing the upper side of the medial meniscus folded in the intercondylar notch. (b) Sagittal view demonstrating horizontal and vertical peripheral tear.

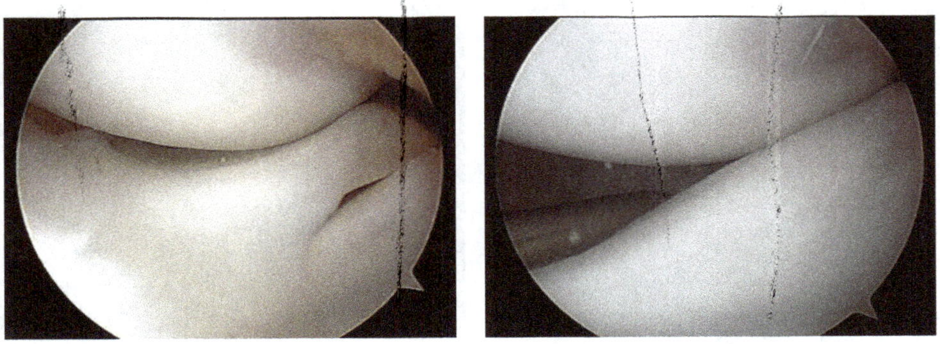

(a) (b)

FIGURE 6: Arthroscopic image of the medial femorotibial compartment of the left knee from the anterolateral portal. (a) A medial discoid meniscus is shown. (b) The upper side of the meniscus is easily displaced into the intercondylar notch with a probe.

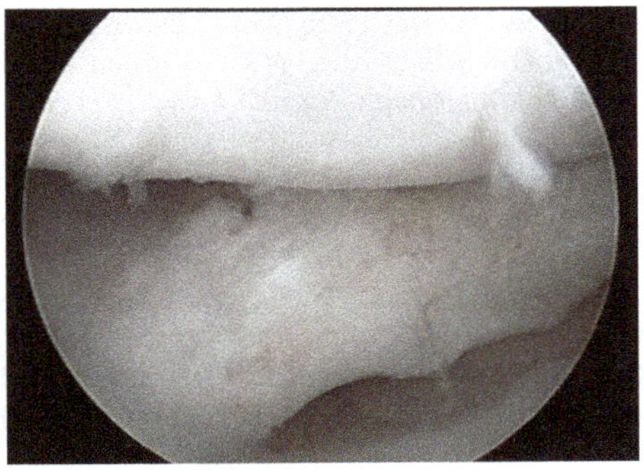

FIGURE 7: Arthroscopic image of the medial femorotibial compartment of the left knee from the anterolateral portal. Medial discoid meniscus shown after saucerization and suture.

In the MRI images done two years after the surgery for follow-up there was a reduction of menisci size and increased intensity in T2 signal. We consider that this changes could be caused by radiofrequency saucerization. Wasser et al. reported that, in 6 of the 20 symptomatic discoid meniscus they treated, on the postoperative MRI they found a high signal intensity in T2-weight signal. They considered this finding to be related to the healing process of the sutured discoid meniscus although there was no relation between neither the hypersignal and the surgery performed nor between hypersignal and clinical results [15].

4. Conclusion

There is an increasing amount of literature supporting meniscus repair as the treatment of discoid menisci tears in red zone although more long-term follow-up studies need to be done to get better evidence about this subject. The development of different surgical techniques and surgical devices has facilitated this procedure. Suture and saucerization of torn discoid menisci have yielded excellent clinical results, even

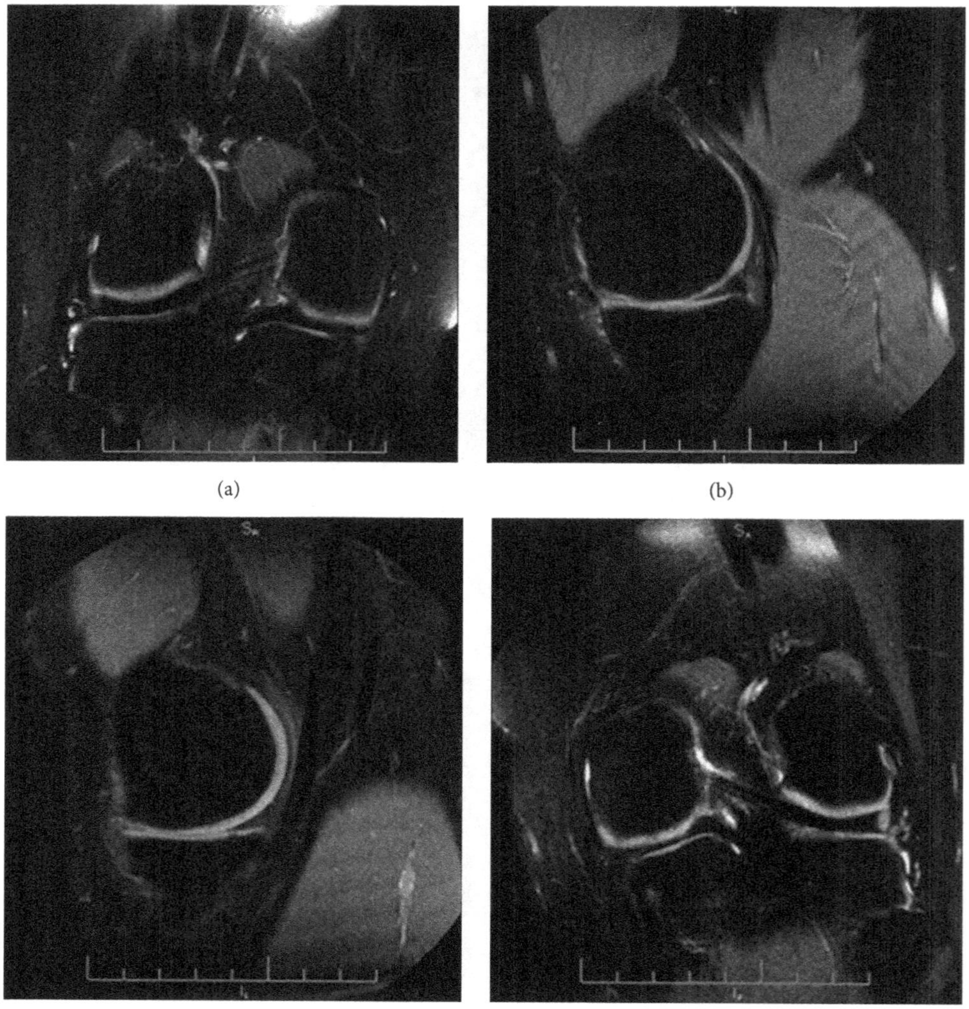

(a) (b) (c) (d)

FIGURE 8

in meniscal tears difficult to repair, when properly indicated [20]. To the best of our knowledge this is the first case published of bilateral medial discoid menisci tear treated with arthroscopic repair and saucerization in the same patient.

Disclosure

Level of evidence is IV.

Competing Interests

The authors declare that they have no competing interests.

References

[1] H. Ikeuchi, "Arthroscopic treatment of discoid lateral meniscus. Technique and long-term results," *Clinical Orthopaedics and Related Research*, vol. 167, pp. 19–28, 1982.

[2] J. M. Dickason, W. Del Pizzo, M. E. Blazina, J. M. Fox, M. J. Friedman, and S. J. Snyder, "A series of ten discoid medial menisci," *Clinical Orthopaedics and Related Research*, vol. 168, pp. 75–79, 1982.

[3] I. Kushare, K. Klingele, and W. Samora, "Discoid meniscus: diagnosis and management," *Orthopedic Clinics of North America*, vol. 46, no. 4, pp. 533–540, 2015.

[4] S. G. Kini, P. Walker, and W. Bruce, "Bilateral symptomatic discoid medial meniscus of the knee-case report and review of literature," *Archives of Trauma Research*, vol. 4, no. 1, 2015.

[5] M. Watanabe, S. Takeda, and H. Ikeuchi, Atlas of arthroscopy, 1979.

[6] M. R. Jordan, "Lateral meniscal variants: evaluation and treatment," *Journal of the American Academy of Orthopaedic Surgeons*, vol. 4, no. 4, pp. 191–200, 1996.

[7] A. Espejo-Baena, V. Urbano-Labajos, M. J. R. del Pino, and I. Peral-Infantes, "A simple device for inside-out meniscal suture," *Arthroscopy*, vol. 20, no. 8, pp. e85–e87, 2004.

[8] N. M. Patel, S. R. Cody, and T. J. Ganley, "Symptomatic bilateral discoid menisci in children: a comparison with unilaterally

symptomatic patients," *Journal of Pediatric Orthopaedics*, vol. 32, no. 1, pp. 5–8, 2012.

[9] M. E. Marchetti, D. C. Jones, D. A. Fischer, J. L. Boyd, and H. M. Fritts, "Bilateral discoid medial menisci of the knee," *The American Journal of Orthopedics*, vol. 36, no. 6, pp. 317–321, 2007.

[10] L.-X. Chen, Y.-F. Ao, J.-K. Yu et al., "Clinical features and prognosis of discoid medial meniscus," *Knee Surgery, Sports Traumatology, Arthroscopy*, vol. 21, no. 2, pp. 398–402, 2013.

[11] W. K. Auge II and C. C. Kaeding, "Bilateral discoid medial menisci with extensive intrasubstance cleavage tears: MRI and arthroscopic correlation," *Arthroscopy*, vol. 10, no. 3, pp. 313–318, 1994.

[12] R. D. Vandermeer and F. K. Cunningham, "Arthroscopic treatment of the discoid lateral meniscus: results of long-term follow-up," *Arthroscopy*, vol. 5, no. 2, pp. 101–109, 1989.

[13] O. Kose, M. Celiktas, O. F. Egerci, F. Guler, S. Ozyurek, and Y. Sarpel, "Prognostic factors affecting the outcome of arthroscopic saucerization in discoid lateral meniscus: a retrospective analysis of 48 cases," *Musculoskeletal Surgery*, vol. 99, no. 2, pp. 165–170, 2015.

[14] T. J. Fairbank, "Knee joint changes after meniscectomy," *The Journal of Bone & Joint Surgery—American Volume*, vol. 30, no. 4, pp. 664–670, 1948.

[15] L. Wasser, J. Knörr, F. Accadbled, A. Abid, and J. Sales De Gauzy, "Arthroscopic treatment of discoid meniscus in children: clinical and MRI results," *Orthopaedics and Traumatology: Surgery and Research*, vol. 97, no. 3, pp. 297–303, 2011.

[16] B. Chedal-Bornu, V. Morin, and D. Saragaglia, "Meniscoplasty for lateral discoid meniscus tears: long-term results of 14 cases," *Orthopaedics and Traumatology: Surgery and Research*, vol. 101, no. 6, pp. 699–702, 2015.

[17] W. J. Yoo, W. Y. Jang, M. S. Park et al., "Arthroscopic treatment for symptomatic discoid meniscus in children: midterm outcomes and prognostic factors," *Arthroscopy*, vol. 31, no. 12, pp. 2327–2334, 2015.

[18] R. Becker, D. Wirz, C. Wolf, B. Göpfert, W. Nebelung, and N. Friederich, "Measurement of meniscofemoral contact pressure after repair of bucket-handle tears with biodegradable implants," *Archives of Orthopaedic and Trauma Surgery*, vol. 125, no. 4, pp. 254–260, 2005.

[19] P. Johal, A. Williams, P. Wragg, D. Hunt, and W. Gedroyc, "Tibio-femoral movement in the living knee. A study of weight bearing and non-weight bearing knee kinematics using 'interventional' MRI," *Journal of Biomechanics*, vol. 38, no. 2, pp. 269–276, 2005.

[20] J. H. Ahn, S. H. Lee, J. C. Yoo, Y. S. Lee, and H. C. Ha, "Arthroscopic partial meniscectomy with repair of the peripheral tear for symptomatic discoid lateral meniscus in children: results of minimum 2 years of follow-up," *Arthroscopy*, vol. 24, no. 8, pp. 888–898, 2008.

36

Valgus Slipped Capital Femoral Epiphysis in Patient with Hypopituitarism

Yoshihiro Kotoura,[1] Yasuhiro Fujiwara,[1] Tatsuro Hayashida,[1] Koji Murakami,[1] Satoshi Makio,[1] Yuichi Shimizu,[1] Yoshinobu Oka,[2] Wook-Choel Kim,[2] Taku Ogura,[1] and Toshikazu Kubo[2]

[1] *Department of Orthopaedic Surgery, Nantan General Hospital, Nantan, Japan*
[2] *Department of Orthopaedics, Graduate School of Medical Science, Kyoto Prefectural University of Medicine, Kyoto, Japan*

Correspondence should be addressed to Yoshihiro Kotoura; ykotoura@gmail.com

Academic Editor: Hitesh N. Modi

Slipped capital femoral epiphysis (SCFE) is a common disease of adolescent and the epiphysis is positioned more posteromedially in relation to the femoral neck shaft with varus SCFE; however, posterolateral displacement of the capital epiphysis, valgus SCFE, occurs less frequently. We report a case of valgus SCFE in a 17-year-old boy with hypopituitarism. After falling down, he experienced difficulty in walking. The radiographs were inconclusive; however three-dimensional computed tomography images showed lateral displacement of the epiphysis on the right femoral head. Valgus SCFE was diagnosed. The patient underwent in situ pinning of both sides. In situ pinning on the left side was performed as a prophylactic pinning because of endocrine abnormalities. At the 1-year follow-up, he could walk without any difficulty and there were no signs of pain. The epiphysis is commonly positioned more posteromedially in relation to the femoral neck shaft with most SCFE, but, in this case, the epiphysis slipped laterally. Differential diagnosis included femoral neck fracture (Delbet-Colonna type 1); however, this was less likely due to the absence of other clinical signs. Therefore, we diagnosed the patient as SCFE. When children complain of leg pain and limp, valgus SCFE that may not be visualized on anteroposterior radiographs needs to be considered.

1. Introduction

Acute posttraumatic limp is a common reason for children's hospitalization; however the diagnosis is not always easy for trauma physicians, because sometimes the signs are not specific and its diagnostic images are unclear. Many of these causes are not dangerous, but sometimes there are conditions requiring more serious treatment. One of these conditions is slipped capital femoral epiphysis (SCFE) and the treatment is emergent. SCFE is a common disease of adolescent and the epiphysis is usually positioned more posteromedially in relation to the femoral neck shaft with varus SCFE. Varus SCFE is not uncommon; however posterolateral displacement of the capital epiphysis, valgus SCFE, is uncommon. A definitive diagnosis can be difficult but there should be a high degree of clinical suspicion. We report a case of valgus SCFE in a 17-year-old boy with hypopituitarism.

2. Case Report

The patient was a 17-year-old boy with hypopituitarism, autism, and a history of septooptic dysplasia with whom communication was difficult. He was receiving treatment with dexamethasone 100 μg and Levothyroxine sodium 1 mg per day. One month before admission, he experienced a fall, which resulted in difficulty in walking. At the first visit to the physician, because he could not describe any symptoms, only knee radiography was performed and there were no abnormalities. The pain in his right leg progressively worsened and he presented to our outpatient clinic after one month.

On physical examination, the patient was slightly obese with a height of 161 cm and weight of 63 kg noted. His right leg was externally rotated, and he hesitated to stand up. The passive range of motion of the right hip was limited, especially in

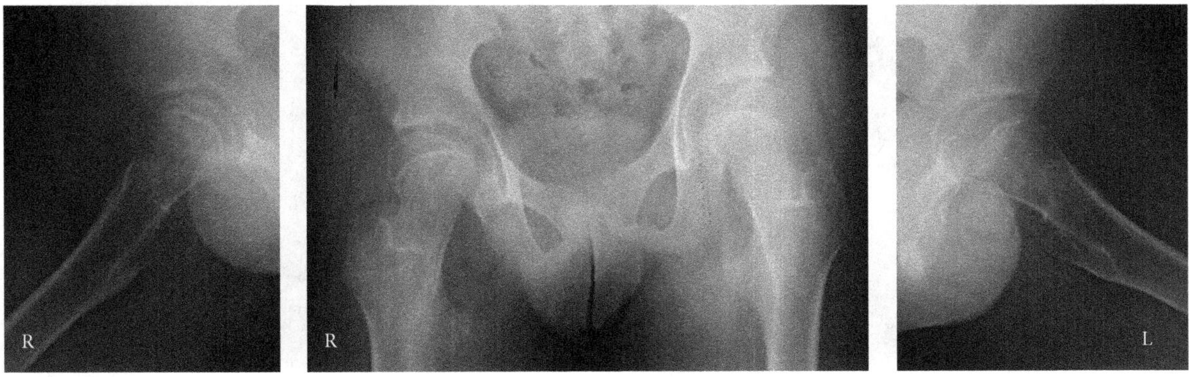

FIGURE 1: (a) Frog-lateral radiograph of the right hip joint showing almost normal. (b) Anteroposterior radiograph of the right hip joint showing lateral displacement of the right epiphysis and valgus neck shaft angles bilaterally. (c) Frog-lateral radiograph of left hip showing normal.

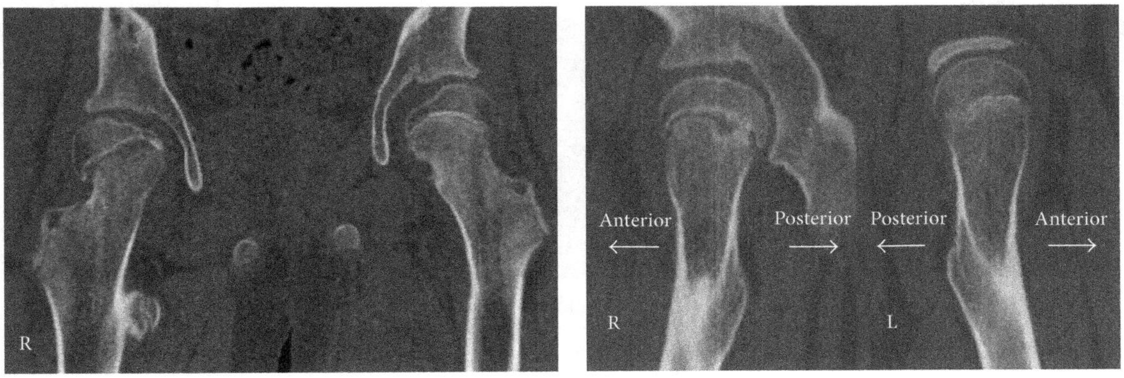

FIGURE 2: Reconstruction coronal (a) and sagittal (b) CT images of the right hip showing lateral displacement of the epiphysis.

adduction and internal rotation (right/left; flexion 90°/120°, extension 10°/10°, abduction 45°/45°, adduction 0°/30°, external rotation 60°/45°, and internal rotation 10°/30°). Serum insulin-like growth factor-1 and insulin-like growth factor-binding protein 3 levels were low, but free triiodothyronine, free thyroxine, and adrenocorticotropic hormone levels were almost normal. The radiographs of the hip joints showed a right atypical slippage of the epiphysis (Figure 1). Both neck shaft angles were large (right/left; 160°/155°) and lateral tilts of the physis were normal on intact side (right/left; 35° lateral/13° medial). Three-dimensional computed tomography (3D CT) images showed lateral epiphyseal displacement on the right femoral head (Figures 2 and 3), indicating valgus SCFE.

The patient underwent in situ pinning of the hip on both sides. On the right side, the procedure was performed through a limited 5 cm longitudinal incision, positioned medially on the thigh (frog position), posterior to the femoral neurovascular bundle. A single φ5.5 mm partially threaded cannulated screw (Meira, Japan) was placed across the physis. In situ pinning on the left side was performed as a prophylactic pinning because of endocrine abnormalities (Figure 4). Postoperatively, we had difficulty in limiting weight bearing due to communication difficulties.

One month after surgery, he could walk better than before the operation. At the 1-year follow-up, he could walk without difficulty and there were no signs of pain. The passive range of motion of the right hip joint was slightly improved in flexion, adduction, and internal rotation (100°, 20°, and 20°, resp.). Radiographs showed no signs of avascular necrosis or chondrolysis of the epiphysis; the physis showed no signs of early partial closure.

3. Discussion

SCFE is an adolescent hip disorder. Clinically, the patient with SCFE may have hip pain, thigh pain or knee pain, an acute or insidious onset of a limp, and decrease of the range of motion of the hip. The condition is associated with obesity and growth surge and it is occasionally associated with endocrine disorders such as hypothyroidism, growth hormone deficiency, hypopituitarism, and hyperparathyroidism. In most SCFE cases, the capital femoral epiphysis is displaced

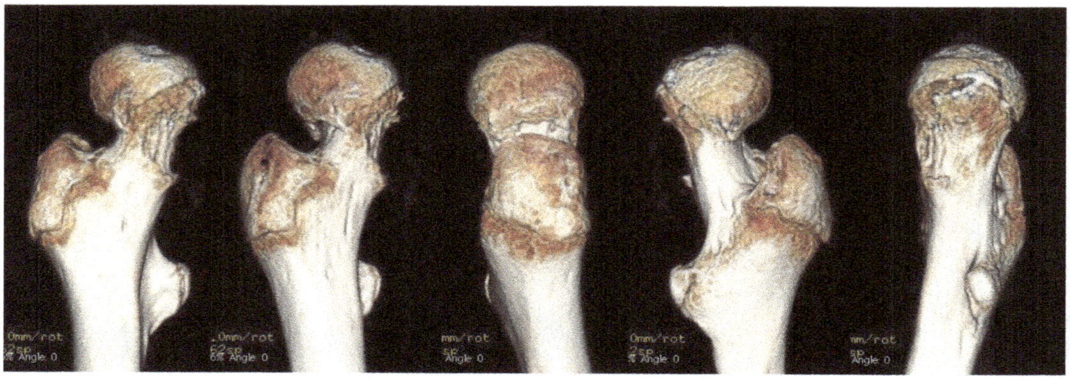

FIGURE 3: 3D CT images showed the right epiphyseal displacement was laterally.

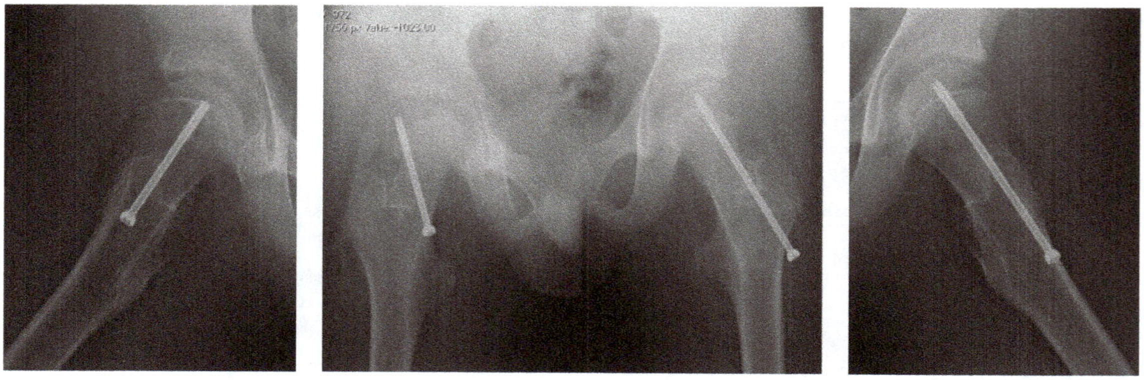

(a) (b) (c)

FIGURE 4: Postoperative (a) frog-lateral radiograph of the right hip joint. (b) Anteroposterior radiograph showing the screw for the valgus SCFE was placed more medially than for a typical varus SCFE. (c) Frog-lateral radiograph of the left hip joint.

posterior and medial relative to the femoral neck. The medial displacement shows a varus appearance on anteroposterior radiographs. Lateral displacement of the femoral head is a rare case and is referred to as "valgus" SCFE. Müller first described valgus SCFE in 1926 [1]. Fewer than 100 cases have been reported to date, and these case reports have not described the specific criteria [2] used in the diagnosis of valgus SCFE. Loder et al. estimated the prevalence of valgus slip to be 1.9% by taking into account all the reported cases in literature until 2006 [3]. This indicated approximately 1-2% of all idiopathic SCFE cases were probably due to a valgus slip. Yngve et al. reported that the valgus neck shaft angles and lateral tilt of the physis were risk factors for valgus SCFE [4]. According to the report by Loder et al., there were significant differences between valgus and varus SCFE for symptom duration, body mass index, and sex: 76% of valgus SCFE occurred in girls [5].

The delayed skeletal maturation is a common finding in endocrine disorders and the risk factor for SCFE. According to the report by Loder et al., 5.2 to 6.9% of patients with SCFE are associated with endocrine disorders [6]. They assessed 85 patients with SCFE and known endocrine disorders. The most common primary endocrine diagnosis was hypothyroidism in 34 patients (40%) and growth hormone deficiency in 21 patients (25%) and 30 patients (35%) had other endocrinopathies such as hypogonadism, hypopituitarism, hyperparathyroidism, and growth hormone excess. Yngve et al. reported on the association between endocrine disorders and valgus SCFE, 2 patients with underdeveloped genitalia and 1 with panhypopituitarism in a series of 7 patients with valgus patients [4]. In a review by Shank et al., four of the 12 valgus patients suffered from panhypopituitarism and they indicated the association between hypopituitarism and valgus SCFE [2]. In this case, the valgus neck shaft angles and hypopituitarism resulting in growth hormone deficiency and hypothyroidism were consistent with those previously reported.

The Klein line has been reported to be an early indicator of varus SCFE. Klein et al. used the line along the superior aspect of the femoral neck as an index of SCFE [7]. In valgus SCFE, however, the line will always be normal and this has emphasized the need for lateral radiographs to be performed in all children with hip pain [3]. In our case, the Klein line was normal on anteroposterior radiograph. In addition, the lateral view was almost normal on lateral radiograph. 3D CT images were helpful and clearly showed that the direction of the epiphyseal displacement was laterally. Venkatadass et al. reported that 3D CT images showed slippage direction of the femoral head and needed for appropriate treatment selection [8]. Differential diagnoses included femoral neck fracture (Delbet-Colonna type 1 [9]) and coxofemoral dysplasia; however these were less likely because of the patient's age and absence of other clinical signs.

Segal et al. have described the importance of appropriate screw placement when considering treatment options [10]. In a valgus slip, the slippage is further posterior and hence the entry point for the screw must be more medial [8]. Both Segal and Loder reported that the proximity of the neurovascular bundle increases the risk associated with the medial approach and recommended an open surgery to protect the neurovascular structures. In this case, a mini-incision, which was positioned medially on the thigh (frog position), was performed. We also used in situ pinning through the medial femoral metaphysis. During surgery, a three-dimensional imaging system (ARCADIS Orbic 3D®, Siemens, Munich, Germany) was used to visualize the direction of slippage and to guide the appropriate placement of screws.

In conclusion, acute posttraumatic limp and leg pain in the adolescent boy was diagnosed as valgus SCFE. It might be associated with valgus neck shaft angles and endocrine disorders. 3D CT images were useful in establishing diagnosis. For appropriate and safe in situ pinning, we made a limited open incision and used three-dimensional imaging system to protect the femoral neurovascular bundle. When children complain of leg pain, valgus SCFE which may not be visualized on anteroposterior radiographs needs to be considered.

Competing Interests

Each author certifies that he has no commercial associations (e.g., consultancies, stock ownership, equity interest, and patent/licensing arrangements) that might pose a conflict of interest in connection with the submitted manuscript.

Acknowledgments

The authors are deeply grateful to Dr. Joseph Oxendine and Dr. Asako Oxendine for their great support of this study. And they express gratitude to their families for the moral support and warm encouragement.

References

[1] W. Müller, "Die Entstehung von Coxa valga durch Epiphysenverschiebung," *Beitrage Zur Klinischen Chirurgie*, vol. 137, pp. 148–164, 1926.

[2] C. F. Shank, E. J. Thiel, and K. E. Klingele, "Valgus slipped capital femoral epiphysis: prevalence, presentation, and treatment options," *Journal of Pediatric Orthopaedics*, vol. 30, no. 2, pp. 140–146, 2010.

[3] R. T. Loder, P. W. O'Donnell, W. P. Didelot, and K. J. Kayes, "Valgus slipped capital femoral epiphysis," *Journal of Pediatric Orthopaedics*, vol. 26, no. 5, pp. 594–600, 2006.

[4] D. A. Yngve, D. L. Moulton, and E. B. Evans, "Valgus slipped capital femoral epiphysis," *Journal of Pediatric Orthopaedics Part B*, vol. 14, no. 3, pp. 172–176, 2005.

[5] P. Koczewski, "Valgus slipped capital femoral epiphysis: subcapital growth plate orientation analysis," *Journal of Pediatric Orthopaedics B*, vol. 22, no. 6, pp. 548–552, 2013.

[6] R. T. Loder, B. Wittenberg, and G. DeSilva, "Slipped capital femoral epiphysis associated with endocrine disorders," *Journal of Pediatric Orthopaedics*, vol. 15, no. 3, pp. 349–356, 1995.

[7] A. Klein, R. J. Joplin, J. A. Reidy, and J. Hanelin, "Slipped capital femoral epiphysis; early diagnosis and treatment facilitated by normal roentgenograms," *The Journal of Bone and Joint Surgery*, vol. 34, no. 1, pp. 233–239, 1952.

[8] K. Venkatadass, A. P. Shetty, and S. Rajasekaran, "Valgus slipped capital femoral epiphysis: report of two cases and a comprehensive review of literature," *Journal of Pediatric Orthopaedics Part B*, vol. 20, no. 5, pp. 291–294, 2011.

[9] P. C. Colonna, "Fracture of the neck of the femur in childhood," *Annals of Surgery*, vol. 88, no. 5, pp. 902–907, 1928.

[10] L. S. Segal, P. P. Weitzel, and R. S. Davidson, "Valgus slipped capital femoral epiphysis. Fact or fiction?" *Clinical Orthopaedics and Related Research*, no. 322, pp. 91–98, 1996.

37

INFIX/EXFIX: Massive Open Pelvic Injuries and Review of the Literature

Rahul Vaidya,[1,2] Kerellos Nasr,[1] Enrique Feria-Arias,[1] Rebecca Fisher,[2] Marvin Kajy,[2] and Lawrence N. Diebel[2]

[1]*Detroit Medical Center, 4D University Health Center, Detroit Receiving Hospital, 4201 Street Antoine Boulevard, Detroit, MI 48201, USA*
[2]*4D University Health Center, Detroit Receiving Hospital, Wayne State University, 4201 Street Antoine Boulevard, Detroit, MI 48201, USA*

Correspondence should be addressed to Rahul Vaidya; rvaidya@dmc.org

Academic Editor: Arul Ramasamy

Introduction. Open pelvic fractures make up 2–5% of all pelvic ring injuries. Their mortality has been reported to be as high as 50%. During Operation Enduring Freedom protocols for massive open pelvic injuries lead to the survival of injuries once thought to be fatal. The INFIX is a subcutaneous anterior fixator for pelvic stabilization which is stronger than external fixation. The purpose of this paper is to describe the use of INFIX and modern algorithms for massive open pelvic injuries. *Methods*. An IRB approved retrospective review describes 4 cases in civilian practice with massive open pelvic injuries. We also review the modern literature on open pelvic injures. *Discussion*. Key components in the care of massive open pelvic injuries include hemorrhage control by clamping of the aorta or REBOA when necessary and fecal/urinary diversion. The INFIX can be used internally, as a partial INFIX partial EXFIX, or as an EXFIX. Its low profile allows for easy application of wound vacs and wound care and when subcutaneous avoids pin tract infections. *Conclusion*. Massive open pelvic injuries are a difficult problem. Following modern protocols can help prevent mortality.

1. Introduction

Open pelvic fractures make up 2–5% [1–6] of all pelvic ring injuries and their mortality has been reported to be as high as 50% [1, 2, 7–9].

One of the most complex open pelvic fracture injury patterns is the high-energy improvised explosive device blast suffered by a dismounted soldier presenting with traumatic bilateral lower extremity amputations including pelvic and perineal involvement. During Operation Enduring Freedom protocols for the care of these individuals lead to survival of injuries once thought to be fatal [10]. These lessons have advanced the care of massive open pelvic fractures and extremity injuries and can be applied to civilian injuries as well.

The INFIX is an Anterior Subcutaneous Pelvic Fixation Device which is biomechanically stronger than an external fixator due to its internal profile, has the advantage of improved patient comfort/mobility, eliminates pin tract infections, and can serve as temporary and then definitive fixation once the posterior pelvis is stabilized [11–17]. We think this is the ideal tool for stabilization out of war and disaster zones where temporary stabilization often remains the method of treatment for several weeks or as definitive treatment. It can be used as an INFIX, as a partial INFIX partial EXFIX (INFIX/EXFIX), and as an EXFIX as it is biomechanically stronger than a 2-pin supra-acetabular EXFIX due to its low profile [15, 18].

The purpose of this paper is to describe (1) the use of pelvic INFIX in complex open pelvic injuries; (2) the use of a complex open pelvic fracture protocol developed in OEF in civilian practice; and (3) review the literature for open pelvic injuries.

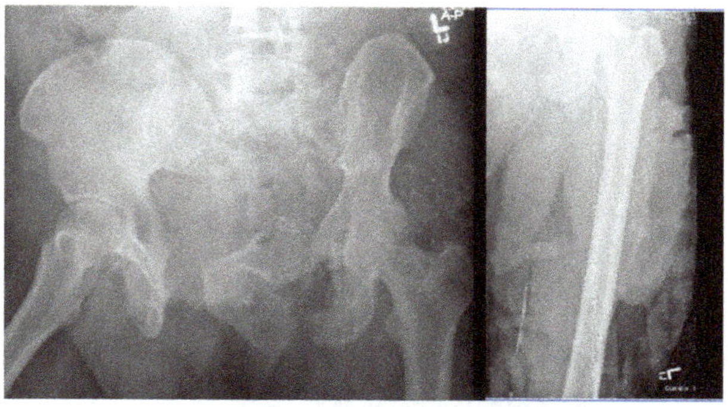

FIGURE 1: (Case 1) 41 yo male crushed by fork lift. APC 3 massive open pelvic ring injury and mangled left lower extremity arrived in extremis. The left leg with a vascular injury was debrided, had an above knee amputation, and eventually resulted in a hip disarticulation.

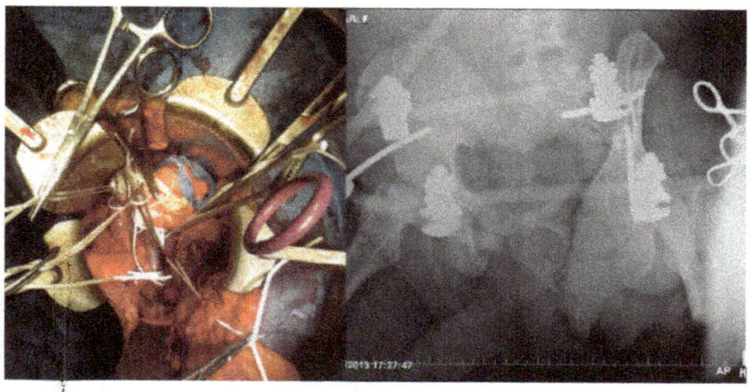

FIGURE 2: Laparotomy was performed where intra-abdominal bleeding was controlled and then the aorta and IVC clamped low in the abdomen to stop the blood loss from his pelvis and left lower extremity.

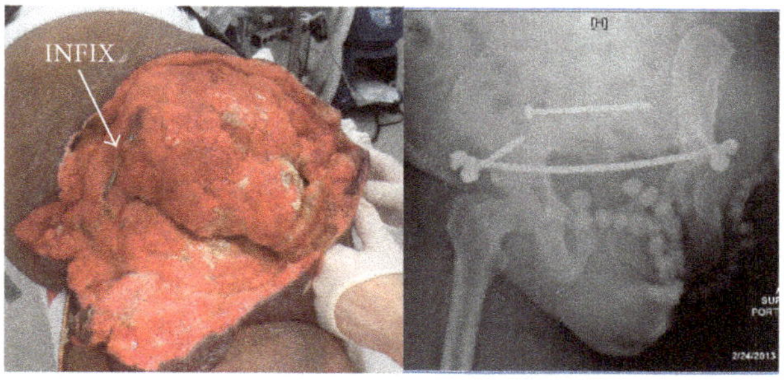

FIGURE 3: INFIX/EXFIX, as well as a percutaneous SI joint screw to stabilize the pelvis then antibiotic beads and wound vacs to combat the soft tissue injury.

2. Methods

An IRB approved retrospective study was performed on 4 open pelvic fractures that had significant soft tissue injury. All were treated by the ATLS protocol, pelvic INFIX device, and laparotomy with control of the vessels to the lower limbs when indicated. Two case examples are given. We also reviewed the available literature on open pelvic fractures and with regard to acute care; initial surgical procedure; hemorrhage control; soft tissue care; bowel injury; urogenital injuries; definitive pelvic stabilization; and the INFIX device.

3. Case Examples

3.1. Case 1. A 41-year-old healthy male was crushed by a fork-lift and brought to our ER in hemorrhagic shock. He suffered a massive open injury to his left leg and pelvis (Figure 1). ATLS protocol was followed, the massive transfusion protocol was activated, and a pelvic binder applied for his APC 3 pelvic injury. He was transferred to the OR for intra-abdominal bleeding identified on FAST exam and a lack of response to transfusion. A laparotomy was performed where intra-abdominal bleeding was eventually controlled and then the aorta and IVC were clamped low in the abdomen to stop the bleeding from his pelvis and left lower extremity. During this time the left leg wound was debrided and irrigated, and it was realized that a high above knee amputation was required as the leg was nonviable. A pelvic EXFIX was placed, and the patient was given a high diverting colostomy. Urology placed a suprapubic catheter and removed an avulsed devascularized left testicle. Once the vessels were ligated distally, the aorta and vena cava were released (Figure 2). He was transferred to the ICU. He received 31 units of PRBC, 18 units of FFP, 25 units of platelets, and 5 units of cryoprecipitate over the first 24 hrs and stabilized hemodynamically.

The patient underwent serial debridement because of ongoing and progressive tissue necrosis in the stump, treated with negative pressure wound vacs and antibiotic beads. The above-the-knee amputation was converted to a hip disarticulation but the patient still had a massive wound over his pelvis and his lower abdomen. The wound vacs were difficult to apply with the external fixator and the pelvis was still relatively unstable so the external fixator was removed and reduction of his pelvic ring injury was performed with a subcutaneous anterior internal fixator, as well as one percutaneous SI joint screw (Figure 3). This presented somewhat a challenge given the extent of the patient's open wounds on the left hemipelvis leaving part of the internal fixator exposed to air on the left side. The construct stabilized the injury and the low profile of the INFIX allowed easy application of the wound vac.

The wound and patient stabilized, and skin grafts were applied to the defect once good granulation tissue was apparent around the pelvic INFIX (Figure 4).

The patient underwent removal of his suprapubic catheter and eventual reanastomosis of the bowel once all the wounds had healed. He was fortunate to have functional return of his urethra.

The traumatized area under the skin grafts has had formation of heterotopic bone which required removal on 2 occasions due to pain with prosthetic fitting. This is finally underway 2 years after the injury.

3.2. Case 2. This is a 62-year-old male who was involved in a motor vehicle accident. His open injury was missed initially when he arrived in extremis and developed a massive pelvic

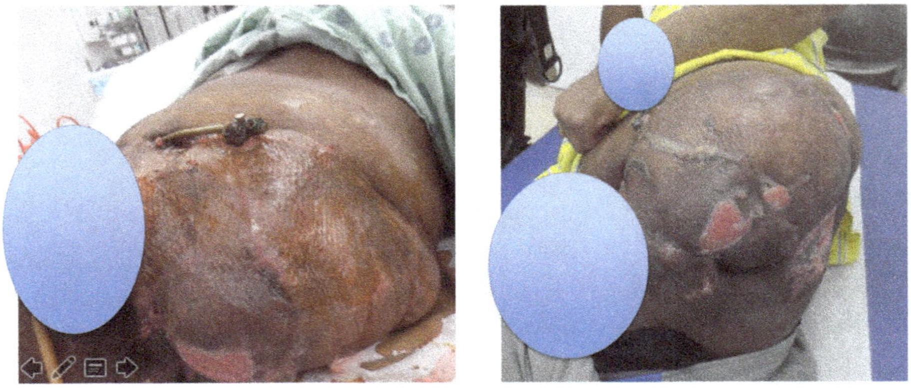

(a) (b)

FIGURE 4: (a) Wound healing and (b) the fixator removed.

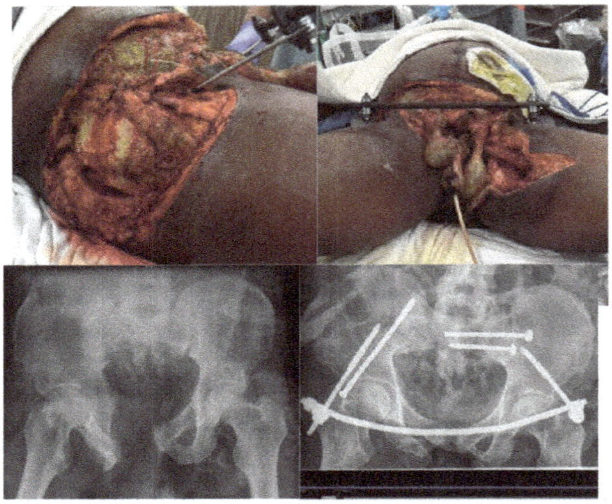

FIGURE 5: This is a 62-year-old male who was involved in a motor vehicle accident. His open injury was missed initially when he arrived in extremis and developed a massive pelvic soft tissue infection requiring debridement over the first 3 days.

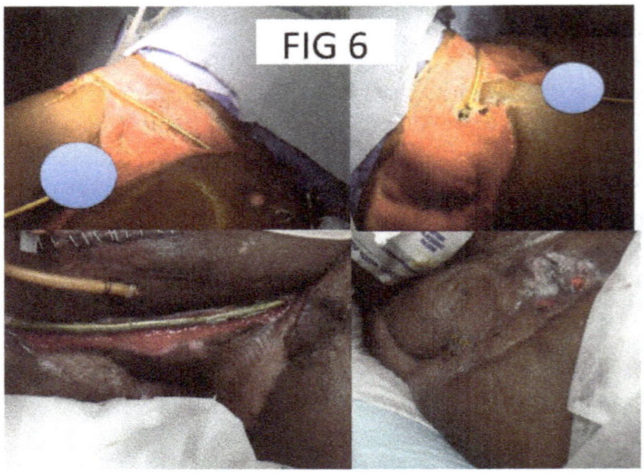

FIGURE 6: After fixation bowel and urinary diversion and wound management.

soft tissue infection requiring debridement over the first 3 days. He had a colostomy, superpubic catheter, percutaneous reduction of his iliac wing, SI screws, and an anterior INFIX. His testicles were implanted under the medial thigh and he had extensive wound care (Figures 5 and 6). This was followed by a long ICU course and dressing changes daily. The wound granulated in and the INFIX was removed once we felt that there was adequate healing (5 months). The patient had skin grafts and still has a colostomy.

3.3. Case 3. A 23 yo male was involved in an MVA where his pelvis was impaled by a pole. ATLS protocol was initiated and he was taken emergently to the OR to stabilize his bleeding. The aorta was clamped, the pelvis packed and antishock SI screws with a EXFIX using low profile INFIX implants were applied, and a colostomy was performed. The aorta was released and right iliac vessel ligated but bleeding persisted despite packing and angiography. The patient was given a massive transfusion with 30 PRBC's 25 units platelets and 30 u plasma but expired on POD #3 in the ICU due to head injury and ARDS.

3.4. Case 4. A 21 yo male was involved in a motorcycle accident where he hit his perineum hard on the motorcycle gas tank and suffered an APC 3 injury with herniation of his bowels. He was hemodynamically stable after ATLS protocol with resuscitation. He went to the OR for an I and D, a colostomy, suprapubic urinary catheter, and stabilization of his pelvis with an INFIX and SI screws. He did well postoperatively and at latest follow-up had his colostomy reconnected and urethra reconstructed (see Table 1).

4. Discussion

Pelvic fractures are a major cause of mortality among trauma patients. These fractures often result from a high-energy

Table 1: Case summaries.

Case	Injury	General surgery	Urology	Orthopaedics	Outcome
1 41 yo forklift- crush ISS 20	APC 3 massive open injury Crushed pelvis Extremis	Pelvic packing, temporary Aortic control clamp, colostomy	Suprapubic, orchiectomy	INFIX/EXFIX posterior SI screw, hip disarticulation	Survived to prosthetic fitting, bowel hooked up, Complication with heterotopic bone prosthetic fitting
2 62 yo MVA ISS 18	LC3 open Massive anterior open injury Extremis	Colostomy, debridement, implanted testicles in thigh	Suprapubic	INFIX/EXFIX, iliac screw posterior SI screws	Wound healed, pelvis healed, skin healing
3 21 yo MVA pelvis impaled by a pole ISS 45	APC3 open Massive anterior and posterior wounds, extremis	Colostomy, aortic control clamp packing	Suprapubic	INFIX antishock SI screws	Patient died in ICU POD #3 Rt tibia open fx, Rib fx pneumothorax bilateral pulmonary contusion
4 21 yo MVA motorcycle ISS 18	APC3 massive perineal wound with bowel hernia	Colostomy laparotomy	Suprapubic catheter	INFIX SI screws	Survived hooked up doing fine

trauma and cause injury to other parts of the body. Associated injuries are therefore common and may affect outcomes in patients with a pelvic fracture. Mortality in patients sustaining pelvic fractures has been reported to be 4–15% [19–24]. Early deaths are attributed to hemorrhage or injuries of the central nervous system, and delayed deaths are reportedly due to sepsis and multiple organ failure [8, 25–29]. Various risk factors for mortality have been observed including increasing age, shock on initial presentation (as defined by a systolic blood pressure <90 mmHg) [19, 20, 23, 25, 27, 30, 31], severity of associated injuries [20, 24, 32, 33], and open pelvic fractures. Open pelvic fractures make up 2–5% [1–6] of all pelvic ring injuries and their mortality rate has been reported to be as high as 50% [1, 2, 7–9]. Mortality is usually related to the same causes as closed pelvic fractures. Over the last 30 years, the mortality rate from pelvic fractures has decreased due to the implementation of multidisciplinary protocols, improved hemorrhage management [27], identification of open injuries, advances in critical care medicine, aggressive fracture management, and early fecal/urinary diversion for open pelvic injuries.

5. The Initial Surgical Procedure Open Pelvic Fracture

Hemorrhage control, surgical debridement, and pelvic volume reduction plus stabilization are the priorities of the index operation. Secondary priorities are stabilization of long bone fractures through external fixation, bladder repair, potential colonic diversion, and irrigation and debridement of open injuries. A multidisciplinary team approach using general, orthopaedic, and urologic surgeons working simultaneously is the most effective method for care of these unstable patients. Emergency pelvic stabilization can be accomplished with a pelvic binder in the trauma bay, which should be converted intraoperatively to an anterior external frame or c-clamp in centers that utilize this device. The patients require massive transfusions with packed red blood cells, plasma, and platelets in what has deemed to be the optimum ratio of 1 : 1 : 1.

6. Hemorrhage Control

Hemorrhage control is accomplished by laparotomy where intra-abdominal bleeding is present. When bleeding is not controlled with these maneuvers, the addition of retroperitoneal pelvic packing (if this expertise is available) is indicated [34, 35]. With communication to the outside (open injury), the bleeding often continues as there is no contained compartment. At this point a decision needs to be made whether or not to clamp or ligate the internal iliac artery, clamp the aorta [10], or use Resuscitative Endovascular Balloon Occlusion of the Aorta (REBOA) [36]. In patients with severe open pelvic or abdominal injuries, temporizing proximal vascular control of the iliac vessels or aorta via a celiotomy or the retroperitoneal approach is an option. The final level of vascular control is a balance of preventing exsanguination and still advancing temporary vascular control to the most distal and viable level. This is critically important in cases requiring hip disarticulation or hemipelvectomy [10], where it is difficult to control bleeding more distally as the vessels often retract into the pelvis.

Angiography and embolization have been shown to be highly effective but should be reserved for those patients who continue to bleed after laparotomy and the index surgical procedure. In institutions where pelvic packing expertise is not yet available, it is the next step after laparotomy and temporary pelvic fixation. If laparotomy is not indicated, angiography is the next step after reduction of pelvic volume with a binder, external fixation, or c-clamp. Angiography may be time consuming and is only useful for arterial bleeding [37].

Once bleeding control is achieved other surgical procedures can proceed.

7. Soft Tissue Care

Adequate index surgical debridement is a critical step in preventing later risks of infection. Systematic sharp debridement of all foreign material, nonviable skin, subcutaneous tissue, fascia, periosteum, and bone is performed back to viable, healthy tissue. Subsequently a meticulous washout, possibly utilizing the pulsed lavage technique, is necessary [10, 37–39]. This is followed either by open wound treatment or vacuum sealed dressings, which allow adequate drainage of the wound. It is important to note that with large fresh wounds the use of a wound vac can lead to excessive hemorrhage. We often refrain from using these devices until the second I and D procedure and once bleeding has stopped. One can expect to be involved in multiple debridement as tissue ischemia continues to evolve over several days. Daily or every second day serial debridement may be necessary [10].

In massive injuries, where amputation of a leg is necessary, one can harvest skin from the amputated extremity for later use. Healthy flaps of skin, subcutaneous tissue, and muscle are kept as attached flaps for later coverage. Wounds can be closed at a later time by delayed primary closure. If the wounds are clean, they can be closed by secondary intention and covered with STSG or rotational myocutaneous flaps.

8. Bowel Injury

Early diverting colostomy or ileostomy and distal rectal washout of residual faeces has been the widely accepted treatment for all open pelvic fractures [37]. It has significantly reduced infective complications and consequently reduced mortality [4, 38–41]. Fecal diversion is preferably performed as a loop but can also be performed as an end colostomy [4, 38–41]. Potential sites of subsequent orthopaedic incisions, external fixator pins, and suprapubic cystostomy should be borne in mind when locating the stoma [1, 42]. Open perineal wounds involving the rectum require fecal diversion with early sphincter repair and local open wound management [43, 44].

9. Urogenital Injuries

If there is any evidence of urethral injury or a positive cystourethrogram, a suprapubic Foley catheter needs to be inserted during the index procedure to ensure the diversion of urine. This is to prevent sepsis from infected urine and to monitor flow for resuscitation. Realignment of the urethra can be accomplished if the patient is stable and the expertise is available; otherwise once diversion is accomplished, realignment can wait [45]. This is accomplished with fluoroscopy or urethroscopy, and both antegrade imaging and retrograde imaging are required to realign the urethra prior to passing a Foley catheter. Reduction of the anterior pelvic ring is helpful for urethral realignment [37].

Intraperitoneal bladder ruptures should be repaired early while extraperitoneal bladder ruptures can be diverted or repaired. In complicated extraperitoneal bladder ruptures (if the patient is stable and the expertise is available) immediate repair may be important especially if an anterior fracture has to be instrumented. These are recommendations by the American Urological Society based on the available evidence [45].

In vaginal lacerations, early definitive repair of the lesion with absorbable sutures is recommended in order to prevent abscess formations. Care must be taken to close the tear while not injuring the uterine arteries, which lie along the lateral borders of the vaginal vault [37, 38].

Scrotal and perineal lacerations should be debrided and irrigated. Like other soft tissue injuries, they can be closed if the wound beds are good. Evaluation of testicular viability should be performed by the urologic or general surgeon [45]. When there is lack of soft tissue coverage, they can be implanted under viable areas like the inner thigh until coverage is possible.

10. Definitive Pelvic Stabilization

Eventually the pelvic ring has to be reconstructed in a patient who is now stable and has survived the initial trauma using damage control orthopaedics. The principles of fixation are the same as for closed fractures except for the soft tissue injury [37, 39, 44]. Posterior fixation can be placed percutaneously after reduction using sacroiliac screws and lumbopelvic fixation for comminuted posterior injuries. Iliac wing fractures can be fixed with plates and screws if soft tissue allows, as external and percutaneous options are not as effective. The anterior pelvic ring, where most soft tissue injuries occur, can be stabilized with definitive external fixation [37, 39, 44] or an anterior internal fixator which we have used as an INFIX/EXFIX. In massive injuries this facilitates the use of vacuum assisted closure techniques as the INFIX can be completely covered with this [11].

The pelvic INFIX was developed for indications where anterior external fixation is commonly used [11]. We feel it is a good replacement for any anterior fixation where one might otherwise use a plate, an EXFIX, or ramus screws [11–18]. It is made with custom pedicle screws (long lengths 80–120 mm) of 7 or 8 mm diameter and sits under the skin in an area we call the "Bikini Line" [13]. It is more stiff than an anterior external fixator [15, 18] that allows patients increased mobility and is particularly useful in obese patients [17]. We have found it particularly useful in conjunction with a laparotomy, in combination with internal fixation as an acetabular fracture, and feel it could be important in patient transportation with pelvic injuries as external fixation pins get infected when left in place for 2 weeks or longer. The INFIX can be loosened allowing definitive reduction and fixation for the posterior pelvic injury and then reused to stabilize the anterior pelvis definitively. We have used this device as an internal fixator, INFIX/EXFIX, partially covered and partially exposed as we have demonstrated in this paper, and as an external fixator when there is no soft tissue coverage. Its low profile makes it much stiffer than an external fixator and it is easy to cover under a wound vac when needed. Originally we did not use INFIX during damage control as the parts were not readily available so we converted external fixators to INFIXs when necessary.

However as sets become available or as in our case we have an INFIX set in our OR, we often will do an INFIX as the index and definitive procedure. We recommend the use of INFIX with the appropriate posterior fixation and have only used it as a standalone device during transport or on certain APC2 injuries with symphyseal disruption.

The complications of INFIX have been previously described and include heterotopic ossification which is usually asymptomatic and implant loosening or failure which is rare and often related to technique [17]. Lateral femoral nerve irritation is common but often goes away once the implant is removed [17]. There have been reports of femoral nerve palsy with the INFIX procedure [46]. We have not seen it in our series and feel it is related to sinking the screws too far into the bone. The ideal scenario is to leave the rod very superficial and fix the pedicle screw height so that the rod sits right at pedicle screw head level. The technique is freely available as a video at the OTA video gallery online [47].

11. Conclusion

Hemorrhage control in massive open pelvic fractures can be difficult because of communication to the outside. Bleeding may continue after pelvic volume is reduced and the pelvis stabilized as there is no contained compartment. Clamping of the aorta or REBOA may be necessary. Early recognition of the open injury with fecal/urinary diversion has resulted in increased survival. The INFIX is a tool to stabilize the pelvis which is stronger than anterior external fixation. Its low profile allows for easy application of wound vacs for wound care, can hold the pelvic stable, and when placed internally for transport avoids infected pin tracks.

Competing Interests

Drs. Kerellos Nasr, Lawrence N. Diebel, Enrique Feria-arias, and Marvin Kajy have no competing interests. Dr. Rahul Vaidya is a consultant for Depuy Synthes Johnson and Johnson and for Smith and Nephew to develop an FDA approved INFIX device. This is not any of the devices shown in this paper which are common pedicle screw devices constructed with off-the-shelf pedicle screw systems with extralong screws.

References

[1] F. D. Brenneman, D. Katyal, B. R. Boulanger, M. Tile, and D. A. Redelmeier, "Long-term outcomes in open pelvic fractures," *Journal of Trauma*, vol. 42, no. 5, pp. 773–777, 1977.

[2] B. S. Davidson, G. T. Simmons, P. R. Williamson, and C. A. Buerk, "Pelvic fractures associated with open perineal wounds: a survivable injury," *Journal of Trauma-Injury, Infection & Critical Care*, vol. 35, no. 1, pp. 36–39, 1993.

[3] P. C. Ferrera and D. A. Hill, "Good outcomes of open pelvic fractures," *Injury*, vol. 30, no. 3, pp. 187–190, 1999.

[4] P. B. Hanson, J. C. Milne, and M. W. Chapman, "Open fractures of the pelvis. Review of 43 cases," *Journal of Bone and Joint Surgery—Series B*, vol. 73, no. 2, pp. 325–329, 1991.

[5] J. P. Perry, "Pelvic open fractures," *Clinical Orthopaedics and Related Research*, vol. 151, pp. 41–45, 1980.

[6] D. Rothenberger, R. Velasco, R. Strate, R. P. Fischer, and J. F. Perry, "Open pelvic fracture: a lethal injury," *The Journal of Trauma*, vol. 18, no. 3, pp. 184–187, 1978.

[7] J. Raffa and N. M. Christensen, "Compound fractures of the pelvis," *The American Journal of Surgery*, vol. 132, no. 2, pp. 282–286, 1976.

[8] K. I. Maull, C. R. Sachatello, and C. B. Ernst, "The deep perineal laceration—an injury frequently associated with open pelvic fractures: a need for aggressive surgical management a report of 12 cases and review of the literature," *The Journal of Trauma*, vol. 17, no. 9, pp. 685–696, 1977.

[9] C. J. Dente, D. V. Feliciano, G. S. Rozycki et al., "The outcome of open pelvic fractures in the modern era," *American Journal of Surgery*, vol. 190, no. 6, pp. 830–835, 2005.

[10] C. N. Mamczak and E. A. Elster, "Complex dismounted IED blast injuries: the initial management of bilateral lower extremity amputations with and without pelvic and perineal involvement," *Journal of Surgical Orthopaedic Advances*, vol. 21, no. 1, pp. 8–14, 2012.

[11] R. Vaidya, R. Colen, J. Vigdorchik, F. Tonnos, and A. Sethi, "Treatment of unstable pelvic ring injuries with an internal anterior fixator and posterior fixation: initial clinical series," *Journal of Orthopaedic Trauma*, vol. 26, no. 1, pp. 1–8, 2012.

[12] C. Moazzam, A. A. Heddings, P. Moodie, and P. A. Cole, "Anterior pelvic subcutaneous internal fixator application: an anatomic study," *Journal of Orthopaedic Trauma*, vol. 26, no. 5, pp. 263–268, 2012.

[13] R. Vaidya, B. Oliphant, R. Jain et al., "The bikini area and bikini line as a location for anterior subcutaneous pelvic fixation: an anatomic and clinical investigation," *Clinical Anatomy*, vol. 26, no. 3, pp. 392–399, 2013.

[14] D. J. Merriman, W. M. Ricci, C. M. McAndrew, and M. J. Gardner, "Is application of an internal anterior pelvic fixator anatomically feasible?" *Clinical Orthopaedics and Related Research*, vol. 470, no. 8, pp. 2111–2115, 2012.

[15] J. M. Vigdorchik, A. O. Esquivel, X. Jin, K. H. Yang, N. A. Onwudiwe, and R. Vaidya, "Biomechanical stability of a supra-acetabular pedicle screw Internal Fixation device (INFIX) vs External Fixation and plates for vertically unstable pelvic fractures," *Journal of Orthopaedic Surgery and Research*, vol. 7, no. 1, article 31, 2012.

[16] M. J. Gardner, S. Mehta, A. Mirza, and W. M. Ricci, "Anterior pelvic reduction and fixation using a subcutaneous internal fixator," *Journal of Orthopaedic Trauma*, vol. 26, no. 5, pp. 314–321, 2012.

[17] R. Vaidya, E. N. Kubiak, P. F. Bergin et al., "Complications of anterior subcutaneous internal fixation for unstable pelvis fractures: a multicenter study," *Clinical Orthopaedics and Related Research*, vol. 470, no. 8, pp. 2124–2131, 2012.

[18] J. M. Vigdorchik, A. O. Esquivel, X. Jin, K. H. Yang, and R. Vaidya, "Anterior internal fixator versus a femoral distractor and external fixation for sacroiliac joint compression and single stance gait testing: a mechanical study in synthetic bone," *International Orthopaedics*, vol. 37, no. 7, pp. 1341–1346, 2013.

[19] K. H. Chong, T. DeCoster, T. Osler, and B. Robinson, "Pelvic fractures and mortality," *The Iowa Orthopaedic Journal*, vol. 17, pp. 110–114, 1997.

[20] J. H. Holstein, U. Culemann, and T. Pohlemann, "What are predictors of mortality in patients with pelvic fractures?"

Clinical Orthopaedics and Related Research, vol. 470, no. 8, pp. 2090–2097, 2012.

[21] K. Lunsjo, A. Tadros, A. Hauggaard, R. Blomgren, J. Kopke, and F. M. Abu-Zidan, "Associated injuries and not fracture instability predict mortality in pelvic fractures: a prospective study of 100 patients," *Journal of Trauma—Injury, Infection and Critical Care*, vol. 62, no. 3, pp. 687–691, 2007.

[22] D. P. O'Brien, F. A. Luchette, S. J. Pereira et al., "Pelvic fracture in the elderly is associated with increased mortality," *Surgery*, vol. 132, no. 4, pp. 710–715, 2002.

[23] A. K. Sathy, A. J. Starr, W. R. Smith et al., "The effect of pelvic fracture on mortality after trauma: an analysis of 63,000 trauma patients," *Journal of Bone and Joint Surgery—Series A*, vol. 91, no. 12, pp. 2803–2810, 2009.

[24] O. P. Sharma, M. F. Oswanski, J. Rabbi, G. M. Georgiadis, S. K. Lauer, and H. A. Stombaugh, "Pelvic fracture risk assessment on admission," *The American Surgeon*, vol. 74, no. 8, pp. 761–766, 2008.

[25] Z. Balogh, K. L. King, P. Mackay et al., "The epidemiology of pelvic ring fractures: a population-based study," *Journal of Trauma-Injury, Infection and Critical Care*, vol. 63, no. 5, pp. 1066–1072, 2007.

[26] P. V. Giannoudis, M. R. W. Grotz, C. Tzioupis et al., "Prevalence of pelvic fractures, associated injuries, and mortality: the United Kingdom perspective," *Journal of Trauma—Injury, Infection and Critical Care*, vol. 63, no. 4, pp. 875–883, 2007.

[27] R. Pfeifer, I. S. Tarkin, B. Rocos, and H.-C. Pape, "Patterns of mortality and causes of death in polytrauma patients: has anything changed?" *Injury*, vol. 40, no. 9, pp. 907–911, 2009.

[28] K. Søreide, A. J. Krüger, A. L. Vårdal, C. L. Ellingsen, E. Søreide, and H. M. Lossius, "Epidemiology and contemporary patterns of trauma deaths: changing place, similar pace, older face," *World Journal of Surgery*, vol. 31, no. 11, pp. 2092–2103, 2007.

[29] R. Vaidya, A. N. Scott, F. Tonnos, I. Hudson, A. J. Martin, and A. Sethi, "Patients with pelvic fractures from blunt trauma. What is the cause of mortality and when?" *American Journal of Surgery*, vol. 211, no. 3, pp. 495–500, 2016.

[30] B. J. Gabbe, R. de Steiger, M. Esser, A. Bucknill, M. K. Russ, and P. A. Cameron, "Predictors of mortality following severe pelvic ring fracture: results of a population-based study," *Injury*, vol. 42, no. 10, pp. 985–991, 2011.

[31] R. B. Gustilo, V. Corpuz, and R. E. Sherman, "Epidemiology, mortality and morbidity in multiple trauma patients," *Orthopedics*, vol. 8, no. 12, pp. 1523–1528, 1985.

[32] A. Gänsslen, T. Pohlemann, C. Paul, P. Lobenhoffer, and H. Tscherne, "Epidemiology of pelvic ring injuries," *Injury*, vol. 27, supplement 1, pp. SA13–SA20, 1996.

[33] J. G. Parreira, R. Coimbra, S. Rasslan, A. Oliveira, M. Fregoneze, and M. Mercadante, "The role of associated injuries on outcome of blunt trauma patients sustaining pelvic fractures," *Injury*, vol. 31, no. 9, pp. 677–682, 2000.

[34] A. Tötterman, J. E. Madsen, N. O. Skaga, and O. Røise, "Extraperitoneal pelvic packing: a salvage procedure to control massive traumatic pelvic hemorrhage," *The Journal of Trauma*, vol. 62, no. 4, pp. 843–852, 2007.

[35] C. C. Cothren, P. M. Osborn, E. E. Moore, S. J. Morgan, J. L. Johnson, and W. R. Smith, "Preperitonal pelvic packing for hemodynamically unstable pelvic fractures: a paradigm shift," *The Journal of Trauma*, vol. 62, no. 4, pp. 834–839, 2007.

[36] A. Stannard, J. L. Eliason, and T. E. Rasmussen, "Resuscitative endovascular balloon occlusion of the aorta (REBOA) as an adjunct for hemorrhagic shock," *Journal of Trauma—Injury, Infection and Critical Care*, vol. 71, no. 6, pp. 1869–1872, 2011.

[37] M. R. W. Grotza, M. K. Allamia, P. Harwooda, H. C. Papeb, C. Krettekb, and P. V. Giannoudisa, "Open pelvic fractures: epidemiology, current concepts of management and outcome," *Injury*, vol. 36, no. 1, pp. 1–13, 2005.

[38] A. L. Jones, J. N. Powell, J. F. Kellam, R. G. McCormack, W. Dust, and P. Wimmer, "Open pelvic fractures: a multicenter retrospective analysis," *Orthopedic Clinics of North America*, vol. 28, no. 3, pp. 345–350, 1997.

[39] L. K. Cannada, R. M. Taylor, R. Reddix, B. Mullis, E. Moghadamian, and M. Erickson, "The Jones-Powell classification of open pelvic fractures: a multicenter study evaluating mortality rates," *Journal of Trauma and Acute Care Surgery*, vol. 74, no. 3, pp. 901–906, 2013.

[40] L. P. Leenen, C. van der Werken, F. Schoots, and R. J. Goris, "Internal fixation of open pelvic fractures," *Journal of Trauma*, vol. 35, pp. 220–225, 1993.

[41] V. Ghaemmaghami, J. Sperry, M. Gunst et al., "Effects of early use of external pelvic compression on transfusion requirements and mortality in pelvic fractures," *American Journal of Surgery*, vol. 194, no. 6, pp. 720–723, 2007.

[42] P. D. Faringer, R. J. Mullins, P. D. Feliciano et al., "Selective fecal diversion in complex open pelvic fractures from blunt trauma," *Archives of Surgery*, vol. 129, no. 9, pp. 958–964, 1994.

[43] A. David, G. Mollenhoff, C. Josten, and G. Muhr, "Perineal injuries in complicated pelvic trauma," *Swiss Surgery Journal*, vol. 1, pp. 4–9, 1996.

[44] M. L. C. Routt Jr., S. E. Nork, and W. J. Mills, "High-energy pelvic ring disruptions," *Orthopedic Clinics of North America*, vol. 33, no. 1, pp. 59–72, 2002.

[45] A. F. Morey, S. Brandes, D. D. Dugi III et al., American Urological Association (AUA) Guideline, 2016, https://www.auanet.org/education/guidelines/urotrauma.cfm.

[46] D. Hesse, U. Kandmir, B. Solberg et al., "Femoral nerve palsy after pelvic fracture treated with INFIX: a case series," *Journal of Orthopaedic Trauma*, vol. 29, no. 3, pp. 138–143, 2015.

[47] F. T. Rahul Vaidya, K. Nasr, P. Kanneganti, and C. Gannon, The Anterior Pelvic Internal Fixator 'INFIX' Technique. OTA Video Library 2016, https://vimeo.com/147862715.

38

A Scaphoid Stress Fracture in a Female Collegiate-Level Shot-Putter and Review of the Literature

Jessica M. Kohring,[1] Heather M. Curtiss,[2] and Andrew R. Tyser[1]

[1]Department of Orthopaedic Surgery, University of Utah, Salt Lake City, UT 84108, USA
[2]Marshfield Clinic, Department of Sports Medicine, Physical Medicine & Rehabilitation, University of Wisconsin-Stevens Point, Marshfield, WI 54449, USA

Correspondence should be addressed to Jessica M. Kohring; jessica.kohring@hsc.utah.edu

Academic Editor: Bayram Unver

Scaphoid stress fractures are rare injuries that have been described in young, high-level athletes who exhibit repetitive loading with the wrist in extension. We present a case of an occult scaphoid stress fracture in a 22-year-old female Division I collegiate shot-putter. She was successfully treated with immobilization in a thumb spica splint for 6 weeks. Loaded wrist extension activities can predispose certain high-level athletes to sustain scaphoid stress fractures, and a high index of suspicion in this patient population may aid prompt diagnosis and management of this rare injury.

1. Introduction

Scaphoid fractures are common in young adults and athletes and can lead to significant morbidity even with early diagnosis and appropriate treatment. While scaphoid fractures are most commonly associated with acute wrist trauma, it is notable that chronic repetitive loaded wrist extension can lead to scaphoid stress fractures [1].

Although rare, scaphoid stress fractures have been described in young, high-level athletes who exhibit repetitive loading with the wrist in extension, most commonly in gymnasts [2–7]. With increasing participation in high-level athletics at an earlier age, there has been a perceived increase in the incidence of pediatric and young adult stress fractures occurring in the upper extremity [5, 8]. Given the well-recognized challenges in diagnosing and managing scaphoid fractures, prompt recognition of these injuries—both acute and chronic varieties—is critical. Here we present a case of an occult scaphoid stress fracture in a 22-year-old female Division I collegiate shot-putter who was successfully treated nonsurgically and returned to sport.

2. Case Report

A 22-year-old female Division I collegiate right-hand dominant shot-putter initially presented with a two-month history of progressive, activity-related right wrist pain, with no report of prior trauma. She noted worsening pain with wrist extension during throwing the shot-put but had no complaints of pain or dysfunction with the discus nor with activities of daily living. The patient had been training for three to four hours per day, five times per week, alternating between the shot-put and discus as well as doing Olympic-style weight lifting for seven years prior to presentation.

Physical exam revealed tenderness to palpation at the anatomic snuffbox and the scaphoid tuberosity. Wrist flexion, extension, and supination were symmetric, but painful with loaded terminal extension in the dominant wrist. Radiographs of the affected wrist at the time of presentation, demonstrated −1 mm ulnar negative variance, with no evidence of abnormality (Figures 1, 2, and 3). Due to a high level of suspicion, a noncontrast 1.5-Tesla MRI of the wrist was obtained. The MRI demonstrated an incomplete stress

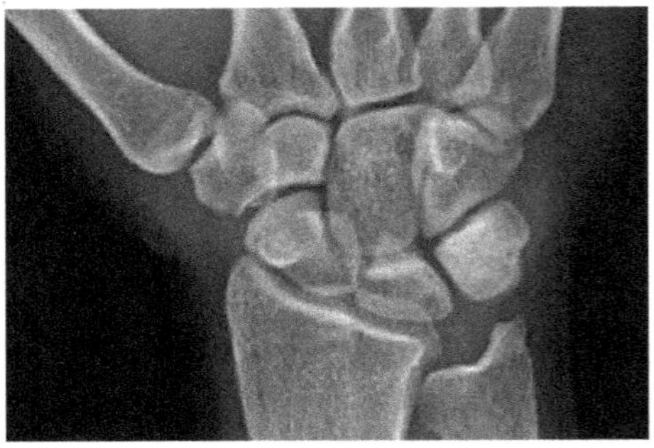

FIGURE 1: Posteroanterior radiographic view of the wrist at the time of initial evaluation that shows no abnormality in the scaphoid.

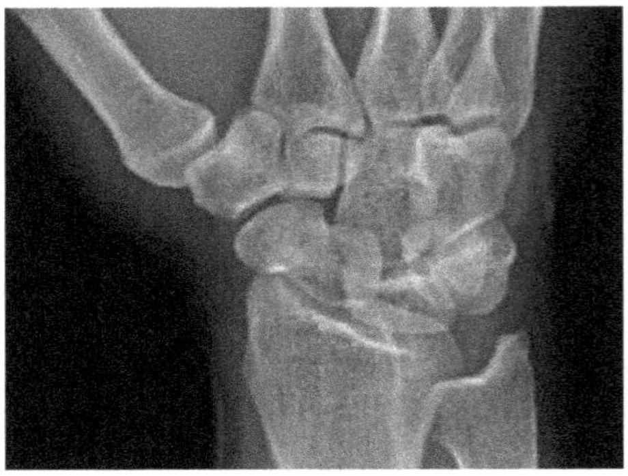

FIGURE 2: An oblique radiographic view at the time of initial evaluation without evidence of abnormality of the scaphoid.

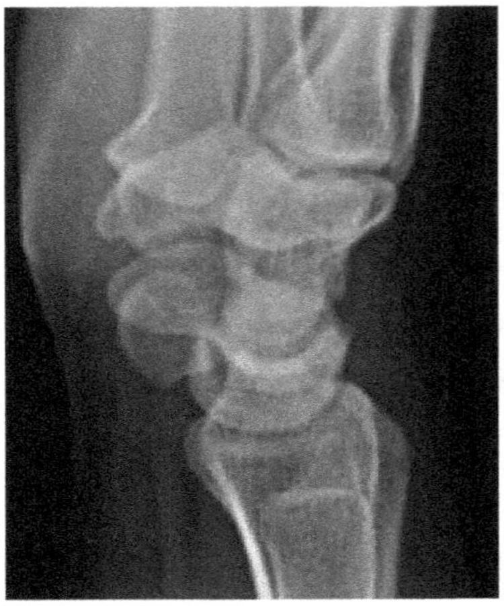

FIGURE 3: A lateral view of the wrist at the time of initial evaluation without radiographic abnormality of the scaphoid.

fracture at the scaphoid waist with associated bone edema and no cortical breakthrough, best seen on the T2 sagittal cut (Figure 4).

The patient was placed in a removable thumb spica wrist splint and was instructed to avoid any loaded extension of the wrist, including throwing the shot-put and weight-training. She was allowed to throw discus as it did not cause any pain. After three weeks, the patient reported no symptoms or pain with wrist extension. Radiographs obtained at 6 weeks after thumb spica immobilization were negative for any evidence of scaphoid fracture (Figures 5, 6, and 7). On physical exam, the patient had no tenderness to palpation in the anatomic snuffbox. The patient was released back to full activity without restrictions and returned to full participation in Division I shot-put without symptoms thereafter. At follow-up three years after her diagnosis, she reported no pain and no limitations in wrist or hand use.

3. Discussion

Scaphoid stress fractures are very rare injuries, with only case reports available for analysis in the peer-reviewed literature. In each reported case, the patients were competitive, high-level athletes training for multiple hours per day for several years prior to their presentation (Table 1). While gymnasts have been the athletes most commonly affected [2–7], others have also experienced these rare injuries: divers, soccer goalkeepers, shot-putters, badminton, cricket, and tennis players [3, 9–16].

Common to all of these athletic activities is the act of repetitive loaded wrist extension. Although the exact factors that lead to stress fractures of the scaphoid remain unclear, it has been suggested that repetitive stress and microtrauma to the bone can exceed native osseous repair mechanisms [3]. In each clinical case of a scaphoid stress fracture reported in the literature to date, including this one, the scaphoid waist was the location of the stress fracture.

Loaded wrist extension creates stresses that are typically centered at the scaphoid waist. In a cadaver study, Weber and Chao reported that 460 to 960 pounds of force applied to an extended wrist was required to acutely fracture the scaphoid, at the waist [17]. A more recent biomechanical study performed by Majima et al. found that loading the wrist in extension transmits force primarily through the scaphoid waist [18]. Handstands and other static maneuvers that require maximum wrist extension have been reported to exert considerable force across the scaphoid waist, but not to the extent needed to cause acute fracture [17].

Interestingly, the majority of scaphoid stress fractures have been reported in young male athletes, with 14 male and only 2 female patients reported in the available literature. The exact mechanism for this apparent gender discrepancy remains unclear but may be related to males reaching skeletal maturity at a later age than females, as adolescence appears to be a risk factor for suffering a scaphoid stress fracture. Similarly, while a direct link to age, sex, and athletic participation remains speculative, scaphoid stress fractures may be in part due to more intense participation in higher-level, longer-duration athletic training during adolescence.

Importantly, many of the published case reports regarding scaphoid stress fractures have noted a delay in diagnosis with this injury, with the majority of cases being recognized only after the fracture became apparent on plain radiographs [2, 3, 5]. Several case reports obtained bone scans to aid in their diagnosis of a scaphoid stress fracture [2–4], but more recently advanced imaging such as MRI and/or CTs

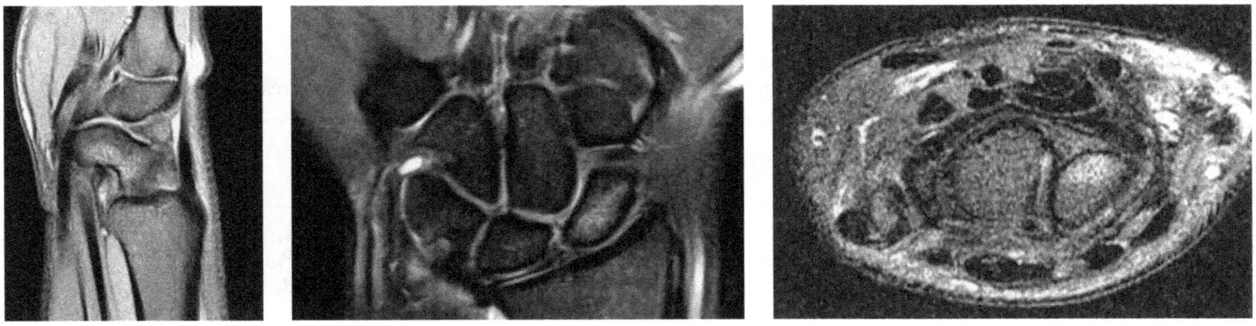

(a) (b) (c)

FIGURE 4: (a) A 1.5-Tesla MRI T2 sagittal cut demonstrating palmar scaphoid waist bone edema consistent with incomplete scaphoid waist stress fracture obtained at the time of initial presentation. (b) A 1.5-Tesla MRI T2 coronal cut showing scaphoid waist bone edema consistent with incomplete scaphoid waist stress fracture obtained at the time of initial presentation. (c) A 1.5-Tesla MRI T2 axial cut showing palmar scaphoid waist bone edema consistent with incomplete scaphoid waist stress fracture obtained at the time of initial presentation.

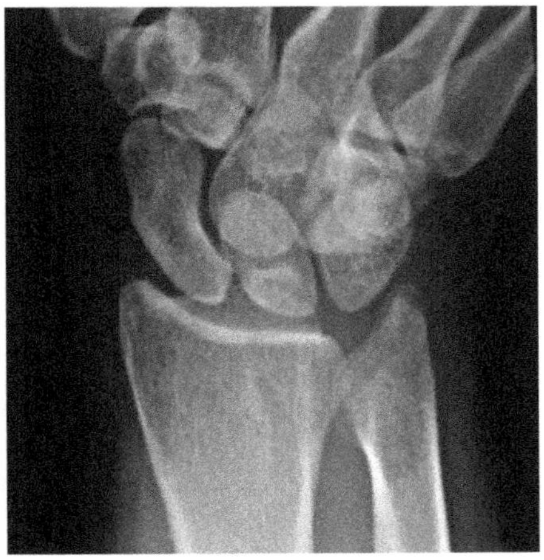

FIGURE 5: A scaphoid view obtained 6 weeks after presentation without radiographic evidence of a scaphoid waist fracture.

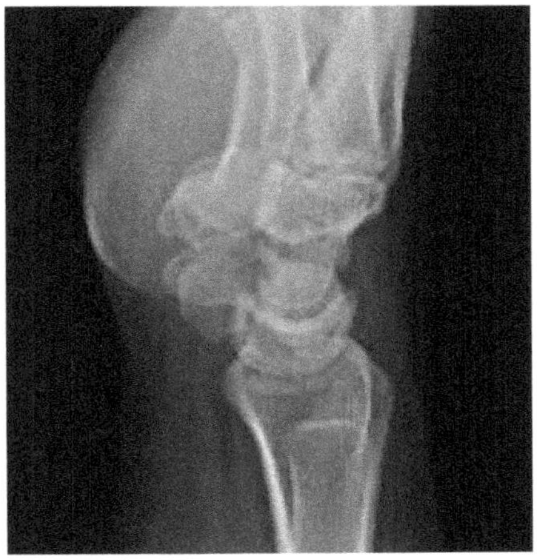

FIGURE 7: A lateral radiographic view obtained at 6 weeks after initial presentation showing a normal appearing scaphoid.

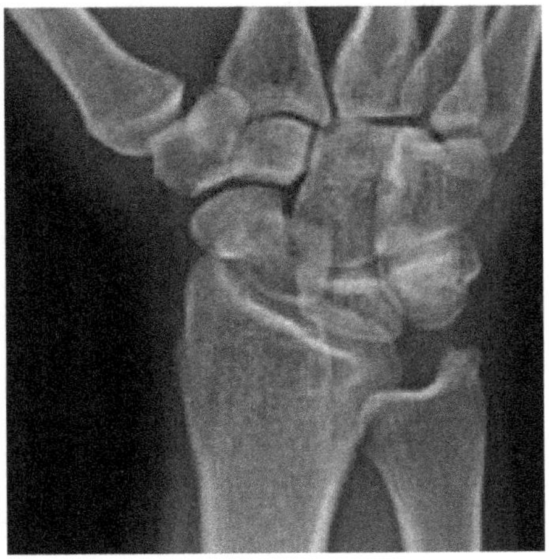

FIGURE 6: An oblique radiographic view obtained 6 weeks after presentation with no radiographic abnormality of the scaphoid.

has been utilized to diagnose or confirm scaphoid stress fractures [6, 7, 11, 13, 15, 16]. Several patients with negative presenting radiographs had the fracture only later diagnosed on repeat radiographs or advanced imaging [2, 3, 6]. In the case presented here, the presenting radiographs were negative, and an MRI was essential for making the diagnosis.

There are no current guidelines specific to the treatment of scaphoid stress fractures. However, for displaced or chronic scaphoid fractures or nonunions, surgical intervention is typically recommended. For nondisplaced or incomplete fractures, as in this case, nonsurgical treatment with immobilization is usually appropriate. Of the cases described in the literature, nine of the cases were treated nonoperatively [2, 3, 5, 9, 15, 16], two cases were initially treated nonoperatively but their patients had ongoing pain and evidence of nonunion requiring surgical intervention [6, 10], and five cases were treated with open reduction and internal fixation [7, 11–13]. For all patients treated with surgery, either a Herbert screw

TABLE 1: Clinical characteristics, imaging evaluation, and treatment method for scaphoid stress fractures published in the literature.

Author	Sport	Age (years)/ gender	Laterality	Pain duration	Time to diagnosis after presentation	Imaging presentation	Treatment	Scaphoid fracture location
Manzione and Pizzutillo [2]	Gymnast	16 M	Left	6 weeks	2 weeks	Negative XR; positive bone scan	Thumb spica cast ×10 weeks	Waist
Hanks et al. [3]	Shot-putter	19 M	Right	1.5 years	2 months	Negative initial XR; positive repeat XR at 2 months	Thumb spica cast/splint ×11 weeks	Waist
	Gymnast*	18 M	Left	2 years	1 year, 2 weeks	Positive XR; positive bone scan prior to XR	Thumb spica cast ×4 months	Waist
			Right	3 weeks	No delay	Positive bone scan; negative XR	Thumb spica cast ×6 weeks	Waist
	Gymnast	18 M	Left	2 months	No delay	Positive bone scan; negative XR	Thumb spica cast ×6 weeks	Waist
Engel and Feldner-Busztin [4]	Gymnast	18 M	Bilateral	1 year	Not mentioned	Positive bone scan & XR	Not mentioned	Waist
Inagaki and Inoue [9]	Badminton	16 M	Right	7 weeks	No delay	Positive XR	Thumb spica cast ×8 weeks	Waist
Matzkin and Singer [5]	Gymnast	13 F	Right	3 months	3 months	Negative initial XR; positive XR 3 months later	Long arm spica ×8 weeks, short arm thumb spica ×4 weeks	Waist
Brutus and Chahidi [10]	Badminton	23 M	Right	8 weeks	No delay	Positive XR	Thumb spica cast ×8 weeks and then ORIF: Herbert screw & graft	Waist
Hosey et al. [11]	Diver	13 F	Right	2 months	No delay	Positive XR; confirmed on MRI	ORIF: Herbert screw	Waist
Rethnam et al. [12]	Cricketer	38 M	Right	2 years	No delay	Positive XR	ORIF: Herbert screw & graft	Waist
Yamagiwa et al. [6]	Gymnast	18 M	Right	Not mentioned	No delay	Positive MRI; negative XR	Thumb spica cast ×8 weeks and then ORIF: Herbert screw	Waist
Nakamoto et al. [7]	Gymnast	18 M	Right	3 months	No delay	Positive XR; confirmed on MRI	ORIF: Herbert screw	Waist
Pidemunt et al. [13]	Goalkeeper	13 M	Bilateral	2 years	No delay	Positive XR; confirmed on CT	ORIF: graft & Herbert screw	Waist
Mohamed Haflah et al. [14]	Diver	16 M	Bilateral	18 months (right)	1 year (right), no delay (left)	Positive XR R wrist (nonunion); incidental positive XR L wrist	ORIF: headless compression screw & graft	Waist
Saglam et al. [15]	Goalkeeper	19 M	Bilateral	4 years	No delay	Positive XR; confirmed on MRI	Thumb spica cast ×12 weeks	Waist
Kohyama et al. [16]	Tennis	18 M	Right	4 months	No delay	Positive XR; confirmed on CT & MRI	Thumb spica cast/splint ×12 weeks	Waist
Kohring et al. (current report)	Shot-putter	22 F	Right	2 months	No delay	Negative XR; positive MRI	Thumb spica splint ×6 weeks	Waist

*Same patient with two different presentations.

or a headless compression screw was used with the majority of cases also using bone autograft [6, 7, 10–13]. All patients reported had successful treatment outcomes regardless of the intervention with return to athletic activities and no reports of recurrence of pain, reinjury, nonunion, or malunion at longer-term follow-up.

In summary, stress fractures of the scaphoid are exceedingly rare but potentially devastating if not recognized and treated promptly. Clinicians should have a high index of suspicion when evaluating an athlete or patient who presents with an insidious onset of activity-related wrist pain and snuffbox tenderness and who is involved in a sport that requires repetitive loaded wrist extension. While the majority of cases described have involved male athletes, scaphoid stress fractures also occur in females. A low-threshold to obtain advanced imaging when radiographs appear negative for scaphoid pathology may aid in the early diagnosis of this rare entity, avoid fracture nonunion, and reduce the need for complex surgical intervention.

Competing Interests

The authors declare that there are no competing interests regarding the publication of this paper.

References

[1] R. L. Linscheid and J. H. Dobyns, "Athletic injuries of the wrist," *Clinical Orthopaedics and Related Research*, vol. 198, pp. 141–151, 1985.

[2] M. Manzione and P. D. Pizzutillo, "Stress fracture of the scaphoid waist: a case report," *The American Journal of Sports Medicine*, vol. 9, no. 4, pp. 268–269, 1981.

[3] G. A. Hanks, A. Kalenak, L. S. Bowman, and W. J. Sebastianelli, "Stress fractures of the carpal scaphoid: a report of four cases," *The Journal of Bone & Joint Surgery—American Volume*, vol. 71, no. 6, pp. 938–941, 1989.

[4] A. Engel and H. Feldner-Busztin, "Bilateral stress fracture of the scaphoid: a case report," *Archives of Orthopaedic and Trauma Surgery*, vol. 110, no. 6, pp. 314–315, 1991.

[5] E. Matzkin and D. I. Singer, "Scaphoid stress fracture in a 13-year-old gymnast: a case report," *Journal of Hand Surgery*, vol. 25, no. 4, pp. 710–713, 2000.

[6] T. Yamagiwa, H. Fujioka, H. Okuno et al., "Surgical treatment of stress fracture of the scaphoid of an adolescent gymnast," *Journal of Sports Science and Medicine*, vol. 8, no. 4, pp. 702–704, 2009.

[7] J. C. Nakamoto, M. Saito, G. Medina, and B. Schor, "Scaphoid stress fracture in high-level gymnast: a case report," *Case Reports in Orthopedics*, vol. 2011, Article ID 492407, 3 pages, 2011.

[8] C. M. Coady and L. J. Micheli, "Stress fractures in the pediatric athlete," *Clinics in Sports Medicine*, vol. 16, no. 2, pp. 225–238, 1997.

[9] H. Inagaki and G. Inoue, "Stress fracture of the scaphoid combined with the distal radial epiphysiolysis," *British Journal of Sports Medicine*, vol. 31, no. 3, pp. 256–257, 1997.

[10] J. P. Brutus and N. Chahidi, "Could this unusual scaphoid fracture occurring in a badminton player be a stress fracture?" *Chirurgie de la Main*, vol. 23, no. 1, pp. 52–54, 2004.

[11] R. G. Hosey, J. M. Hauk, and M. R. Boland, "Scaphoid stress fracture: an unusual cause of wrist pain in a competitive diver," *Orthopedics*, vol. 29, no. 6, pp. 503–505, 2006.

[12] U. Rethnam, R. S. U. Yesupalan, and T. M. Kumar, "Non union of scaphoid fracture in a cricketer—possibility of a stress fracture: a case report," *Journal of Medical Case Reports*, vol. 1, article 37, 2007.

[13] G. Pidemunt, R. Torres-Claramunt, A. Ginés, S. De Zabala, and J. Cebamanos, "Bilateral stress fracture of the carpal scaphoid: report in a child and review of the literature," *Clinical Journal of Sport Medicine*, vol. 22, no. 6, pp. 511–513, 2012.

[14] N. H. Mohamed Haflah, N. F. Mat Nor, S. Abdullah, and J. Sapuan, "Bilateral scaphoid stress fracture in a platform diver presenting with unilateral symptoms," *Singapore Medical Journal*, vol. 55, no. 10, pp. e159–e161, 2014.

[15] F. Saglam, D. Gulabi, Ö. Baysal, H. I. Bekler, Z. Tasdemir, and N. Elmali, "Chronic wrist pain in a goalkeeper; Bilateral scaphoid stress fracture: a case report," *International Journal of Surgery Case Reports*, vol. 7, pp. 20–22, 2015.

[16] S. Kohyama, A. Kanamori, T. Tanaka, Y. Hara, and M. Yamazaki, "Stress fracture of the scaphoid in an elite junior tennis player: a case report and review of the literature," *Journal of Medical Case Reports*, vol. 10, no. 1, article 8, 2016.

[17] E. R. Weber and E. Y. Chao, "An experimental approach to the mechanism of scaphoid waist fractures," *Journal of Hand Surgery*, vol. 3, no. 2, pp. 142–148, 1978.

[18] M. Majima, E. Horii, H. Matsuki, H. Hirata, and E. Genda, "Load transmission through the wrist in the extended position," *Journal of Hand Surgery*, vol. 33, no. 2, pp. 182–188, 2008.

A Ruptured Digital Epidermal Inclusion Cyst: A Sinister Presentation

Iain Bohler, Phillip Fletcher, Amanda Ragg, and Andrew Vane

Orthopaedic Department, Tauranga Hospital, Cameron Road, Tauranga, Bay of Plenty 3112, New Zealand

Correspondence should be addressed to Iain Bohler; iain.bohler@doctors.net.uk

Academic Editor: Mark K. Lyons

Epidermal inclusion cysts are benign cutaneous lesions caused by dermal or subdermal implantation and proliferation of epidermal squamous epithelium as a result of trauma or surgery. They are typically located on the scalp, face, trunk, neck, or back; however they can be found anywhere on the body. Lesions are asymptomatic unless complicated by rupture, malignant transformation to squamous cell carcinoma, or infection at which point they can clinically appear as more sinister pathologies. We present the case of a 45-year-old laborer with a ruptured epidermal inclusion cyst, manifesting clinically and radiographically as a malignancy. Following MRI, definitive surgical management may appear to be a logical progression in management of the patient. This case however is a good example of why meticulously following surgical protocol when evaluating an unknown soft tissue mass is imperative. By following protocol, an alternate diagnosis was made and the patient has since gone on to a make a full recovery without life transforming surgery.

1. Introduction

A 45-year-old male presented to the orthopaedic outpatient department with an 18-month history of a gradually growing mass on the middle finger of his right dominant hand. The mass had grown at an increased rate over the previous 6 months culminating in self-referral to the emergency department after acute pain affecting his ability to complete work as a laborer at the local port. The patient identified a crush injury to his fingers involving a fridge approximately 6 months earlier; concluding the mass had extended in size from this time. After a failed attempt at aspiration the patient was discharged on oral antibiotics with orthopaedic follow-up. He reports no significant past medical history; however he smokes 10–15 cigarettes per day.

On examination, a fusiform swelling of his right middle finger was present centred on a tender mass on the radio-volar aspect of the middle phalanx. There was no evidence of infection or vascular disturbance; however paraesthesia was noted distal to the mass on the ulnar aspect of his finger. Flexion at the interphalangeal and metacarpophalangeal joints was restricted secondary to pain and mass effect of the lesion.

X-ray demonstrated a radial soft tissue swelling without bony involvement (Figure 1) whilst an ultrasound scan demonstrated marked subcutaneous oedema and thickening of the flexor tendon with synovial thickening of the PIPJ. No drainable focal fluid collection or foreign body was demonstrated.

Urgent magnetic resonance imaging (MRI) with contrast was requested demonstrating an extensive poorly defined infiltrating soft tissue mass around the middle phalanx, of intermediate T1 signal (Figures 2 and 3) and high T2 signal (Figures 4 and 5). The large hemicircumferential component abutting the flexor tendon is noted whilst a central tongue extends distally. A lobulated proximal extension is also noted extending just short of the 2nd web space. There was moderate enhancement with significant areas of central nonenhancement, most in keeping with malignancy. The differential diagnosis includes synovial sarcoma or epithelioid sarcoma. There was increased vascularity to the lesion (Figure 6). There was no bone or joint involvement.

The patient proceeded with incisional biopsy prior to likely ray amputation. A mid-lateral radial incision was made over the middle phalanx and four large pieces of tan coloured, friable, abnormal tissue were resected and sent for histology.

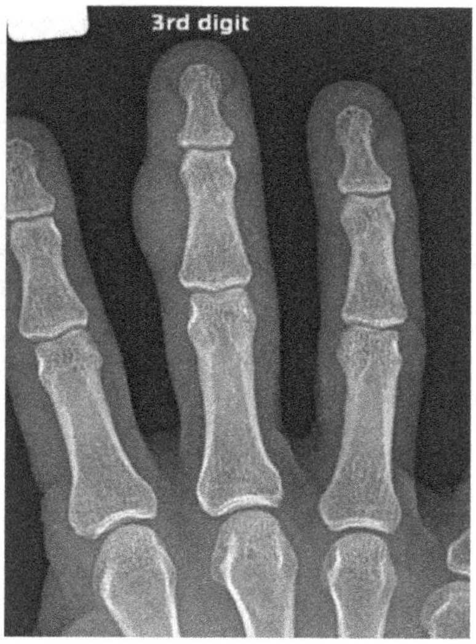

FIGURE 1: AP radiograph showing large fusiform soft tissue swelling of right middle finger at a level of the middle phalanx.

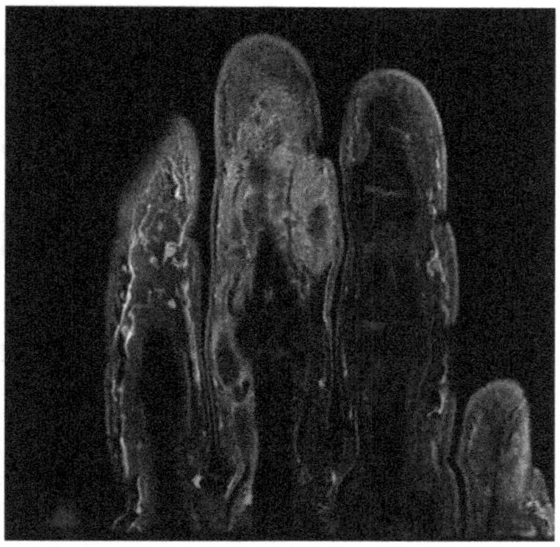

FIGURE 2: Proton density fat saturated coronal image showing a poorly defined lesion extending to the web space.

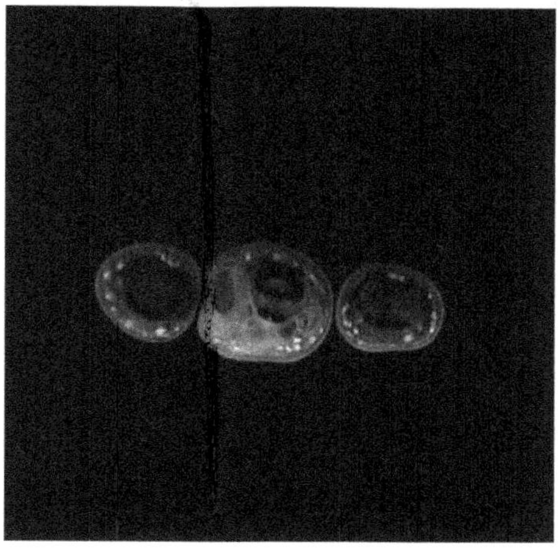

FIGURE 3: Axial proton density fat saturated sequence showing a mass extending hemicircumferentially around the flexor tendon of the middle phalanx.

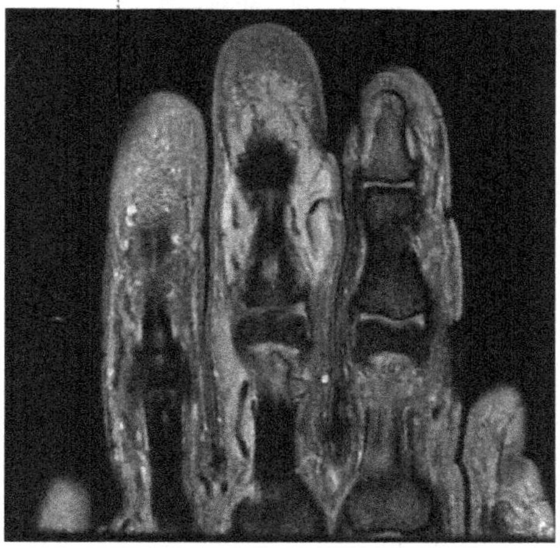

FIGURE 4: Coronal T1 fat saturated image after contrast showing central area of nonenhancement (necrosis/cystic content) and web space extension.

Wound swabs and a small amount of necrotic tissue was sent for microscopy, culture, and sensitivity. Staging computed tomography (CT) of chest, abdomen, and pelvis showed no evidence of metastases. Microbiology samples identified light growths of *Staphylococcus warneri*, *Staphylococcus capitis*, and *Staphylococcus epidermidis* susceptible to flucloxacillin.

Pathology reports showed sections of fibrovascular connective tissue with a small area of associated hyperkeratotic stratified squamous epithelium. Fragments of calcified debris were visible within an extensive foreign body type granulomatous inflammatory cell infiltrate. Findings were in keeping with a ruptured epidermal inclusion cyst with secondary inflammatory response.

An excision of the soft tissue mass was performed after confirming benign nature of the mass with frozen section analysis. Intraoperatively a 3 mm sharp foreign organic body was identified in the mass, around an area of pus and necrosed tissue (Figure 7).

The patient has since proceeded to make a full recovery and has returned to full time work.

2. Discussion

Epidermal inclusion cysts are subcutaneous lesions caused by dermal or subdermal implantation and proliferation of epidermal squamous epithelium as a result of trauma or surgery. They are typically located on the digits, scalp, face, trunk, neck, or back; however they can be found anywhere on the body. Occlusion of pilosebaceous units, human papilomavirus 57, and HPV 60 infection are rare but significant alternate pathogenesis. Most patients present with an asymptomatic or incidental mass unless complicated by rupture, malignant transformation to squamous cell carcinoma, or infection [1, 2].

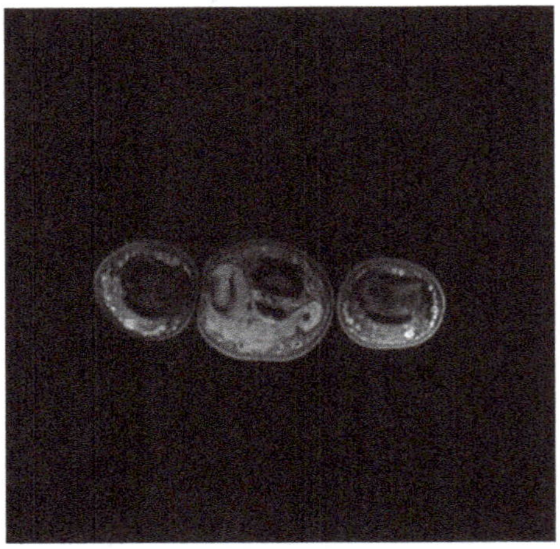

Figure 5: Axial T1 fat saturated after contrast.

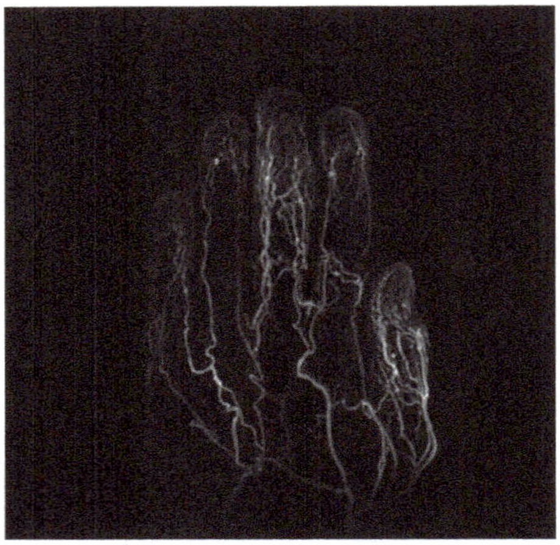

Figure 6: 3D postcontrast Time Resolved Imaging of Contrast Kinetics (TRICKS) angiogram showing vascularity of the lesion.

Sonographically, the cysts usually appear as well as circumscribed hypoechoic masses. MRI scanning is the investigation of choice. T1 weighting shows low or intermediate signal whilst T2 weighting shows high signal. Differential diagnosis should include neurogenic tumours, Myxoid tumours, dermatofibrosarcomas, nodular fasciitis, and ganglion cysts [2].

As with any lesion, it is imperative to meticulously follow surgical protocol in the diagnosis and management stages to minimise adverse outcomes, incomplete resection, seeding, bleeding, and infection. Most errors in management of an unknown lesion occur from incomplete or inappropriate presurgical diagnosis [3].

Initial assessment should begin with comprehensive history and physical examination. Social history of environmental exposures and smoking status can be key whilst systemic features such as fever, weight loss, and malaise are infrequent but unforgiveable if missed.

Large rapidly growing lesions should invoke immediate concern whilst tenderness is often pathognomonic of infection and inflammation or less commonly malignant infiltration. Lesions that are superficial, cystic, or less than 5 cm in size are likely to be benign whilst deep lesions larger than 5 cm have a higher malignant potential. Lymph node examination is imperative [3].

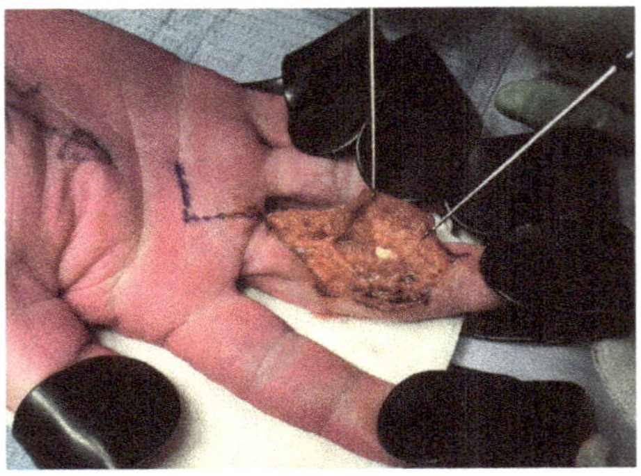

Figure 7: A central area of white pus can be seen whilst the necrotic tissue of the mass on the radial aspect of the digit extends into the web space.

Biplanar radiographs and ultrasound are suitable and cost effective initial investigations; however, magnetic resonance imaging is the imaging investigation of choice should any concerning features be raised. Biopsy and pathological evaluation should remain the last events in the evaluation of a soft tissue mass. It is good practice to discuss the biopsy procedure with pathology and radiology specialists prior to procedure to avoid tumour seeding and consideration of limb salvage procedures. Biopsy whether open or closed should be performed adhering to the following principles [3]:

(1) Careful consideration of approach to avoid further neurovascular or compartmental contamination.

(2) Lesions extending to bone which should be sampled from soft tissue to avoid increasing the risk of pathological fractures.

(3) The track which should be excisable en bloc with the tumour.

(4) Avoidance of haematoma collection.

CT staging of malignant lesions should be undertaken with chest, abdomen, and pelvic imaging to investigate metastases and is useful as an adjuvant to MRI for delineating tumour matrix and cortical destruction [3].

3. Conclusion

It is likely that the small thorn-like structure identified on removal of the mass was responsible for an unnoticed penetrating injury to the finger some time earlier, implanting dermis deep in the digit. The incident with the fridge may have resulted in rupture of the ensuing epidermal inclusion cyst, propagating its extension along the length of the finger. This rupture in combination with chronic low grade infection secondary to foreign body and constant aggravation due to the physical nature of the patient's job resulted in the semiacute deterioration in symptoms and presentation.

Complication of epidermal inclusion cysts with rupture, infection, or malignant transformation compounds clinical diagnosis. This case is a good example of why meticulously following surgical protocol when evaluating a soft tissue mass is imperative. Following MRI, definitive surgical management may appear to be a logical progression in management of the patient. In this case, a clinically and radiographic diagnosis of synovial sarcoma would have resulted in ray amputation extending into the hand. By following protocol, an alternate diagnosis was made and the patient has since made a full recovery without life transforming surgery.

Consent

The patient provided signed consent for use and reproduction of clinical images, which are anonymized.

Disclosure

All surgeons are affiliated to the Bay of Plenty District health board, a public health board in New Zealand.

Competing Interests

The authors confirm absolutely no conflict of interests.

References

[1] W. Jin, N. R. Kyung, Y. K. Gou, C. K. Hyun, H. L. Jae, and S. P. Ji, "Sonographic findings of ruptured epidermal inclusion cysts in superficial soft tissue: emphasis on shapes, pericystic changes, and pericystic vascularity," *Journal of Ultrasound in Medicine*, vol. 27, no. 2, pp. 171–176, 2008.

[2] S. H. Hong, H. W. Chung, J. Y. Choi et al., "MRI findings of subcutaneous epidermal cysts: emphasis on the presence of rupture," *American Journal of Roentgenology*, vol. 186, no. 4, pp. 961–966, 2006.

[3] J. Pretell-Mazzini, M. D. Barton, S. A. Conway, and H. T. Temple, "Current concepts review—unplanned excision of soft-tissue sarcomas: current concepts for management and prognosis," *The Journal of Bone & Joint Surgery—American Volume*, vol. 97, no. 7, pp. 597–603, 2015.

40

Knee-Extension Training with a Single-Joint Hybrid Assistive Limb during the Early Postoperative Period after Total Knee Arthroplasty in a Patient with Osteoarthritis

Tomokazu Yoshioka,[1,2] Hisashi Sugaya,[1,2] Shigeki Kubota,[1,2] Mio Onishi,[2] Akihiro Kanamori,[2] Yoshiyuki Sankai,[3] and Masashi Yamazaki[2]

[1]*Division of Regenerative Medicine for Musculoskeletal System, Faculty of Medicine, University of Tsukuba, 1-1-1 Tennodai, Tsukuba, Ibaraki 305-8575, Japan*
[2]*Department of Orthopedic Surgery, Faculty of Medicine, University of Tsukuba, 1-1-1 Tennodai, Tsukuba, Ibaraki 305-8575, Japan*
[3]*Faculty of Systems and Information Engineering, University of Tsukuba, 1-1-1 Tennodai, Tsukuba, Ibaraki 305-8577, Japan*

Correspondence should be addressed to Tomokazu Yoshioka; yoshioka@md.tsukuba.ac.jp

Academic Editor: Werner Kolb

The knee range of motion is an important outcome of total knee arthroplasty (TKA). According to previous studies, the knee range of motion temporarily decreases for approximately 1 month after TKA due to postoperative pain and quadriceps dysfunction following surgical invasion into the knee extensor mechanism. We describe our experience with a knee-extension training program based on a single-joint hybrid assistive limb (HAL-SJ, Cyberdyne Inc., Tsukuba, Japan) during the acute recovery phase after TKA. HAL-SJ is a wearable robot suit that facilitates the voluntary control of knee joint motion. A 76-year-old man underwent HAL-SJ-based knee-extension training, which enabled him to perform knee function training during the acute phase after TKA without causing increased pain. Thus, he regained the ability to fully extend his knee postoperatively. HAL-SJ-based knee-extension training can be used as a novel post-TKA rehabilitation modality.

1. Introduction

The knee range of motion is an important outcome of total knee arthroplasty (TKA), a procedure commonly used to treat osteoarthritis of the knee [1]. According to previous studies, the knee range of motion decreases temporarily for approximately 1 month after TKA due to postoperative pain and quadriceps dysfunction following surgical invasion of the knee extensor mechanism. These previous studies have also indicated that this decrease in the knee range of motion correlates significantly with decreases in joint function and the patient's degree of satisfaction [2, 3]. Currently, no joint function exercises intended to maintain the range of passive knee extension obtained through surgery can be performed without pain, even when using active extension. Therefore, a new treatment strategy is needed to prevent the prolongation of extension lag after TKA.

The single-joint hybrid assistive limb (HAL) (HAL-SJ, Cyberdyne Inc., Tsukuba, Japan) is a wearable robot suit that facilitates the voluntary control of knee joint motion (Figure 1). With this suit, signals from muscle action potentials are detected through electrodes on the surface of the skin and processed through a computer, after which the patient is provided with assisted joint motions. The power unit on the knee joint comprises angular sensors and actuators, and the control system comprises a cybernetic voluntary control (CVC) and cybernetic autonomous control (CAC) system [4]. The HAL has been reported to be effective in the functional recovery of various mobility disorders [5–8]. Although studies have reported successful outcomes for acute

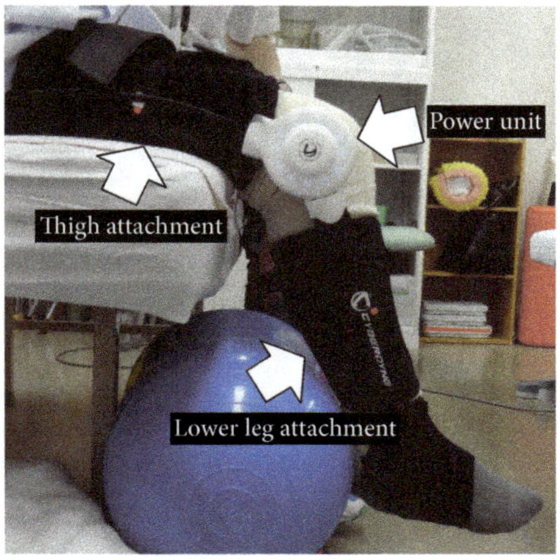

Figure 1: Lateral image of the single-joint hybrid assistive limb on the patient's right knee joint. Thigh and lower leg attachments are adjusted to the patient's body and connected by a power unit.

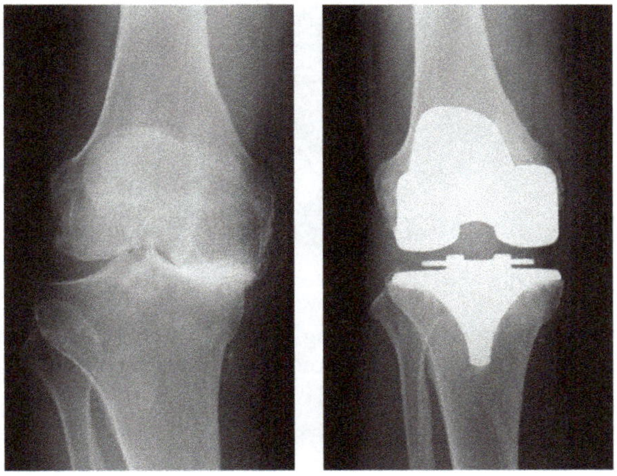

(a) (b)

Figure 2: Preoperative (a) and postoperative (b) frontal radiographs of the knee.

or chronic mobility disorders, there have been no reports on the use of HAL-SJ for degenerative joint diseases or related postoperative recovery to date. Accordingly, we describe our experience with a HAL-SJ-based knee-extension training program during the acute recovery phase after TKA.

2. Case Presentation

A 76-year-old man underwent right TKA (Vanguard, Zimmer Biomet Inc., Warsaw, IN, USA) for grade 4 (Kellgren-Lawrence scale) osteoarthritis of the knee (Figures 2 and 3). The HAL treatment program was divided into the following five phases.

2.1. Preoperative Observation Phase (Day of Hospital Admission to the Day of Surgery). The patient's thigh circumference and lower leg length were measured preoperatively, thus allowing us to adjust the HAL-SJ to the patient's size to ensure accurate training (Figure 1). We palpated the patient's quadriceps muscles (vastus medialis, rectus femoris, and vastus lateralis) and attached electrodes to each muscle to detect the bioelectric potentials of the long axes along the belly of each muscle. Then, we instructed the patient to perform knee-extension exercises and contract his quadriceps. We asked the patient to simulate the knee-extension training exercises, which were to be performed postoperatively, by performing 10 knee extensions with HAL-SJ assistance; the muscle that exhibited the highest bioelectric potential amplitude was used. The patient sat with his lower leg hanging down naturally, and we adjusted the height of the chair so his feet were not in contact with the floor (Figure 1).

2.2. Surgery Phase (Day of Surgery). TKA was performed through a longitudinal incision with a medial parapatellar approach. We cemented the femoral and tibial components using the modified gap technique and a posterior stabilized-type device.

2.3. Postoperative Observation Phase (Postoperative Days 1–7). On the first day after surgery, the patient was able to place full body weight on his leg; subsequently, he began rehabilitation (sitting, standing, and walking training; joint range of motion training; muscle strength maintenance; and muscle strengthening training) under the guidance of a physical therapist. Until discharge, he engaged in rehabilitation exercises for 20–40 min 5 days per week. Continuous passive motion (CPM) training began on the second postoperative day after the intra-articular drain was removed, and it was performed for 1 hour per day until discharge. On the seventh postoperative day, we attached electrodes to the quadriceps muscle again to detect the bioelectric potential along the long axis of the rectus femoris muscle belly (Figure 4(a)). Then, the patient was instructed to perform active knee-extension exercises to contract his quadriceps and thus simulate training with the HAL-SJ (Figure 4(b)).

2.4. HAL-SJ Therapy Phase (Postoperative Day 8 to Discharge). After 1 week of postoperative observation, we confirmed that his general condition had stabilized, and we decided to initiate HAL-SJ therapy. The CVC mode of the HAL-SJ, which was used in this study, can support a patient's voluntary motion according to the voluntary muscle activity and assistive torque provided to the knee joint [7]. This mode also allows the operator to adjust the degree of physical support to achieve patient comfort while gradually reducing support as training progresses. In addition to conventional rehabilitation (Figure 5(a)), the patient also performed HAL-SJ-assisted knee-extension exercises in a seated position at a frequency of 10 exercises/set for 5 sets twice weekly (HAL-SJ range of motion: 0–120°; Figure 5(b)). Training was performed 3 times (postoperative days 8, 10, and 17). The mean duration of a HAL-SJ training session was 26 min, which included the total time for which the HAL-SJ was worn and the duration of training (39, 22, and 17 min on postoperative days 8, 10, and 17, resp.).

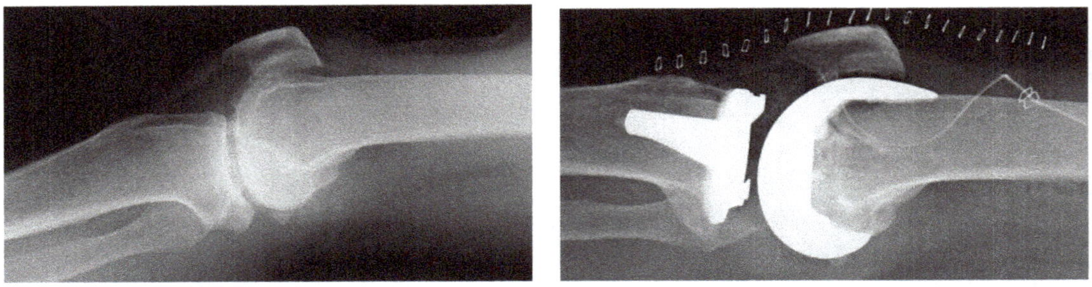

(a) (b)

Figure 3: Lateral radiographs of the knee. (a) Preoperative passive knee extension without anesthesia. (b) Passive extension under postoperative anesthesia immediately postoperatively. Full knee extension was restricted preoperatively but it was possible immediately postoperatively.

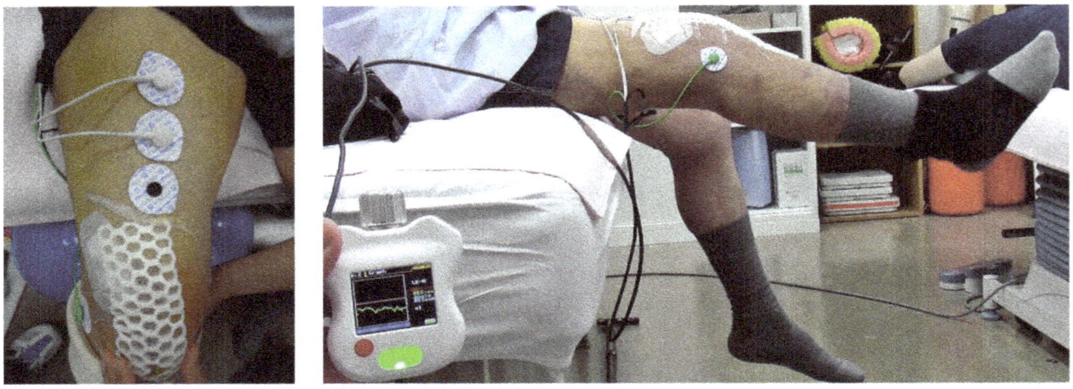

(a) (b)

Figure 4: Bioelectric potential detection and simulation before single-joint hybrid assistive limb training. Electrodes were attached to the muscle belly of the quadriceps (a), and rectus femoris simulation (b) was performed. Electrodes were placed to avoid surgical wound.

2.5. Post-HAL-SJ Therapy Observation Phase (Discharge to 3 Months after the End of HAL-SJ Therapy). There were no adverse effects related to HAL-SJ training. The patient was able to walk using a T cane, and he was discharged on postoperative day 21. Posttherapy assessments were conducted on an outpatient basis at 1 and 3 months after the end of the third HAL-SJ therapy session.

The following assessments were conducted: extension lag (maximum knee joint extension angle during passive exercise and that during active exercise), knee pain (visual analog scale, VAS), and isometric knee-extension muscle strength (IKEMS) before surgery, before and after HAL-SJ training, and at 1 and 3 months after training ended. The knee range of motion was measured using goniometry at accuracy of up to 1.0°, as goniometric measurements of range of motion have been reported to be more reliable than visual observation [9]. The measurement landmarks were the greater trochanter of the femur, proximal head of the fibula, and lateral malleolus. The maximal IKEMS of the operated leg was assessed while the patient was seated with 90° flexion in the hips and knees. Two measurements were taken using a μTas F-1 handheld dynamometer (Anima Corp., Tokyo, Japan) that was fixed to the chair. Each trial lasted for 3–5 s, with a 30-second rest period between trials. The higher of the two valid measurements was recorded. All measurements were performed by a single trained physical therapist to eliminate interobserver variability.

The extension lag, VAS, and IKEMS results are shown in Table 1. The extension lag was 15° preoperatively; this value decreased gradually over time to 1° at 3 months after therapy, indicating improvement. Comparisons before and after HAL-SJ therapy indicated that the 3 intervention sessions yielded respective improvements of 5°, 9°, and 5°. The VAS decreased from 55 mm before surgery to 17 mm at 3 months after the end of HAL-SJ therapy. Notably, training was not stopped because of increased knee pain from the HAL-SJ intervention. The maximum IKEMS value of 35.2 kgf was recorded before surgery. This value decreased markedly postoperatively and was measured as 18.3 kgf at 3 months after the end of the third HAL-SJ therapy session. Although this final value did not indicate recovery to the preoperative level, our comparison of IKEMS before and after HAL-SJ therapy indicated a slight improvement over the 3 intervention sessions (0.4, 0.0, and 1.8 kgf, resp.).

Clinical outcomes were assessed using the Japanese Orthopedic Association score [10]. The preoperative score of 55 points (pain, walking ability: 15 points; pain, ability to ascend/descend stairs: 5 points; flexion angle: 25 points;

TABLE 1: Chronological changes in EL, VAS, and IKEMS.

	Preoperative	First HAL-SJ (***POD 8)		Second HAL-SJ (POD 10)		Third HAL-SJ (POD 17)		At discharge (POD 21)	Following the end of the third HAL-SJ	
		*IPO	**IFO	IPO	IFO	IPO	IFO		1 month	3 months
EL (degrees)	15	10	5	12	3	10	5	4	4	1
VAS (mm)	55	28	4	20	20	32	46	40	18	17
IKEMS (kg)	35.2	8.7	9.1	5.6	5.6	10.7	12.5	16.9	16.9	18.3

EL: extension lag; VAS: visual analog scale; IKEMS: isometric knee-extension muscle strength; HAL-SJ: single-joint hybrid assistive limb.
*IPO: immediately before the intervention.
**IFO: immediately following the intervention.
***POD: postoperative day.

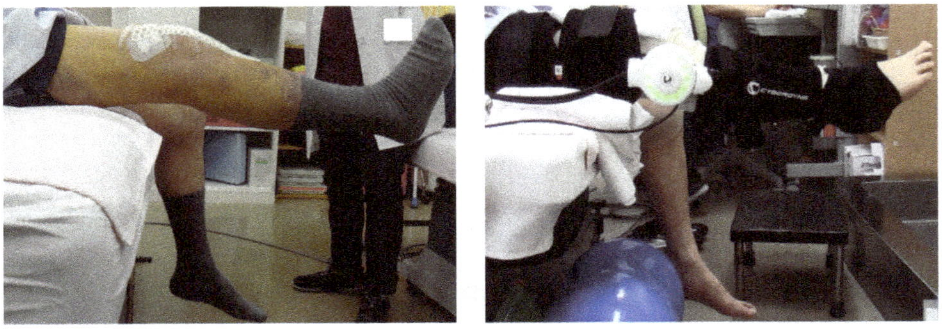

(a) (b)

FIGURE 5: Knee-extension training on postoperative day 8. Active knee extension (a) did not result in full extension, whereas extension with single-joint hybrid assistive limb assistance resulted in full knee extension (b).

swelling: 10 points) improved to 90 points (pain, walking ability: 30 points; pain, ability to ascend/descend stairs: 20 points; flexion angle: 30 points; swelling: 10 points) at 3 months after the end of HAL-SJ therapy.

3. Discussion

The patient's clinical course described herein has yielded two important clinical findings. First, knee-extension training with HAL-SJ, performed as part of the acute phase of post-TKA rehabilitation, resulted in immediate improvements in extension lag. Second, knee-extension training with HAL-SJ could be performed without increased pain.

We will first address the immediate improvement in extension lag. According to a recent review, CPM with a knee-range-of-motion training device commonly used for acute post-TKA rehabilitation resulted in early improvements in the knee flexion range of motion, compared to not using CPM; however, neither the range of active nor that of passive knee extension improved with CPM [11]. Restricted post-TKA knee extension (decreased or poor extension range) has been significantly correlated with decreases in the Oxford Knee Score and clinical outcomes related to standing, as indicated by the Short Form-36 physical component score [2]. Therefore, maintenance of the improved knee-extension range obtained through surgery is extremely important to improving knee function. In the present study, HAL-SJ-based knee-extension training led to an immediate improvement in extension lag even though the quadriceps did not exhibit significant strengthening. This result suggests that this improvement resulted from the facilitation of the muscular and neural functions of the quadriceps by HAL-SJ, which allowed the knee to extend fully because of the presence of a bioelectric potential in the quadriceps and the degree of feedback strength.

As mentioned before, HAL-SJ-based knee-extension training, even during the acute postoperative stage, did not cause an increase in knee pain. Although isometric quadriceps training is performed during the acute post-TKA phase to address decreased or dysfunctional knee extension related to surgical invasion of the knee-extension mechanism, it is difficult for patients to sufficiently perform knee-extension training because of pain and swelling caused by the operation [2, 11, 12]. HAL-SJ-based knee-extension training, however, can be performed during the acute post-TKA phase without increased pain. We believe that this is due to the knee-assistive function of HAL-SJ.

Two case reports on postoperative interventional training using HAL have been published in the field of orthopedic surgery. Both reports described improvements in walking ability when HAL was used in patients with thoracic vertebra ossification of the posterior longitudinal ligament [8, 13]. In contrast, the present study is the first to report on the use of HAL-SJ knee-extension training during the acute phase following TKA for osteoarthritis of the knee.

In conclusion, HAL-SJ-based knee-extension training allows the performance of knee function training during the acute post-TKA phase without causing increased pain, thus maintaining the patient's surgically recovered ability to fully extend the knee. Although inability to fully extend the knee is a cause of reduced knee function and decreased satisfaction in patients after TKA, there is currently no effective modality for the recovery of knee-extension function. Therefore, HAL-SJ-based knee-extension training can be used as a novel post-TKA rehabilitation modality. Reduced medical costs can also be anticipated, as early recovery of knee function would reduce hospital stays and the nursing care burden consequent to improved patient independence. However, the mechanism underlying the immediate improvement in extension lag remains unknown; therefore, further study from a neurophysiological perspective is required.

Ethical Approval

The study was carried out in accordance with the Declaration of Helsinki and within the appropriate ethical framework.

Consent

Written informed consent was obtained from the patient for publication of this case report and any accompanying images.

Competing Interests

A commercial party having a direct financial interest in the results of the research supporting this article has conferred or will confer a financial benefit on one of the authors. Yoshiyuki Sankai is CEO of Cyberdyne Inc., Ibaraki, Japan. Cyberdyne is the manufacturer of the robot suit (hybrid assistive limb). Cyberdyne was not directly involved in the study design; collection, analysis, or interpretation of data; writing the report; or the decision to submit the paper for publication. No commercial party having a direct financial interest in the results of the research supporting this article has or will confer a benefit on the authors or on any organization with which the authors are associated (Tomokazu Yoshioka, Hisashi Sugaya, Shigeki Kubota, Mio Onishi, Akihiro Kanamori, and Masashi Yamazaki).

References

[1] K. Y. Chiu, T. P. Ng, W. M. Tang, and W. P. Yau, "Review article: knee flexion after total knee arthroplasty," *Journal of Orthopaedic Surgery*, vol. 10, no. 2, pp. 194–202, 2002.

[2] Z. Zhou, K. S. A. Yew, E. Arul et al., "Recovery in knee range of motion reaches a plateau by 12 months after total knee arthroplasty," *Knee Surgery, Sports Traumatology, Arthroscopy*, vol. 23, no. 6, pp. 1729–1733, 2015.

[3] R. L. Mizner, S. C. Petterson, and L. Snyder-Mackler, "Quadriceps strength and the time course of functional recovery after total knee arthroplasty," *The Journal of Orthopaedic and Sports Physical Therapy*, vol. 35, no. 7, pp. 424–436, 2005.

[4] H. Kawamoto and Y. Sankai, "Power assist method based on phase sequence and muscle force condition for HAL," *Advanced Robotics*, vol. 19, no. 7, pp. 717–734, 2005.

[5] H. Kawamoto, K. Kamibayashi, Y. Nakata et al., "Pilot study of locomotion improvement using hybrid assistive limb in chronic stroke patients," *BMC Neurology*, vol. 13, article 141, 2013.

[6] S. Kubota, Y. Nakata, K. Eguchi et al., "Feasibility of rehabilitation training with a newly developed wearable robot for patients with limited mobility," *Archives of Physical Medicine and Rehabilitation*, vol. 94, no. 6, pp. 1080–1087, 2013.

[7] M. Aach, O. Cruciger, M. Sczesny-Kaiser et al., "Voluntary driven exoskeleton as a new tool for rehabilitation in chronic spinal cord injury: A pilot study," *Spine Journal*, vol. 14, no. 12, pp. 2847–2853, 2014.

[8] K. Fujii, T. Abe, S. Kubota et al., "The voluntary driven exoskeleton Hybrid Assistive Limb (HAL) for postoperative training of thoracic ossification of the posterior longitudinal ligament: a case report," *The Journal of Spinal Cord Medicine*, 2016.

[9] A. F. Lenssen, E. M. van Dam, Y. H. F. Crijns et al., "Reproducibility of goniometric measurement of the knee in the in-hospital phase following total knee arthroplasty," *BMC Musculoskeletal Disorders*, vol. 8, article 83, 2007.

[10] M. Okuda, S. Omokawa, K. Okahashi, M. Akahane, and Y. Tanaka, "Validity and reliability of the Japanese Orthopaedic Association score for osteoarthritic knees," *Journal of Orthopaedic Science*, vol. 17, no. 6, pp. 750–756, 2012.

[11] J. B. Mistry, E. D. Elmallah, A. Bhave et al., "Rehabilitative guidelines after total knee arthroplasty: a review," *Journal of Knee Surgery*, vol. 29, no. 3, pp. 201–217, 2016.

[12] Y.-H. Pua, "The time course of knee swelling post total knee arthroplasty and its associations with quadriceps strength and gait speed," *Journal of Arthroplasty*, vol. 30, no. 7, pp. 1215–1219, 2015.

[13] H. Sakakima, K. Ijiri, F. Matsuda et al., "A newly developed robot suit hybrid assistive limb facilitated walking rehabilitation after spinal surgery for thoracic ossification of the posterior longitudinal ligament: a case report," *Case Reports in Orthopedics*, vol. 2013, Article ID 621405, 4 pages, 2013.

A Method of Using a Pelvic C-Clamp for Intraoperative Reduction of a Zone 3 Sacral Fracture

Daniel H. Wiznia,[1] Nishwant Swami,[2] Chang-Yeon Kim,[1] and Michael P. Leslie[1]

[1] *Department of Orthopaedics and Rehabilitation, Yale University School of Medicine, 800 Howard Avenue, New Haven, CT 06510, USA*
[2] *Yale University, 800 Howard Ave., New Haven, CT, USA*

Correspondence should be addressed to Daniel H. Wiznia; daniel.wiznia@yale.edu

Academic Editor: Athanassios Papanikolaou

It is challenging to properly reduce pelvic ring injuries that involve a zone 3 sacral fracture. Several open and closed reduction methods have been described. Percutaneous reductions are challenging, and improper reductions can have poor long-term outcomes. The pelvic C-clamp is a tool designed to provide emergency stabilization to patients suffering from c-type pelvic ring injuries. We describe a case in which a patient's open book pelvic ring injury with a zone three sacral fracture is reduced intraoperatively with the use of a pelvic C-clamp and stabilized with transsacral screws.

1. Introduction

Zone three sacral fractures are challenging to reduce, and they frequently require open reduction. Open treatment methodologies suffer from the common complication of wound breakdown. Indirect reduction with the use of percutaneous transsacral screws has been shown to be an effective method to fix unstable pelvic ring injuries with lower wound complications [1].

In an emergency setting, the pelvic C-clamp stabilizes pelvic ring injuries and controls hemorrhage [2]. With an assembly time of approximately ten minutes, the C-clamp staunches bleeding by applying compression indirectly to fracture surfaces and the veins of the presacral plexus [2–4]. Instruments similar to the C-clamp can be traced to Germany from reports published in the 1960s. The C-clamp in its current form came into wider use after reports were published by Ganz et al. in 1991 and Buckle et al. in 1994 [3, 5]. In contrast to other tools available for compression of pelvic ring injuries, the C-clamp allows for unrestricted access to the abdomen, pelvis, and proximal femur. These properties make the C-clamp ideal to be used intraoperatively to obtain compression of the posterior pelvic ring.

In this paper, we describe a patient who suffered an open book pelvic ring injury with a zone 3 sacral fracture. We describe a surgical technique in which the pelvic C-clamp was used nontraditionally intraoperatively as a reduction modality with the patient in the prone position in conjunction with percutaneous transsacral screw fixation. We have obtained the written informed consent of the patient for print and electronic publication, as well as permission for the use of radiographs. Potential conflicts of interest do not exist for any of the authors.

2. Case Report

A 44-year-old man suffered a pelvic ring injury and a comminuted proximal humerus fracture-dislocation in a motorcycle collision. The patient was transferred from an outside hospital where he had been intubated and placed in a pelvic binder and fluid resuscitated. At the time of presentation at our facility, the patient was deemed hemodynamically stable with a GCS of 11. A pelvic hematoma could be seen on the outside hospital CT. The pelvic ring injury consisted of a pubic symphysis disruption and a markedly displaced complete zone 3 sacral fracture from S1 through the coccyx (Figures 1 and 2). On exam, he was noted to have left lower extremity weakness but intact sensation.

On hospital day 3, the patient was brought to the operating room for fixation of the anterior and posterior pelvic

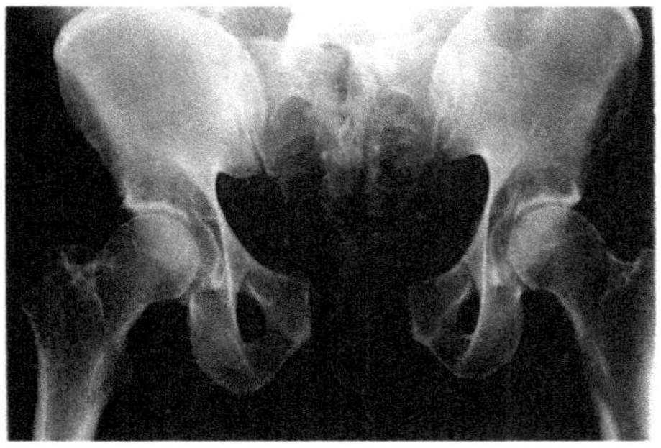

FIGURE 1: Presenting pelvis injury X-ray.

ring injuries. First, he underwent open reduction and internal fixation of his anterior pelvic ring injury. While the patient was positioned supine, the pubic symphysis was reduced with a Farabeuf clamp and stabilized with a 6-hole symphyseal plate with 3.5 mm screw fixation. The posterior ring was then compressed with S1 and S2 transsacral screws compressing the zone 3 sacral fracture.

On hospital day 4, postoperative radiographs demonstrated unacceptable residual displacement of his sacrum through the zone 3 fracture site (Figures 3(a) and 3(b)). This displacement of the sacrum was thought to be secondary to tension banding of the anterior pelvic ring preventing the posterior ring reduction. The patient returned to the operating room on hospital day 12 for revision in the prone position. Transsacral guide wires were placed through the S1 and S2 transsacral cannulated screws. Both screws were removed. A pelvic C-clamp was then applied over the S2 transsacral wire. Radiographs demonstrated an anatomic reduction. With the C-clamp holding the sacral fracture reduction, S1 transsacral screw was engaged into the far ilium allowing for more compression across the fracture site. An additional guide wire was passed at the S2 level for further stability. Another transsacral screw was placed across the fracture utilizing one of the S2 guide wires (Figures 3(c) and 3(d)).

The patient's hospital course was complicated by pneumonia and a deep vein thrombosis. The patient was discharged to short term rehabilitation on hospital day 30, with restrictions not to bear more than 25 pounds to the left lower extremity. At the patient's 8-week follow-up appointment, he complained of burning and numbness over the buttocks. At the patient's three-month follow-up, he complained of sacral and bilateral buttock pain, as well as sexual dysfunction. At a recent 3-year follow-up the patient is weight bearing as tolerated without restriction. He has returned to motorcycling.

3. Discussion

To our knowledge, no published case describes the use of a pelvic C-clamp in a nonemergency setting for the stabilization and reduction of a zone 3 sacral fracture. In addition, very little has been described in terms of using the pelvic C-clamp in nonemergent settings to achieve intraoperative reduction of pelvic ring injuries.

The following paragraph provides a historical perspective regarding the C-clamp. Pneumatic antishock garments (PASG) and medical antishock trousers (MAST) were used in the 1960s and 1970s to stabilize patients with severe pelvic trauma and hemorrhage [6, 7]. To improve upon the limited abdominal access of these methods as well as to provide improved stability to posteriorly unstable fractures, Mohanty et al. designed the sliding bar C-clamp and Buckle et al. designed the curved arm ratchet gear pelvic stabilizer [7, 8]. The C-clamp was found to provide significant compression to the posterior ring [9], allowed access to the abdomen, and could be retained as a temporary measure while definitive fixation was achieved [5, 10, 11]. The use of the pelvic C-clamp has decreased as C-clamp related complications have become more recognized and with the routine use of pelvic binders at the scene of the injury [11]. The C-clamp is currently manufactured and sold by DePuy Synthes Trauma division, West Chester, Pennsylvania [12].

It should be noted that the current version of the DePuy Synthes C-clamp is cannulated, which allows the C-clamp cannulated nails to be placed over a guidewire. This feature allowed the application of the C-clamp over the guide wire inserted through the previously placed S2 screw.

The patient in our case report suffered a pelvic ring injury that consisted of a pubic symphysis disruption and a complete zone 3 sacral fracture. The patient's pelvic ring injury can be classified as an anterior-posterior compression type 3 pelvic ring injury. The complete zone 3 sacral fracture acts as though there has been disruption of the anterior and posterior sacroiliac ligaments. This rare type of anterior-posterior compression pelvic ring injury is described by Bellabarba et al. in a case series of 10 patients. The pelvis is externally rotationally displaced and is vertically stable, with unilateral, partial disruption of the posterior arch [13].

In their case series of 10 patients who suffered open book pelvis injuries with zone 3 sacral fractures, Bellabarba et al. describe eight patients treated with open reduction and internal fixation. Regarding patient outcomes, Bellabarba et al. described three out of ten patients who complained of sexual dysfunction. We observed this complication in our patient. Bellabarba et al. also describe one patient who required a suprapubic catheter because of a urethral stricture. None of the patients in the series suffered motor or sensory neurologic compromise [13].

We attribute the challenge to reduce this patient's sacrum as secondary to his supine positioning and tension banding of the anterior ring. In addition, the patient's obesity (BMI 37) made the reduction challenging. During the second operation, by positioning the patient in the prone position, the patient's weight may have acted to provide a compressive force to the posterior ring, and the C-clamp provided additional compression across the fracture.

It should be noted that while the surgical team's use of intraoperative fluoroscopy ensured a safe path for the SI screws during the primary procedure, the malreduction was not identified, likely because the quality of the intraoperative fluoroscopy was deteriorated by the patient's obesity. A more critical review by the surgical team may have been able to identify the malreduction intraoperatively and provided an opportunity to revise the reduction.

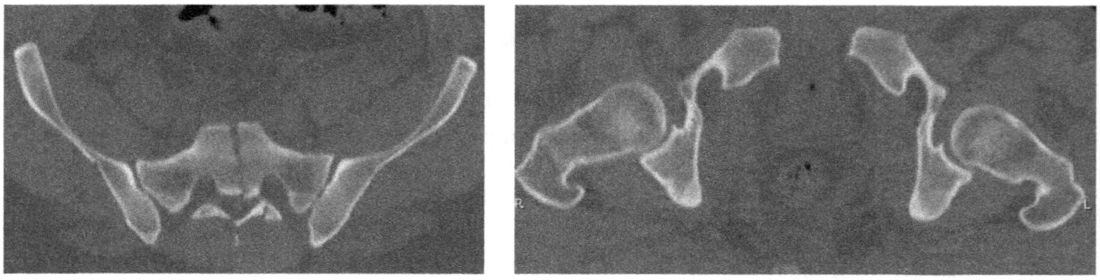

(a) (b)

Figure 2: Presenting injury CT scan axial cuts ((a) and (b)).

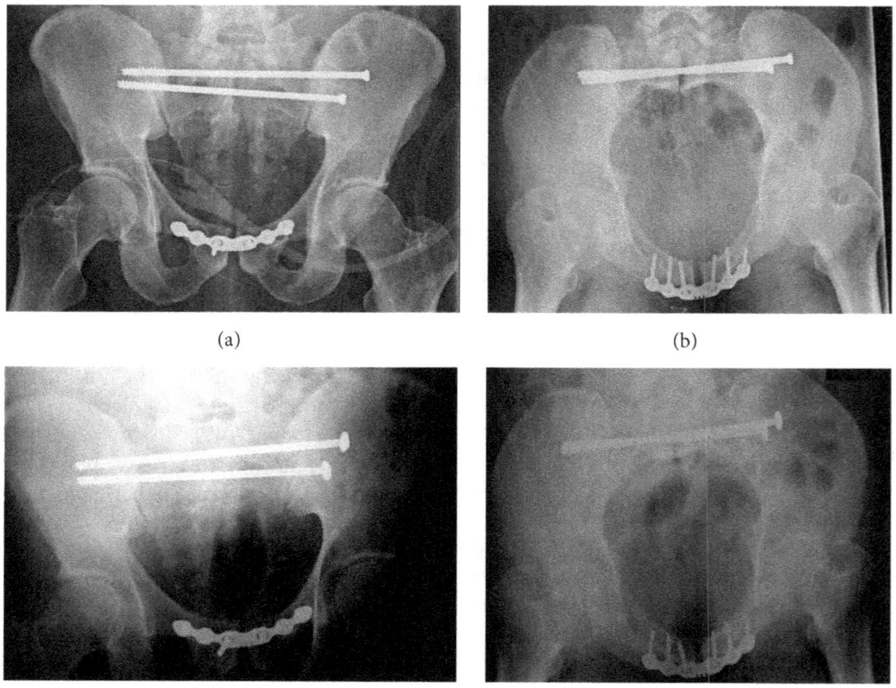

(a) (b) (c) (d)

Figure 3: Pelvis (a) anteroposterior and (b) inlet views before using C-clamp and pelvis (c) anteroposterior and (d) inlet views after using C-clamp.

Figure 3 demonstrates the degree of the malreduction after the first surgery (Figures 3(a) and 3(b)) and the degree in which the diastasis was compressed after the second surgery (Figures 3(c) and 3(d)). In biomechanical studies, C-clamps have been shown to apply some of the highest compressive loads on the posterior pelvic ring [14]. Figures 4(a), 4(b), and 4(c) demonstrate the healed pelvis with multiple broken screws two years postoperatively.

There are two studies which describe the use of the C-clamp to reduce Denis zone 2 sacral fractures. Wright et al. describe successful reduction and fixation of a sacroiliac joint dissociation associated with a contralateral Denis classification zone 2 sacral fracture in a 26-year-old male using the pelvic C-clamp. The authors describe the use of the C-clamp intraoperatively, which allowed for reduction of the dissociated sacroiliac joint and the placement of transsacroiliac screws [15]. Wright et al. recommend conducting the surgery with the patient in the supine position, obtaining fixation of the anterior pelvic ring injury first, and applying the C-clamp at the S2 level [15]. Quintero et al. describe using the pelvic C-clamp to reduce a Denis classification zone 2 sacral fracture with approximately 5 cm lateral displacement. Their technique describes the intraoperative use of the pelvic C-clamp to obtain definitive fixation with the patient positioned prone [16].

As a note of caution, those who decide to use the C-clamp should be properly trained in its application. There are true risks in incorrectly inserting the pins such as breaching the iliac wing, the sciatic notch, and the hip joint [17].

In conclusion, the use of the pelvic C-clamp can be considered for patients who have suffered a posterior pelvic ring disruption in which there is a large amount of diastasis without vertical instability. Patient positioning must be

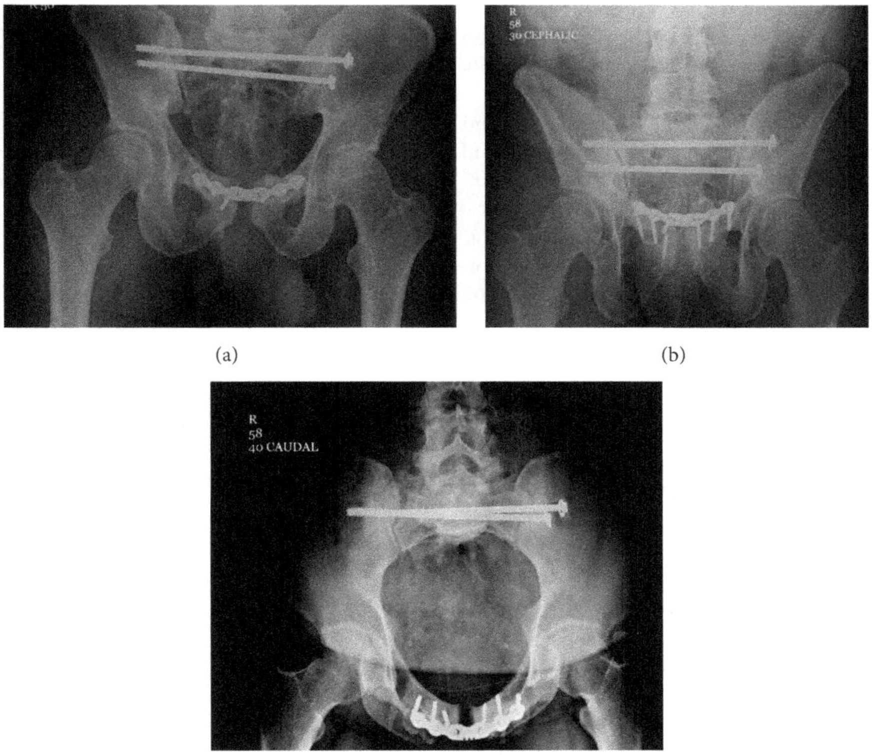

(a) (b) (c)

Figure 4: (a) Pelvis AP, (b) outlet, and (c) inlet views at two-year follow-up.

considered preoperatively given how critical it can be to the success of reduction maneuvers.

Ethical Approval

The Human Research Protection Program approved this retrospective chart review.

Consent

The authors have obtained the patients' written informed consent for print and electronic publication of the report, as well as permission for the use of photographs.

Disclosure

This manuscript is an original work that has not been previously published and is not under consideration for publication elsewhere. All authors accept responsibility for the manuscript's contents.

Competing Interests

The authors declare that there is no conflict of interests regarding the publication of this paper. There was no financial or technical support for this article.

Authors' Contributions

All authors have read and approved the manuscript and agree the work is ready for submission.

References

[1] K. Yinger, J. Scalise, S. A. Olson, B. K. Bay, and C. G. Finkemeier, "Biomechanical comparison of posterior pelvic ring fixation," *Journal of Orthopaedic Trauma*, vol. 17, no. 7, pp. 481–487, 2003.

[2] T. Lustenberger, C. Meier, E. Benninger, P. M. Lenzlinger, and M. J. B. Keel, "C-clamp and pelvic packing for control of hemorrhage in patients with pelvic ring disruption," *Journal of Emergencies, Trauma and Shock*, vol. 4, no. 4, pp. 477–482, 2011.

[3] R. Buckle, B. D. Browner, and M. Morandi, "Emergency reduction for pelvic ring disruptions and control of associated hemorrhage using the pelvic stabilizer," *Techniques in Orthopaedics*, vol. 9, no. 4, pp. 258–266, 1994.

[4] W. Ertel, M. Keel, K. Eid, A. Platz, and O. Trentz, "Control of severe hemorrhage using C-clamp and pelvic packing in multiply injured patients with pelvic ring disruption," *Journal of Orthopaedic Trauma*, vol. 15, no. 7, pp. 468–474, 2001.

[5] R. Ganz, R. J. Krushell, R. P. Jakob, and J. Kuffer, "The antishock pelvic clamp," *Clinical Orthopaedics and Related Research*, no. 267, pp. 71–78, 1991.

[6] D. J. Batalden, P. H. Wickstrom, E. Ruiz, and R. B. Gustilo, "Value of the G suit in patients with severe pelvic fracture. Controlling hemorrhagic shock," *Archives of Surgery*, vol. 109, no. 2, pp. 326–328, 1974.

[7] K. Mohanty, D. Musso, J. N. Powell, J. B. Kortbeek, and A. W. Kirkpatrick, "Emergent management of pelvic ring injuries: an update," *Canadian Journal of Surgery*, vol. 48, no. 1, pp. 49–56, 2005.

[8] R. Buckle, B. D. Browner, and M. Morandi, "Controversies and perils: emergency reduction for pelvic ring disruptions and control of associated hemorrhage using the pelvic stabilizer," *Techniques in Orthopaedics*, vol. 9, no. 4, pp. 258–266, 1994.

[9] P. Witschger, P. Heini, and R. Ganz, "Pelvic clamps for controlling shock in posterior pelvic ring injuries. Application, biomechanical aspects and initial clinical results," *Der Orthopade*, vol. 21, no. 6, pp. 393–399, 1992.

[10] M. Schütz, U. Stöckle, R. Hoffmann, N. Südkamp, and N. Haas, "Clinical experience with two types of pelvic C-clamps for unstable pelvic ring injuries," *Injury*, vol. 27, no. 1, pp. SA46–SA50, 1996.

[11] M. Wollgarten, M. J. B. Keel, and H.-C. Pape, "Editorial: emergency fixation of the pelvic ring using the pelvic C clamp—has anything changed?" *Injury*, vol. 46, Article ID 30002, pp. S1–S2, 2015.

[12] Pelvic C-clamp, *DePuy Synthes*, 2016, https://www.depuysynthes.com/hcp/trauma/products/qs/pelvic-c-clamp-1.

[13] C. Bellabarba, J. D. Stewart, W. M. Ricci, T. G. DiPasquale, and B. R. Bolhofner, "Midline sagittal sacral fractures in anterior-posterior compression pelvic ring injuries," *Journal of Orthopaedic Trauma*, vol. 17, no. 1, pp. 32–37, 2003.

[14] R. M. Sellei, P. Schandelmaier, P. Kobbe, M. Knobe, and H.-C. Pape, "Can a modified anterior external fixator provide posterior compression of AP compression type III pelvic injuries?" *Clinical Orthopaedics and Related Research*, vol. 471, no. 9, pp. 2862–2868, 2013.

[15] R. D. Wright, D. A. Glueck, J. B. Selby, and W. J. Rosenblum, "Intraoperative use of the pelvic c-clamp as an aid in reduction for posterior sacroiliac fixation," *Journal of Orthopaedic Trauma*, vol. 20, no. 8, pp. 576–579, 2006.

[16] A. J. Quintero, I. S. Tarkin, and H.-C. Pape, "Case report: the prone reduction of a sacroiliac disruption with a pelvic C-clamp," *Clinical Orthopaedics and Related Research*, vol. 467, no. 4, pp. 1103–1106, 2009.

[17] H. Koller and Z. J. Balogh, "Single training session for first time pelvic C-clamp users: correct pin placement and frame assembly," *Injury*, vol. 43, no. 4, pp. 436–439, 2012.

42

Magnesium-Based Absorbable Metal Screws for Intra-Articular Fracture Fixation

Roland Biber,[1,2] Johannes Pauser,[2] Markus Geßlein,[1,2] and Hermann Josef Bail[1,2]

[1]Nuremberg General Hospital, Paracelsus Medical University, Nuremberg, Germany
[2]Department of Orthopaedics and Traumatology, Nuremberg General Hospital, Nuremberg, Germany

Correspondence should be addressed to Roland Biber; biber@klinikum-nuernberg.de

Academic Editor: Giulio Maccauro

MAGNEZIX® (Syntellix AG, Hanover, Germany) is a biodegradable magnesium-based alloy (MgYREZr) which is currently used to manufacture bioabsorbable compression screws. To date, there are very few studies reporting on a limited number of elective foot surgeries using this innovative implant. This case report describes the application of this screw for osteochondral fracture fixation at the humeral capitulum next to a loose radial head prosthesis, which was revised at the same time. The clinical course was uneventful. Degradation of the magnesium alloy did not interfere with fracture healing. Showing an excellent clinical result and free range-of-motion, the contour of the implant was still visible in a one-year follow-up.

1. Introduction

Fixation of osteochondral fragments has to provide high stability, so that early mobilization and physiotherapy of the treated joint can be ensured. Current implants made of steel or titanium are able to meet these demands. However, in case the implant has to be removed due to complications, for example, the prominence of the head of a screw or if cartilage is lost postoperatively, a revision surgery becomes necessary. Biodegradable materials are an option to overcome this issue. This class of implants commonly consists of polymers, which lack adequate mechanical strength. Degradation of polymers is mostly facilitated by hydrolyses, only in some cases by enzymes. Hydrolyses, however, can result in an acid environment, favouring foreign body reactions and infections [1–3].

Biodegradable magnesium-based implants are an innovative alternative. Here, several alloys have recently been studied in animal experiments [4–9]. In 2013, the MAGNEZIX screw (Syntellix AG, Hannover, Germany) was the first magnesium implant to be approved for application in humans worldwide. The MAGNEZIX 3.2 mm compression screw chemically consists of the magnesium-alloy MgYREZr (i.e., magnesium, yttrium, rare earth metal, and zirconium). It is available in a range of lengths from 10 mm to 40 mm (in 2 mm increments) (Figure 1).

Experimental studies on this material proved biocompatibility and osteoconductivity. Several studies on magnesium implants even revealed an osteogenic potential [1, 2, 4, 10–12]. There seems to be no potential for allergic effects [1]. The expected time until complete degradation is about one year as shown in an animal study [12].

Although more than 15.000 implants have been placed on the market, there are only limited publications about this innovation, mostly in the field of elective orthopaedic surgery. In particular, this experience is limited to foot surgery. One major study reports on fixations of 13 Chevron osteotomies with MAGNEZIX screws. Comparing the results to a control group fixed with titanium alloy screws, no disadvantages were identified [2]. Early results (1-year experience) have recently been published, reporting good clinical outcome after distal metatarsal osteotomies for hallux valgus in the short term and a high patient satisfaction [13]. Up to now, there are no clinical reports whatsoever on trauma applications.

2. Case Presentation

We report the case of a 73-year-old female who suffered two falls within a short period. The first fall resulted in painful loosening of a radial head prosthesis. Waiting for the already scheduled operation, the second fall occurred, resulting in an

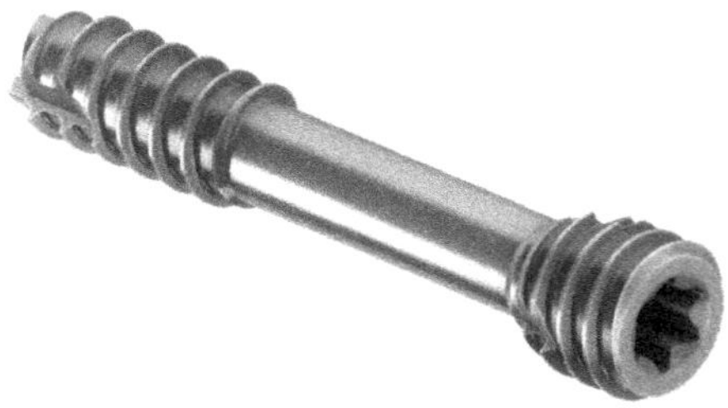

FIGURE 1: The compression screw MAGNEZIX CS resembles a cannulated conventional compression screw. However, it is made of a completely bioabsorbable magnesium alloy (MgYREZr).

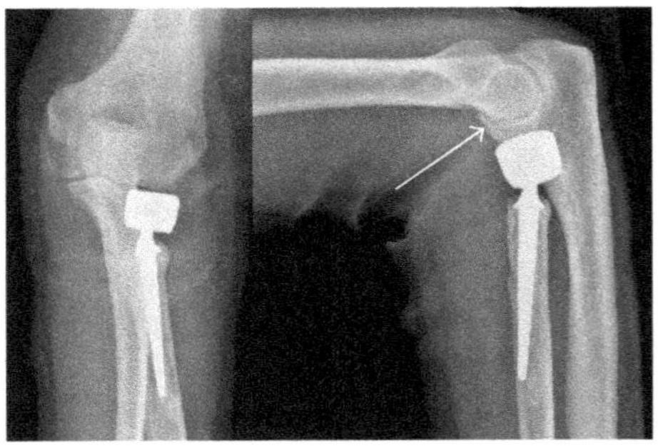

FIGURE 2: Surgery was indicated for both painful loosening of a radial head prosthesis and an osteochondral fracture of the capitulum humeri (white arrow).

additional fracture of the humeral capitulum (Figure 2). Via a lateral approach to the elbow, we performed revision of the radial head prosthesis, exchanging it for a cemented version. The large osteochondral fragment of the capitulum humeri was openly reduced, temporarily fixed by two Kirschner wires, and fixed with a MAGNEZIX compression screw (Ø 3.2 mm, length 32 mm).

Operative technique resembled that of conventional cannulated compression screws with placement of Ø 1.2 mm guide wire, drilling Ø 2.5 mm, countersink Ø 3.5 mm, and Ø 3.2 mm screw insertion; all steps are performed cannulating over guide wire.

Postoperative wound healing was uneventful. For mobilization, range-of-motion (ROM) was unrestricted, and the patient was advised with limited weight bearing (5 kg) for 6 weeks. A cast was applied for two weeks for wound healing protection only.

As the MgYREZr implant appears somewhat radiopaque, postoperatively X-rays allow correct implant placement to be checked without preventing the evaluation of the fracture area (Figure 3).

Further clinical course was uneventful. Physiotherapy was started and continued for 6 weeks, when unrestricted ROM was achieved (extension/flexion 0°-0°-120°). No adverse effects such as wound healing disturbance, swelling, or pain were noted.

At 1-year follow-up, the patient displayed an excellent clinical result, still with unrestricted ROM without pain, swelling, or other functional deficits. The contour of the implant was still visible on plain radiographs, and the surrounding bone and joint structures seemed radiographically undisturbed (Figure 4).

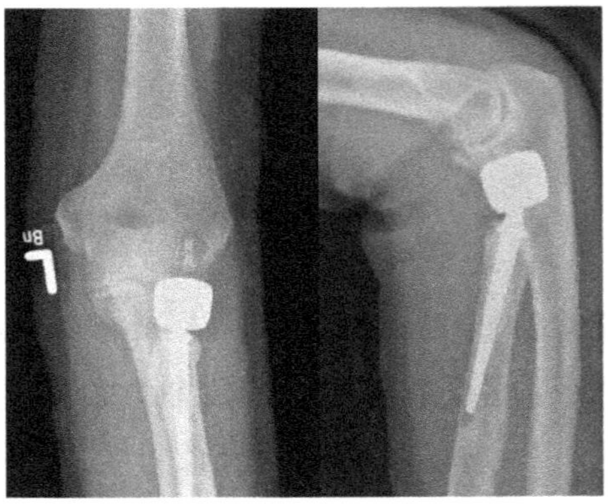

FIGURE 3: On postoperative X-ray, the MAGNEZIX CS can be identified as mildly radiopaque structure.

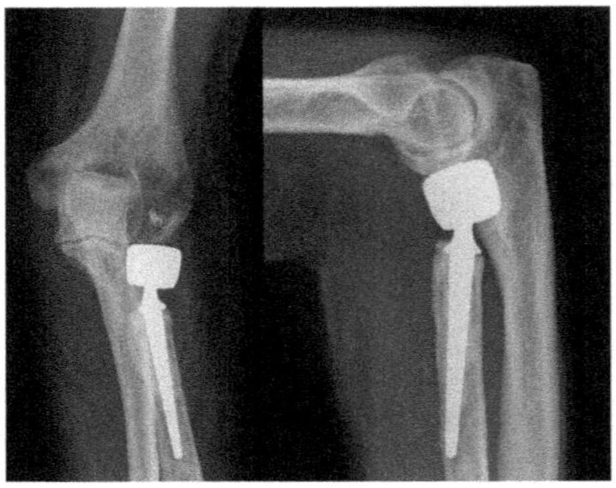

FIGURE 4: At one-year follow-up, the patient showed an excellent clinical result. The contour of the MAGNEZIX CS implant is still clearly visible.

3. Discussion

Metal removal may be challenging especially for small, intra-articular implants inserted below the surface of the cartilage. Considerable field damage may occur; thus, the decision for implant removal is taken with caution nowadays. Earlier publications suggest that steel or titanium alloy screws should be routinely removed, if used for fixation of osteochondral fragments [14, 15]. This suggestion changed over time to remove metal screws only, if complications occur. To further reduce the rate of revision surgery, biodegradable implants have been introduced [16]. The rate of metal implant removal in osteochondral fractures, even in knee joints after patella dislocation, is not exactly known [16, 17]. Aydoğmuş et al. reported in their recent publication a case of patellofemoral implant friction after the refixation of an osteochondral fragment with two headless metal compression screws [18]. For the rare procedure of fixation of osteochondral fragments of the capitellum, only case reports have been identified [19, 20].

Usage of biodegradable, nevertheless stable metal screws would represent a remarkable advantage regarding this issue. Theoretical applications include all kinds of screw fixation in small bones as well as fixation of small fragments including osteochondral flakes. The MAGNEZIX screw is approved for these indications (CE mark, HSA approval (Singapore)). The manufacturer explicitly recommends this implant for intra- and extra-articular fractures, nonunions, bone fusion, bunionectomies, and osteotomies [21].

Up to now, there is limited experience about the clinical application of the MAGNEZIX CS. Reports currently focus on elective foot surgery such as Chevron-type osteotomies of the first metatarsal bone [2, 13]. Our report now expands the application into the field of trauma surgery. After fixation of an intra-articular elbow fracture with a MAGNEZIX CS 3.2, we observed uneventful healing both clinically and radiologically. Radiologic follow-up did not detect any evidence for interference of any implant degradation products with fracture healing.

Our finding of an uneventful consolidation of the osteochondral fracture of the elbow after MAGNEZIX screw fixation is consistent with the studies of Windhagen et al., who also reported normal bone consolidation without any radiographic abnormalities around their Chevron osteotomies [2]. Degradation of magnesium alloys is known to produce hydrogen, which can form cavities within the tissue [10, 22]. Animal experiments with 1-year follow-up, however, indicated no associated bone loss [12]. In our case, no radiolucent zones were detected in the area of the implant. However, a computed tomography (CT) was not performed due to the unnecessary exposure of the patient to radiation.

Operative technique and handling of the MAGNEZIX CS were completely equivalent to conventional metal screws made of titanium. Although magnesium alloys have generally lower Young's Modulus than titanium alloys [6, 10, 12], applied torques and intraoperative stability appeared comparable to titanium implants. Degradation studies showed an implant mass reduction of less than 10% during the first six weeks, with the pull-out forces even increasing after four weeks [5]. In animal experiments, complete degradation of MgYREZr implants takes about one year [12]. Our finding of a radiographically visible screw after one year should not necessarily be interpreted as a fully intact metallic screw. Waizy et al. have shown that after 12 months the screw has turned to an apatite formation possessing a high density [12]. MRI scans after 36 months revealed that the former implants site becomes saturated with bone tissue (partially cancellous or cortical) following the degradation of the implant [23]. Therefore, it can be speculated that the now visible contour of the implant may resemble bone tissue.

4. Conclusion

The MAGNEZIX CS is a fully degradable implant made of magnesium alloy [MgYREZr]. Reports on clinical applications are limited to a relatively small number of Chevron osteotomies in the past. This is the first report on a trauma application, where the implant was used for an intra-articular fracture fixation in the elbow. The clinical and radiological course was uneventful. On one-year follow-up, the contour of the implant was still visible on plain radiographs. Further clinical reports are needed in order to describe clinical and radiological outcomes of this innovative implant.

Competing Interests

The authors declare that they have no competing interests.

References

[1] B. J. C. Luthringer, F. Feyerabend, and R. Willumeit-Römer, "Magnesium-based implants: a mini-review," *Magnesium Research*, vol. 27, no. 4, pp. 142–154, 2014.

[2] H. Windhagen, K. Radtke, A. Weizbauer et al., "Biodegradable magnesium-based screw clinically equivalent to titanium screw in hallux valgus surgery: Short term results of the first prospective, randomized, controlled clinical pilot study," *BioMedical Engineering Online*, vol. 12, article 62, 2013.

[3] J.-M. Seitz, M. Durisin, J. Goldman, and J. W. Drelich, "Recent advances in biodegradable metals for medical sutures: a critical review," *Advanced Healthcare Materials*, vol. 4, no. 13, pp. 1915–1936, 2015.

[4] A. Bondarenko, N. Angrisani, A. Meyer-Lindenberg, J. M. Seitz, H. Waizy, and J. Reifenrath, "Magnesium-based bone implants: immunohistochemical analysis of peri-implant osteogenesis by evaluation of osteopontin and osteocalcin expression," *Journal of Biomedical Materials Research—Part A*, vol. 102, no. 5, pp. 1449–1457, 2014.

[5] N. Erdmann, N. Angrisani, J. Reifenrath et al., "Biomechanical testing and degradation analysis of MgCa0.8 alloy screws: a comparative in vivo study in rabbits," *Acta Biomaterialia*, vol. 7, no. 3, pp. 1421–1428, 2011.

[6] N. Erdmann, A. Bondarenko, M. Hewicker-Trautwein et al., "Evaluation of the soft tissue biocompatibility of MgCa0.8 and surgical steel 316 L in vivo: a comparative study in rabbits," *BioMedical Engineering Online*, vol. 9, article 63, 2010.

[7] J. Reifenrath, N. Angrisani, N. Erdmann et al., "Degrading magnesium screws ZEK100: biomechanical testing, degradation analysis and soft-tissue biocompatibility in a rabbit model," *Biomedical Materials*, vol. 8, no. 4, Article ID 045012, 2013.

[8] B. Heublein, R. Rohde, V. Kaese, M. Niemeyer, W. Hartung, and A. Haverich, "Biocorrosion of magnesium alloys: a new principle in cardiovascular implant technology?" *Heart*, vol. 89, no. 6, pp. 651–656, 2003.

[9] E. Aghion, G. Levy, and S. Ovadia, "In vivo behavior of biodegradable Mg-Nd-Y-Zr-Ca alloy," *Journal of Materials Science: Materials in Medicine*, vol. 23, no. 3, pp. 805–812, 2012.

[10] M. P. Staiger, A. M. Pietak, J. Huadmai, and G. Dias, "Magnesium and its alloys as orthopedic biomaterials: a review," *Biomaterials*, vol. 27, no. 9, pp. 1728–1734, 2006.

[11] E. Zhang, L. Xu, G. Yu, F. Pan, and K. Yang, "In vivo evaluation of biodegradable magnesium alloy bone implant in the first 6 months implantation," *Journal of Biomedical Materials Research Part A*, vol. 90, no. 3, pp. 882–893, 2009.

[12] H. Waizy, J. Diekmann, A. Weizbauer et al., "In vivo study of a biodegradable orthopedic screw (MgYREZr-alloy) in a rabbit model for up to 12 months," *Journal of Biomaterials Applications*, vol. 28, no. 5, pp. 667–675, 2014.

[13] C. Plaass, S. Ettinger, L. Sonnow et al., "Early results using a biodegradable magnesium screw for modified chevron osteotomies," *Journal of Orthopaedic Research*, 2016.

[14] Y. Matsusue, T. Nakamura, S. Suzuki, and R. Iwasaki, "Biodegradable pin fixation of osteochondral fragments of the knee," *Clinical Orthopaedics and Related Research*, no. 322, pp. 166–173, 1996.

[15] P. Aichroth, "Osteochondritis dissecans of the knee. A clinical survey," *The Journal of Bone & Joint Surgery—British Volume*, vol. 53, no. 3, pp. 440–447, 1971.

[16] S. J. Walsh, M. J. Boyle, and V. Morganti, "Large osteochondral fractures of the lateral femoral condyle in the adolescent: outcome of bioabsorbable pin fixation," *The Journal of Bone & Joint Surgery—American Volume*, vol. 90, no. 7, pp. 1473–1478, 2008.

[17] J. Kühle, N. P. Südkamp, and P. Niemeyer, "Osteochondral fractures at the knee joint," *Unfallchirurg*, vol. 118, no. 7, pp. 621–634, 2015.

[18] S. Aydoğmuş, T. M. Duymuş, and T. Keçeci, "An unexpected complication after headless compression screw fixation of an osteochondral fracture of patella," *Case Reports in Orthopedics*, vol. 2016, Article ID 7290104, 4 pages, 2016.

[19] C. P. Silveri, S. J. Corso, and J. Roofeh, "Herbert screw fixation of a capitellum fracture. A case report and review," *Clinical Orthopaedics and Related Research*, vol. 300, pp. 123–126, 1994.

[20] J. F. Sodl, E. T. Ricchetti, and G. R. Huffman, "Acute osteochondral shear fracture of the capitellum in a twelve-year-old patient: a case report," *Journal of Bone and Joint Surgery—Series A*, vol. 90, no. 3, pp. 629–633, 2008.

[21] J.-M. Seitz, A. Lucas, and M. Kirschner, "Magnesium-based compression screws: a novelty in the clinical use of implants," *JOM*, vol. 68, no. 4, pp. 1177–1182, 2016.

[22] G. Song and A. Atrens, "Understanding magnesium corrosion—a framework for improved alloy performance," *Advanced Engineering Materials*, vol. 5, no. 12, pp. 837–858, 2003.

[23] C. Modrejewski, C. Plaass, S. Ettinger et al., "Degradation behaviour of Magnesium alloy screws after distal metatarsal osteotomies in MRI," Fuß& Sprunggelenk, 2015.

Permissions

All chapters in this book were first published in CRIO, by Hindawi Publishing Corporation; hereby published with permission under the Creative Commons Attribution License or equivalent. Every chapter published in this book has been scrutinized by our experts. Their significance has been extensively debated. The topics covered herein carry significant findings which will fuel the growth of the discipline. They may even be implemented as practical applications or may be referred to as a beginning point for another development.

The contributors of this book come from diverse backgrounds, making this book a truly international effort. This book will bring forth new frontiers with its revolutionizing research information and detailed analysis of the nascent developments around the world.

We would like to thank all the contributing authors for lending their expertise to make the book truly unique. They have played a crucial role in the development of this book. Without their invaluable contributions this book wouldn't have been possible. They have made vital efforts to compile up to date information on the varied aspects of this subject to make this book a valuable addition to the collection of many professionals and students.

This book was conceptualized with the vision of imparting up-to-date information and advanced data in this field. To ensure the same, a matchless editorial board was set up. Every individual on the board went through rigorous rounds of assessment to prove their worth. After which they invested a large part of their time researching and compiling the most relevant data for our readers.

The editorial board has been involved in producing this book since its inception. They have spent rigorous hours researching and exploring the diverse topics which have resulted in the successful publishing of this book. They have passed on their knowledge of decades through this book. To expedite this challenging task, the publisher supported the team at every step. A small team of assistant editors was also appointed to further simplify the editing procedure and attain best results for the readers.

Apart from the editorial board, the designing team has also invested a significant amount of their time in understanding the subject and creating the most relevant covers. They scrutinized every image to scout for the most suitable representation of the subject and create an appropriate cover for the book.

The publishing team has been an ardent support to the editorial, designing and production team. Their endless efforts to recruit the best for this project, has resulted in the accomplishment of this book. They are a veteran in the field of academics and their pool of knowledge is as vast as their experience in printing. Their expertise and guidance has proved useful at every step. Their uncompromising quality standards have made this book an exceptional effort. Their encouragement from time to time has been an inspiration for everyone.

The publisher and the editorial board hope that this book will prove to be a valuable piece of knowledge for researchers, students, practitioners and scholars across the globe.

List of Contributors

Eisuke Nomura, Hisatada Hiraoka and Hiroya Sakai
Department of Orthopaedic Surgery, Saitama Medical Center, Saitama Medical University, Kawagoe, Saitama, Japan

Benjamin Degeorge, Louis Dagneaux, David Forget, Florent Gaillard and François Canovas
Department of Orthopedic Surgery, Division of Lower Limb Surgery, Lapeyronie University Hospital 371 Avenue du Doyen Gaston Giraud, 34295 Montpellier Cedex 5, France

Jérôme Tirefort
Division of Orthopaedics and Trauma Surgery, Department of Surgery, Geneva University Hospitals, Geneva, Switzerland

Frank C. Kolo
Rive Droite Radiology Center, Geneva, Switzerland

Alexandre Lädermann
Division of Orthopaedics and Trauma Surgery, Department of Surgery, Geneva University Hospitals, Geneva, Switzerland
Faculty of Medicine, University of Geneva, Geneva, Switzerland
Division of Orthopaedics and Trauma Surgery, La Tour Hospital, Geneva, Switzerland

Yunus Oc, Muhammed Sefa Ozcan, Hasan Basri Sezer and Osman Tugrul Eren
Sisli Hamidiye Etfal Training and Research Hospital, 19 Mayıs Mahallesi, Sisli, 34360 Istanbul, Turkey

Bekir Eray Kilinc
Igdir State Hospital Orthopaedics and Traumatology Department, Igdir, Turkey

L. Baverel, K. Messedi, G. Piétu and V. Crenn
1CHU de Nantes, Clinique Chirurgicale Orthopédique et Traumatologique, Hôtel-Dieu, Place A. Ricordeau, 44093 Nantes Cedex, France

F. Gouin
CHU de Nantes, Clinique Chirurgicale Orthopédique et Traumatologique, Hôtel-Dieu, Place A. Ricordeau, 44093 Nantes Cedex, France
LPRO, Inserm UI957, Laboratoire de la Résorption Osseuse et des Tumeurs Osseuses Primitives, Faculté de Médecine, Université de Nantes, 44000 Nantes, France

Celal Bozkurt and Baran Sarikaya
Department of Orthopaedics and Traumatology, Faculty of Medicine, Harran University, Sanliurfa, Turkey

Mette K. Zebis
Department of Physiotherapy and Occupational Therapy, Faculty of Health and Technology, Metropolitan University College, Copenhagen N, Denmark
Human Movement Analysis Laboratory, Copenhagen University Hospital, Amager-Hvidovre, Copenhagen, Denmark

Christoffer H. Andersen
Department of Physiotherapy and Occupational Therapy, Faculty of Health and Technology, Metropolitan University College, Copenhagen N, Denmark

Jesper Bencke
Human Movement Analysis Laboratory, Copenhagen University Hospital, Amager-Hvidovre, Copenhagen, Denmark

Christina Ørntoft
Department of Sports Science and Clinical Biomechanics, SDU Sport and Health Sciences Cluster (SHSC), University of Southern Denmark, Odense M, Denmark

Connie Linnebjerg
Clinic of Sports Medicine, Danish Elite Sports Organization Team Denmark, Copenhagen, Denmark

Per Hölmich and Kristian Thorborg
Sports Orthopedic Research Center-Copenhagen, Arthroscopic Center, Department of Orthopaedic Surgery, Copenhagen University Hospital, Amager-Hvidovre, Copenhagen, Denmark

Per Aagaard
Institute of Sports Science and Clinical Biomechanics, University of Southern Denmark, Odense, Denmark

Lars L. Andersen
National Research Centre for theWorking Environment, Copenhagen, Denmark
Physical Activity and Human Performance, Center for Sensory-Motor Interaction, Department of Health Science and Technology, Aalborg University, Aalborg, Denmark

Artit Boonrod, Sermsak Sumanont and Manusak Boonard
Department of Orthopedics, Faculty of Medicine, Khon Kaen University, 123 Mittraphap Road, Khon Kaen 40002,Thailand

Arunnit Boonrod
Department of Radiology, Faculty of Medicine, Khon Kaen University, 123 Mittraphap Road, Khon Kaen 40002,Thailand

Levent Adiyeke, Tahir Mutlu Duymus and İsmail Emre Ketencı
Haydarpasa Numune Training and Research Hospital, Department of Orthopaedics and Traumatology, İstanbul, Turkey

Emre Bılgın
Tepecik Education and Research Hospital, Department of Orthopaedics and Traumatology, Izmir, Turkey

Meriç Ugurlar
Şişli Etfal Training and Research Hospital, Department of Orthopaedics and Traumatology, İstanbul, Turkey

John S. Hwang, Peter D. Gibson, Jacob Didesch and Irfan Ahmed
Department of Orthopaedic Surgery, Rutgers,The State University of New Jersey, New JerseyMedical School, Newark, NJ 07103, USA

Valerie A. Fitzhugh
Department of Pathology and Laboratory Medicine, Rutgers,The State University of New Jersey, New Jersey Medical School, Newark, NJ 07103, USA

Tsuyoshi Ohishi and Daisuke Suzuki
Department of Orthopaedic Surgery, Enshu Hospital, Hamamatsu, Shizuoka 430-0929, Japan

Masaaki Takahashi
Joint Center, Jyuzen Memorial Hospital, Hamamatsu, Shizuoka 434-0042, Japan

Yukihiro Matsuyama
Department of Orthopaedic Surgery, Hamamatsu University School of Medicine, Hamamatsu, Shizuoka 431-3192, Japan

Eriko Okano
Department of Orthopedic Surgery, Faculty of Medicine, University of Tsukuba, 1-1-1 Tennodai, Tsukuba, Ibaraki 305-8575, Japan

Tomokazu Yoshioka
Department of Orthopedic Surgery, Faculty of Medicine, University of Tsukuba, 1-1-1 Tennodai, Tsukuba, Ibaraki 305-8575, Japan
Division of Regenerative Medicine for Musculoskeletal System, Faculty of Medicine, University of Tsukuba, 1-1-1 Tennodai, Tsukuba, Ibaraki 305-8575, Japan

Takaji Yanai, Sho Kohyama and Toshikazu Tanaka
Department of Orthopaedic Surgery, Kikkoman General Hospital, 100 Miyazaki, Noda, Chiba 278-0005, Japan

Akihiro Kanamori and Masashi Yamazaki
Department of Orthopedic Surgery, Faculty of Medicine, University of Tsukuba, 1-1-1 Tennodai, Tsukuba, Ibaraki 305-8575, Japan

Mirko Velickovic and Thomas Hockertz
Department of Orthopedic Surgery and Traumatology, Städtisches Klinikum Wolfenbüttel, AlterWeg 80, 38302 Wolfenbüttel, Germany

Akihito Nagano, Daichi Ishimaru, Akihiro Hirakawa and Haruhiko Akiyama
The Department of Orthopaedic Surgery, Gifu University School of Medicine, 1-1 Yanagido, Gifu 501-1193, Japan

Takatoshi Ohno
The Department of Orthopaedic Surgery, Japanese Red Cross Gifu Hospital, 3-36 Iwakuracho, Gifu 502-0844, Japan

Koji Oshima
The Department of Orthopaedic Surgery, Ibi Kousei Hospital, 2547-4 Miwa, Ibigawa-cho, Gifu 501-0691, Japan

Yutaka Nishimoto
The Department of Nursing Course, Gifu University School of Medicine, 1-1 Yanagido, Gifu 501-1193, Japan

Yoshiyuki Ohno
The Department of Orthopaedic Surgery, Gifu Municipal Hospital, 7-1 Kashima-cho, Gifu 500-8323, Japan

Tatsuhiko Miyazaki
The Division of Pathology, Gifu University Hospital, 1-1 Yanagido, Gifu 501-1193, Japan

Ingo Schmidt
SRH Poliklinik Gera GmbH, Straße des Friedens 122, 07548 Gera, Germany

Taisei Sako, Yasuaki Iida, Yuichirou Yokoyama, Shintaro Tsuge, Keiji Hasegawa, Akihito Wada and Hiroshi Takahashi
Department of Orthopaedic Surgery, Toho University School of Medicine, Tokyo, Japan

Tetsuo Mikami
Department of Pathology, Toho University School of Medicine, Tokyo, Japan

Fahad H. Abduljabbar and Bayan Ghalimah
Division of Orthopedic Surgery, St. Mary's Hospital Center, McGill University, 3830 Lacombe Avenue, Montreal, QC, Canada H3T 1M5
Department of Orthopedic Surgery, King Abdulaziz University, Abdullah Sulayman St., Al Jamiah District, Jeddah 80200, Saudi Arabia

Lawrence Lincoln
Division of Orthopedic Surgery, St. Mary's Hospital Center, McGill University, 3830 Lacombe Avenue, Montreal, QC, Canada H3T 1M5

Abdulaziz Aljurayyan
Division of Orthopedic Surgery, St. Mary's Hospital Center, McGill University, 3830 Lacombe Avenue, Montreal, QC, Canada H3T 1M5
Department of Orthopedic Surgery, King Saud University, Riyadh 12372, Saudi Arabia

Akinobu Nishimura
Department of Orthopaedic and Sports Medicine, Graduate School of Medicine, Mie University, 2 174 Edobashi, Tsu, Mie 514-8507, Japan

Shigeto Nakazora, Aki Fukuda and Ko Kato
Department ofOrthopaedic Surgery, Suzuka Kaisei Hospital, 112 Kou, Suzuka, Mie 513-8505, Japan

Akihiro Sudo
Department of Orthopaedic Surgery, Graduate School of Medicine,Mie University, 2-174 Edobashi, Tsu,Mie 514-8507, Japan

MasatoshiMorimoto, Kosaku Higashino, Shinsuke Katoh, Tezuka Fumitake, Kazuta Yamashita, Fumio Hayashi, Yoichiro Takata, Toshinori Sakai, Akihiro Nagamachi and Koichi Sairyo
Department of Orthopedics, Institute of Health Biosciences, University of Tokushima Graduate School, Tokushima, Japan

Hiroyuki Obata, Kentaro Futamura, Osamu Obayashi and Atsuhiko Mogami
Department of Orthopaedic Surgery, Juntendo University Shizuoka Hospital, Shizuoka, Japan

Tomonori Baba and Kazuo Kaneko
Department of Orthopaedic Surgery, Juntendo University School of Medicine, Tokyo, Japan

Hideki Tsuji and Yoshiaki Kurata
Orthopaedic Trauma Center, Sapporo Tokushukai Hospital, Sapporo, Japan

Takenori Tomite and Toshiaki Aizawa
Kitaakita Municipal Hospital, 16-29 Shimosugiaza Kamishimizusawa, Kitaakita City, Akita 018-4221, Japan

Hidetomo Saito, Hiroaki Kijima, NaohisaMiyakoshi and Yoichi Shimada
Department of Orthopedic Surgery, Akita University Graduate School of Medicine, Hondou 1-1-1, Akita City, Akita 010-8543, Japan

Mitsuhiko Kubo, Kosuke Kumagai and Shinji Imai
Department of Orthopaedic Surgery, Shiga University of Medical Science, Otsu, Shiga 520-2192, Japan

Susumu Araki
Department of Orthopaedic Surgery, Shiga University of Medical Science, Otsu, Shiga 520-2192, Japan
Public Interest Incorporated Foundation, Toyosato Hospital, No. 12, 8 Moku, Toyosato-cho, Inukami, Shiga 529-1158, Japan

Tadahiko Ohtsuru, Yasuaki Murata, Yuji Morita, Yutaro Munakata and Yoshiharu Kato
Department of Orthopedic Surgery, TokyoWomen's Medical University, 8-1 Kawada-cho, ShinjukuWard, Tokyo 162-8666, Japan

Marie-Aimée Päivi Soro, Thierry Christen and Sébastien Durand
Department of Plastic and Hand Surgery, Lausanne University Hospital, rue du Bugnon 46, 1011 Lausanne, Switzerland

Walid Osman, Meriem Braiki, Nader Naouar and Mohamed Ben Ayeche
Department of Orthopedic Surgery, Sahloul University Hospital, Sousse, Tunisia

Zeineb Alaya
Department of Rheumatology, Farhat Hached University Hospital, Sousse, Tunisia

Thomas Kurien and Richard G. Pearson
Arthritis Research UK Pain Centre, Nottingham University, Nottingham, UK
Academic Orthopaedics, Trauma and Sports Medicine, School of Medicine,The University of Nottingham, Queen's Medical Centre, Derby Road, Nottingham NG7 2UH, UK

Robert Kerslake
Arthritis Research UK Pain Centre, Nottingham University, Nottingham, UK
Nottingham University Hospitals NHS Trust, Queen's Medical Centre, Nottingham NG7 2UH, UK

Brett Haywood
Arthritis Research UK Pain Centre, Nottingham University, Nottingham, UK
Academic Radiology,The University of Nottingham, Queen's Medical Centre, Derby Road, Nottingham NG7 2UH, UK

Brigitte E. Scammell
Arthritis Research UK Pain Centre, Nottingham University, Nottingham, UK
Academic Orthopaedics, Trauma and Sports Medicine, School of Medicine,The University of Nottingham, Queen's Medical Centre, Derby Road, Nottingham NG7 2UH, UK
Nottingham University Hospitals NHS Trust, Queen's Medical Centre, Nottingham NG7 2UH, UK

Konrad Slynarski
Lekmed Hospital for Special Surgery,Warsaw, Poland

Lukasz Lipinski
Lekmed Hospital for Special Surgery,Warsaw, Poland
Orthopedics and Pediatric Orthopedics Clinic, Medical University of Lodz, Lodz, Poland

Joaquim Soares do Brito, Joana Teixeira and José Portela
Orthopaedics and Trauma Department, Centro Hospitalar Lisboa Norte, EPE-Hospital de Santa Maria, 1649-036 Lisboa, Portugal

Koichiro Okuyama and Nobutoshi Seki
Department of Orthopedic Surgery, Akita Rosai Hospital, Odate, Japan

Keiji Kamo
Department of Orthopedic Surgery, Akita Rosai Hospital, Odate, Japan
Akita Hip Research Group (AHRG), Akita, Japan

Hiroaki Kijima, Shin Yamada and Yoichi Shimada
Akita Hip Research Group (AHRG), Akita, Japan
Department of Orthopedic Surgery, Akita University Graduate School of Medicine, Akita, Japan

Naohisa Miyakoshi
Department of Orthopedic Surgery, Akita University Graduate School of Medicine, Akita, Japan

Mirko Velickovic and Thomas Hockertz
Department of Orthopedic Surgery, Sports Traumatology and Trauma Surgery, Städtisches Klinikum Wolfenbüttel (Wolfenbüttel Municipal Hospital), AlterWeg 80, 38302Wolfenbüttel, Germany

Gan Zhi-Wei Jonathan, Hamid Rahmatullah Bin Abd Razak and Mitra Amit Kanta
Singapore General Hospital, Outram Road, Singapore 169608

Jun Suganuma, Tadashi Sugiki and Yutaka Inoue
Department of Orthopaedic Surgery, Hiratsuka City Hospital, 1-19-1 Minamihara, Hiratsuka, Kanagawa 254-0065, Japan

John G. Skedros
Department ofOrthopaedic Surgery, The University of Utah, Salt Lake City, UT,USA
Utah Orthopaedic Specialists, Salt Lake City, UT, USA
Intermountain Medical Center, Salt Lake City, UT, USA

Tanner R. Henrie
Utah Orthopaedic Specialists, Salt Lake City, UT, USA

Taranjit Singh Tung
Division of Orthopaedic Surgery, Boundary Trails Health Centre, P.O. Box 2000, Station Main,Winkler, MB, Canada R6W1H8

Enrique Sevillano-Perez
Department of Orthopaedic Surgery, Regional University Hospital of Málaga, 29010 Málaga, Spain
Hospital Vithas Parque San Antonio, 29016 Málaga, Spain

Alejandro Espejo-Reina
Hospital Vithas Parque San Antonio, 29016 Málaga, Spain
Department of Orthopaedic Surgery, Virgen de la Victoria University Hospital, 29010 Málaga, Spain

María Josefa Espejo-Reina
Hospital Vithas Parque San Antonio, 29016 Málaga, Spain

Yoshihiro Kotoura, Yasuhiro Fujiwara, Tatsuro Hayashida, Koji Murakami, Satoshi Makio, Yuichi Shimizu and Taku Ogura
Department of Orthopaedic Surgery, Nantan General Hospital, Nantan, Japan

Yoshinobu Oka, Wook-Choel Kim and Toshikazu Kubo
2Department of Orthopaedics, Graduate School of Medical Science, Kyoto Prefectural University of Medicine, Kyoto, Japan

Kerellos Nasr and Enrique Feria-Arias
Detroit Medical Center, 4D University Health Center, Detroit Receiving Hospital, 4201 Street Antoine Boulevard, Detroit, MI 48201, USA

Rahul Vaidya
Detroit Medical Center, 4D University Health Center, Detroit Receiving Hospital, 4201 Street Antoine Boulevard, Detroit, MI 48201, USA
4D University Health Center, Detroit Receiving Hospital,Wayne State University, 4201 Street Antoine Boulevard, Detroit, MI 48201, USA

Rebecca Fisher, Marvin Kajy and Lawrence N. Diebel
4D University Health Center, Detroit Receiving Hospital,Wayne State University, 4201 Street Antoine Boulevard, Detroit, MI 48201, USA

Jessica M. Kohring and Andrew R. Tyser
Department of Orthopaedic Surgery, University of Utah, Salt Lake City, UT 84108, USA

Heather M. Curtiss
Marshfield Clinic, Department of Sports Medicine, Physical Medicine & Rehabilitation, University of Wisconsin-Stevens Point, Marshfield,WI 54449, USA

Iain Bohler, Phillip Fletcher, Amanda Ragg and Andrew Vane
Orthopaedic Department, Tauranga Hospital, Cameron Road, Tauranga, Bay of Plenty 3112, New Zealand

Tomokazu Yoshioka, Hisashi Sugaya0 and Shigeki Kubota
Division of Regenerative Medicine for Musculoskeletal System, Faculty of Medicine, University of Tsukuba, 1-1-1 Tennodai, Tsukuba, Ibaraki 305-8575, Japan
Department of Orthopedic Surgery, Faculty of Medicine, University of Tsukuba, 1-1-1 Tennodai, Tsukuba, Ibaraki 305-8575, Japan

Mio Onishi, Akihiro Kanamori and Masashi Yamazaki
Department of Orthopedic Surgery, Faculty of Medicine, University of Tsukuba, 1-1-1 Tennodai, Tsukuba, Ibaraki 305-8575, Japan

Yoshiyuki Sankai
Faculty of Systems and Information Engineering, University of Tsukuba, 1-1-1 Tennodai, Tsukuba, Ibaraki 305-8577, Japan

Daniel H. Wiznia, Chang-Yeon Kim and Michael P. Leslie
Department of Orthopaedics and Rehabilitation, Yale University School of Medicine, 800 Howard Avenue, New Haven, CT 06510, USA

Nishwant Swami
Yale University, 800 Howard Ave., New Haven, CT, USA

Roland Biber, Markus Geßlein and Hermann Josef Bail
Nuremberg General Hospital, Paracelsus Medical University, Nuremberg, Germany

Johannes Pauser
Department of Orthopaedics and Traumatology, Nuremberg General Hospital, Nuremberg, Germany

Index

www.ingramcontent.com/pod-product-compliance
Lightning Source LLC
Chambersburg PA
CBHW080638200326
41458CB00013B/4671
9781632415097